HEALING
WITH
ESSENTIAL
OILS

"A brilliant and informative must-have book for anyone looking for a natural way to heal and restore and create harmony and balance in their life."

SUE STONE, AUTHOR, TV PRESENTER,
AND TRANSFORMATIONAL LEADER OF
THE SUE STONE FOUNDATION

"This highly recommendable book gives grounded scientific knowledge on essential oils and all the practical advice one needs to use them efficiently to restore and maintain health."

CHRISTOPHER VASEY, N.D., AUTHOR OF
NATURAL ANTIBIOTICS AND ANTIVIRALS

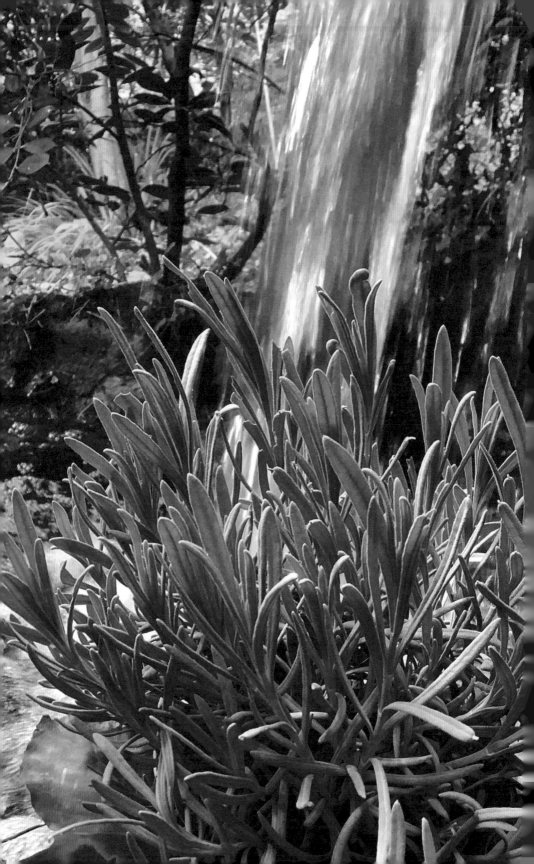

HEALING
WITH
ESSENTIAL
OILS

The Antiviral, Restorative, and
Life-Enhancing Properties of 58 Plants

Heather Dawn Godfrey, PGCE, BSc

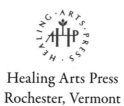

Healing Arts Press
Rochester, Vermont

Healing Arts Press
One Park Street
Rochester, Vermont 05767
www.HealingArtsPress.com

Healing Arts Press is a division of Inner Traditions International

Note to the reader: *This book is intended as an informational guide. The remedies,
approaches, and techniques described herein are meant to supplement, and not to be a
substitute for, professional medical care or treatment. They should not be used to treat a
serious ailment without prior consultation with a qualified health care professional.*

Cataloging-in-Publication Data for this title is available from the Library of Congress

ISBN 978-1-64411-389-9 (print)
ISBN 978-1-64411-390-5 (ebook)

Printed and bound in China by Reliance Printing Co., Ltd.

10 9 8 7 6 5 4 3 2 1

Text design and layout by Virginia Scott Bowman
This book was typeset in Garamond Premier Pro and Gill Sans with Kepler, Hypatia
Sans, and Rockeby used as display typefaces.

To send correspondence to the author of this book, mail a first-class letter to the
author c/o Inner Traditions • Bear & Company, One Park Street, Rochester, VT
05767, and we will forward the communication, or contact the author directly at
www.aromantique.co.uk.

*To my father, Edwin Charles, my childhood
rock and friend. I am so grateful for those moments
we spent talking about the things of life;
my inner compass eased into the light.*

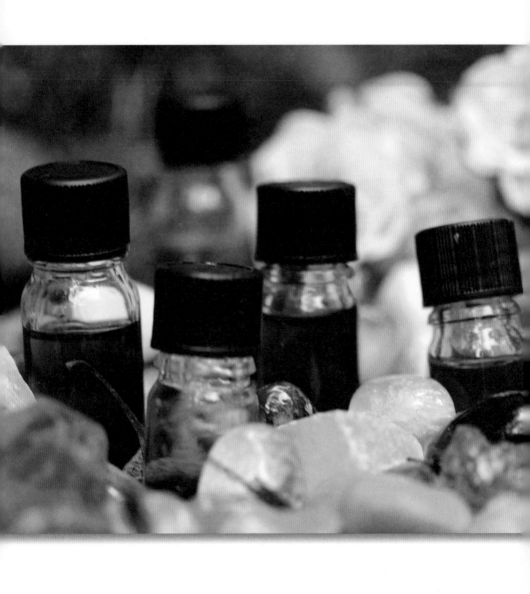

Contents

Foreword by Janey Lee Grace   ix

Acknowledgments   xi

INTRODUCTION
Essential Oils in Context   1

1 What Is an Essential Oil?   5
   A Living Gift from Nature

2 Biodiversity, Botany, and Essential Oils   31
   A Deep Dive into the Plant World

3 Methods of Extraction   77
   From Plant to Bottle

4 Essential Oil Chemistry   109
   A Brief Introduction to the Science of Plant Constituents

5 Using Essential Oils   141
   Optimizing Our Body-Mind-Spirit

6 Essential Oil Profiles   181
   *The Antiviral, Restorative, and Life-Enhancing
   Properties of 58 Plants*

Glossary	317
Bibliography	324
Index	332
About the Author	340

Foreword

Janey Lee Grace

I first became aware of the power of essential oils when I had my first aromatherapy massage. It was the most amazing experience, and I now realize I was fortunate to have found an aromatherapist who really knew her craft. This was very different from a pampering massage experience, and I quickly learned that the different aromas had very different therapeutic effects.

If there were a queen of essential oils, Heather Dawn Godfrey is that person. It's clear that this form of plant medicine is her passion and life purpose, and she is incredibly knowledgeable about how we can all benefit from it.

Essential oils, with their delightful array of scents and intriguing qualities, are found in households throughout the world now. They are present in our food, hygiene products, medicine, beauty and skincare remedies, and incense and perfumes. Essential oils are especially valued for their antimicrobial, skin-care, and psycho-emotional properties. They have been used both therapeutically and aesthetically for thousands of years, as testified in various ancient medicinal canons and scriptures.

But perhaps you have wondered: What exactly is an essential oil, how do essential oils work, what is it about their properties that lends credence to their therapeutic qualities, and why, when they perform similar roles in plants, are their scents so diverse? Heather answers all these questions and more as she invites you to join her in diving deep into this subject to discover why and how essential oils are so much more than just lovely scents. This book provides a comprehensive overview of the properties and qualities of essential oils so that you may effectively hone your use of them and maximize their benefits. You will learn how essential oils evolve within a plant and how the type of plant and the environment that plant grows in determines the chemical composition, qualities, and characteristics of its essential oil. I found this fascinating, as I once had an opportunity to smell lavender oil from lavender grown at high altitude in the Languedoc region of France, and it was quite unlike the lavender oils I had used before.

This book is easy to navigate, too. Information is gathered and summarized in succinct, easy-to-read charts and diagrams, which makes references clear and accessible, so the book is valuable as a practical tool and guide. Heather integrates her own insights and experience, gained through practical application and research, with that of other experts to provide a breadth and depth of knowledge about essential oils, their botany and organic chemistry, and their safe and effective use.

Like Heather's previous books, this book is aimed at those who use essential oils in their everyday life, students and professional practitioners alike. We don't all have the time or resources in our busy, demanding lives to engage in professional training, but here we have a beautifully illustrated, highly accessible resource that provides a sound foundation to support your understanding and use of essential oils.

Essential oils are one of the many gifts provided by nature. They can be used in many ways—as health remedies, to enhance beauty, and in various forms of artistic expression. The aim of this book is to provide a valuable reference to enlighten your awareness of the abundant qualities of essential oils. Whether you already use essential oils at home for your own pleasure, integrate them into your beauty, wellness, or health practice, or use them as artistic and aesthetic ingredients—or if you are simply intrigued by and want to know more about essential oils—this book is for you.

Janey Lee Grace is a well-being presenter and the author of *Happy Healthy Sober,* and she runs the recommendations site www.imperfectlynatural.com.

Acknowledgments

Writing is an insular process, yet it is not achieved in isolation. I could not have written this book without the enduring support and encouragement offered by others: friends and colleagues, incidental acquaintances, strangers I may have found myself chatting with in a café or on a train, as well as teachers, authors, and researchers who so generously shared their own knowledge, experience, and expertise. The list of people I could thank is almost endless. I appreciate everyone, and every situation, for the gifts brought to my perception, perspective, and experience of life and learning. Briefly, but not exclusively, I especially wish to thank Sophie and Simon Olszowski, for their ongoing encouragement and support; Pamela Allsop, for her wise counsel; Vicky Dixon, for the perspective she brings to my endeavors; and as always, my godmother, May Copp, for her sensible, steadying advice and belief in me, and my brother, Stephen Godfrey. I would also like to thank the Inner Traditions team for their professional support and diligence in producing this book from manuscript to printed page. A heartfelt thank you!

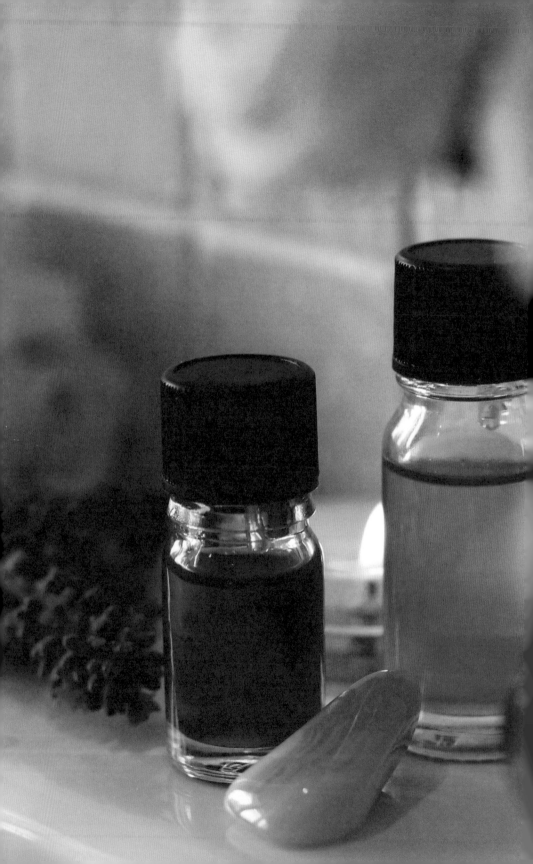

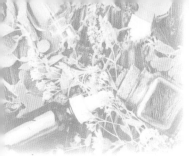

Essential Oils in Context

Life is precious, a gift. Nature is a beautiful expression of this gift. The awe and wonder we experience when we observe a golden red sunset kissing the clouds, a harvest moon suspended in a velveteen starlit sky, or rainbow light reflected in drops of dew glistening in the grass touch and resonate within every cell of our body and in our whole being. Everything in life and in nature is interconnected, like the glistening threads of a spiderweb. Our very first breath as we emerge from our mother's womb fills our lungs with life-sustaining oxygen that in turn awakens our conscious experience of the sensual world into which we are born. We are breathed into life, and with each breath, it seems, we are gifted. Indeed, we are graced with many tools and gifts with which we traverse this life, and in turn we each have gifts to share with one another. And just like a magnificent sunset or a raging waterfall or a pollinating honeybee dancing from flower to flower, we each express and contribute our gifts in our own unique way.

Essential oils straddle the ethereal and the earthly, like a bridge, touching and connecting each shoreline, reassuringly reminding us that one is never far from the other. Observing their scents, we are drawn into the moment, our senses awakened. Essential oils possess qualities that are physically protective and restorative and emotionally grounding and uplifting. Their molecules act as chemical messengers between the cells in plants and plant-consuming animals, a process activated via various mechanisms that involve microscopic informational networks created by the microbiome, the energetic meridian channels, the circulatory systems, and the neural pathways. They instigate responses that defend and stave off intruders while they repair, rejuvenate, and replenish. The rich, sweet scents of blossoms and flowers, for example, are attractive, aphrodisiac, and pleasing, even euphoric. The green scent of leaves is vitalizing. And the earthy scent of bark and roots is protective and grounding. Essential oil molecules radiate in a haze from the plant into the surrounding atmosphere in a way that protects the plant, aids its fertilization, and relays messages to other plants. They also support homeostasis and environmental harmony.

Marguerite Maury (1895–1968), a biochemist, naturopath, and homeopath, in her fascinating book *The Secrets of Life and Youth* (Maury 1989), refers to nature as sovereign, and the plant as a living being with a specific energy potential. Essential oils, in this context, Maury asserts, are a vital force expressed from the very heart of the alchemy of creation. When they are absorbed, the body has "at its disposal a vital and living element to use for its own ends" (Maury, 81), thus rejuvenating the organism, alerting the conscious mind, and enriching the entire being. Used thus, Maury says, rather than simply trying to add years to life, the aim is to add life to years (Maury, 80–81). Of the ethereal and psycho-emotional influences of essential oils, Maury states that the use of odoriferous matter induces a true sentimental and mental liberation; there is a feeling, she observes, of seeing events more objectively and therefore in a truer, clearer perspective (Maury, 82–83). When we experience this liberation, life takes on a magical, wondrous hue; colors and tones seem bright and vibrant, defined and clear.

Born from nature as living beings with specific energy potential, we too are sovereign beings, our body a vessel housing our consciousness, embodying a vital force issuing from the heart of creation. Nature constantly invites us to be consciously alive and aware and present in each moment, while at the same time aiding our survival and our ability to thrive. The gratitude and appreciation we feel are expressions of reverence, which, as Dr. Zach Bush so eloquently states, is the ultimate vessel of love (Bush 2020, May 26).

Healing with Essential Oils complements my two previous books that explore the various qualities and virtues of essential oils. The first book of this trilogy, *Essential Oils for Mindfulness and Meditation,* describes how observation of scent immediately draws our attention to the moment while at the same time instigating a psycho-emotional response via the limbic system that aids focus and alertness and instills a sense of peace and calm in a way that supports meditation and relaxation. *Essential Oils for the Whole Body* goes further, describing how essential oils are physically absorbed and excreted by the body and detailing their valuable characteristics and qualities, from ethereal to practical, with instructions on how to effectively blend essential oils together to create pleasing and effective therapeutic perfumes and remedies.

This book, *Healing with Essential Oils,* dives even deeper, describing and contextualizing the journey of essential oils, from their creation within the plant to the "scentual" substance in the bottle. Comprehending the botanical context of a plant—i.e., the role its oil plays within the plant and within the plant's immediate environment—reveals a great deal about the characteristic properties of an essential oil. You will discover in the following pages how essential oils, once extracted from a plant, then express their own unique traits. Essential oils can be used in many different contexts and in a variety of ways—a phenomenon of their versatility. Thus in these pages (and in the other books too) you have at your disposal a valuable map that leads to these abundant plant treasures.

This book is structured in such a way as to explore the complete journey of essential oils, from plant to bottle:

+ Chapter 1 explains what an essential oil is, how essential oils evolve, and where they are stored within the plant, including the various roles they play, from protecting the plant to aiding its propagation.
+ Chapter 2, "Biodiversity, Botany, and Essential Oils," takes a wider look at essential oil–bearing plants, including their botanical species, habitats, and climatic environments, and explains how plants are identified, categorized, and named.
+ Chapter 3, "Methods of Extraction," explains how essential oils are removed from the plant and how this process formulates the volatile chemical essences we are familiar with.

+ Chapter 4, "Essential Oil Chemistry," identifies the characteristic properties and qualities of the phytochemicals that comprise essential oils and explains how each chemical contributes to and influences their overall scent and therapeutic properties, with particular focus on their antimicrobial value.
+ Chapter 5, "Using Essential Oils," contextualizes the use of essential oils and their integrated remedial role as companions in a healthy lifestyle and includes general advice about safe use and application. This chapter also explores the appropriate use of essential oils for children and the elderly and presents information about which oils are safe to use in this context.
+ Chapter 6, which comprises the second half of this book, provides in-depth profiles of fifty-eight different essential oils. Each profile includes a description of the plant the essential oil is extracted from, the main chemical constituents comprising the oil, and its scent profile, subtle indications, and therapeutic applications—and much more.

The information contained in this book is derived from years of study, research, teaching, and experiential practice (both therapeutic and personal). However, by no means do I know all there is to know about essential oils; the adage "the more I learn, the more I realize how much I don't know" is both humbling and at the same time an exciting truth. I find myself a perpetual traveler in this respect, learning all the time as I discover, and even rediscover, new terrains and landscapes as I journey forth. I trust that the knowledge contained in this book will inform and support you on your journey of discovery and wellness.

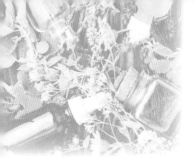

1

What Is an Essential Oil?

A Living Gift from Nature

Essential oils are comprised of volatile terpenes, which along with other chemicals such as alkaloids, bitters, glycosides, gums, saponins, and steroids, are produced in a wide variety of botanical species as a by-product of phytochemical metabolism. The primary role of essential oils is to protect the plant from harm and to aid its propagation. For example, all essential oils are antimicrobial (to varying degrees). They exude a specific fragrance that may attract or repel certain insects and animals. They also regulate the plant's external environment by creating a vaporous haze that influences the ambient temperature and level of humidity of the plant, thus protecting it from adverse atmospheric conditions, among other things. They influence the environment surrounding the plant's roots, particularly the local microbiome, in a way that supports nutrient absorption and proctects the roots from pathogenic invasion. Essential oils contribute to the flavor of edible plants. Indeed, as you will discover, essential oils are one of many threads in nature's intricate, interactive web.

In this chapter we take a closer look at the various processes that lead to the development of essential oils within a plant, beginning with a glimpse at the catalyst influence gifted by the sun's solar rays and the way a plant harnesses this energy to initiate growth and development. You will learn how the conditions of growth influence the content and quality of a plant's essential oil, and how the type of plant and the role its essential oil plays within that plant provides some indication of the oil's characteristic qualities.

PHOTOSYNTHESIS:
THE CONVERSION OF SOLAR ENERGY

The sun provides the primary source of energy, which is received in the form of solar heat and light. Electromagnetic energy radiates from the sun. Upon reaching Earth's atmosphere, these electromagnetic rays are attenuated (a process that reduces the intensity of their flux), primarily by ozone and water vapor, and are then scattered by molecules of air and aerosols in the troposphere surrounding Earth.

Solar heat energy generates movement through energy transfer. This process is easily explained by observing air as it warms. Air becomes less dense as it rises, causing thermal currents and variable atmospheric airflow (wind) as a consequence. Solar heat causes water to evaporate and vaporize as tiny droplets of moisture that rise into the atmosphere, where they are carried and circulated on undulating currents of air to increasingly higher altitudes in the cold troposphere, in the process cooling and condensing to form vaporous clouds that are carried in the ebb and flow of atmospheric currents. As they continue to converge within clouds, the weight and density of these water droplets increases until they succumb to the pull of gravity, at which point they descend again to the ground as drops of rain or clusters of frozen crystals (snow, sleet, or hail, depending on the altitude and temperature). Once earthbound, water continues to descend to the lowest land level, forming springs, streams, and rivers that eventually spill into lakes and oceans.

The momentum created by the movement of solar heat energy generates and perpetuates more energy, which can be captured in momentum and transduced by windmills, water turbines, and wheels that drive hydroelectrical generators and machinery. Thus, solar heat generates a source of renewable energy. Radiant electromagnetic light from the sun (known as *photons*) at the same time similarly scatters and filters through Earth's atmosphere and is absorbed and transduced by plants (and the cells of other receptive organisms, such as algae and cyanobacteria) through a process known as *photosynthesis*. Solar light energy is unstable and cannot be stored until it is converted into stable chemical energy, and photosynthesis is the biological process by which this energy is converted. Photosynthesis occurs when solar light energy makes contact with and is absorbed by plant proteins that contain green chlorophyll; these proteins are found inside organelles called *chloroplasts,* as well as photosynthetic cells. Water plays an important part in this process, too. For example, water is carried to the photosynthetic cell by nonphotosynthetic cells that are found in nongreen parts of the plant, such as the roots, rhizomes, phloem (the living tissue in vascular plants that transports the soluble organic compounds made during photosynthesis), and xylem (the veins on leaves). Stomata, the tiny pores found on the stems and leaves of vascular plants, provide portals where gaseous exchange (oxygen and carbon dioxide) between the plant and the atmosphere takes place. Stomata open during the day to allow gaseous exchange and close at night and in very warm atmospheric conditions to prevent water and gas loss. Most land plants contain both photo- and nonphotosynthetic cells; however, nonphotosynthetic cells rely on photosynthetic cells to provide their energy.

So, light energy (photons) enters the chlorophyll cell (chloroplast) along with carbon dioxide and water transported from the plant's roots. This convergence instigates a complex reaction (photosynthesis) that causes the water molecule to split (a process known as *photolysis*) into hydrogen ions, electrons, and oxygen molecules. The energy released by this process creates an energy-rich bond between ADP (adenosine diphosphate) and Pi (phosphate) to form ATP (adenosine triphosphate), which is the major energy-carrying compound in cells.

Photolysis produces stabilized, storable energy in the form of carbohydrates such as sugars, starch, and cellulose; lipid proteins; and nuecleic acids. Cellulose is used directly by the plant to maintain its structure so it remains stiff and upright, while carbohydrates (sugar and extra starch) are used by all the plant's cells for energy. Excess starch is stored in the roots, rhizomes, and tubers. Unused oxygen is released into the atmosphere.

The compounds produced by this process are vital to the plant's existence and support and sustain its growth and development. These compounds also provide vital nutrients that energize and sustain animals and other life forms when they consume the plant.

light energy photons
↓
water plus carbon dioxide (CO_2) ———→ glucose (carbohydrate) plus oxygen = energy
chloroplasts

Respiration is the term that describes the process by which carbohydrates are broken down within the mitochondria of the photosynthetic cell to produce cellular energy. The plant relies on continual respiration to maintain cellular activity. Without solar light, photosynthesis ceases, and during the light-independent or dark phase, when photons from the sun are not available (for example, at night or when the stomata close to preserve water during the day), the plant reverts to its stored starch reserves to provide the energy needed to maintain respiration and chemical synthesis. During this phase, excess carbon dioxide (CO_2) is released into the atmosphere.

All life on Earth depends on the process of photosynthesis; hence carbohydrates and oxygen are key to life.

Photosynthesis: An Overview

Earth's atmosphere is approximately 79% nitrogen, 20% oxygen, and a 1% mixture of less common gases, including approximately 0.039% carbon dioxide. Green plants create, or synthesize, oxygen and carbon dioxide.

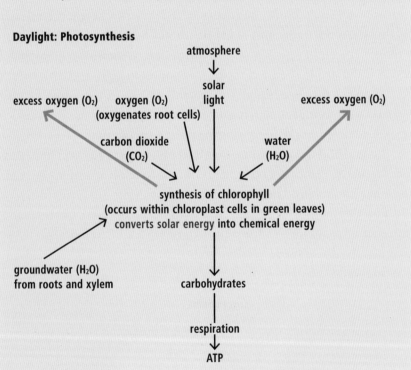

Daylight: Photosynthesis

atmosphere

solar light

excess oxygen (O_2)   oxygen (O_2)
(oxygenates root cells)   excess oxygen (O_2)

carbon dioxide
(CO_2)   water
(H_2O)

synthesis of chlorophyll
(occurs within chloroplast cells in green leaves)
converts solar energy into chemical energy

groundwater (H_2O)
from roots and xylem

carbohydrates

respiration

ATP

DAYTIME PHOTOSYNTHESIS

- Solar light is absorbed by chlorophyll.
- Carbon dioxide (CO_2) is absorbed from the atmosphere.
- Water is transported to chloroplasts through the root system and the xylem.
- Water molecules split into hydrogen ions, electrons, and oxygen (photolysis).
- The bonding of adenosine diphosphate (ADP) and phosphate (Pi) releases energy to form adenosine triphosphate (ATP).
- Carbohydrates (monosaccharides, disaccharides, polysaccharides) are produced.
- Oxygen is released into the atmosphere.

Light-Independent or Dark Phase

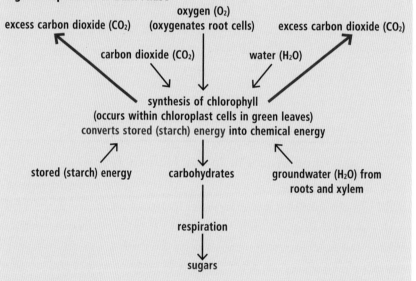

LIGHT-INDEPENDENT OR DARK PHASE

- Carbon dioxide (CO_2) is drawn from the atmosphere.
- Water is transported to chloroplasts through the root system and the xylem.
- Stored starch (mainly found in roots, rhizomes, and tubers), ATP, and hydrogen support and maintain respiration.
- Carbohydrates are produced.
- Excess carbon dioxide is released into the atmosphere.

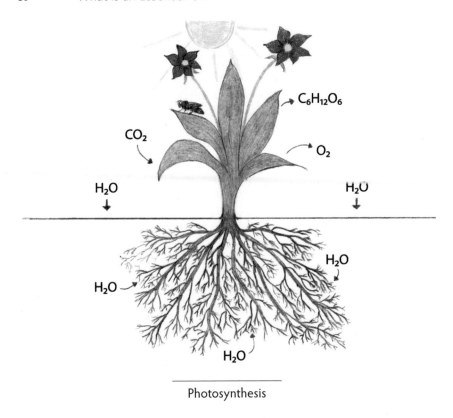

$C_6H_{12}O_6$

CO_2

O_2

H_2O

H_2O

H_2O

H_2O

H_2O

Photosynthesis

Photosynthesis in the Human Animal

Light (photons) absorbed by water in animal cells creates a similar photosynthetic reaction as in plants, splitting water molecules into positively and negatively charged components. Briefly, negatively charged components repel one another and generate energy in the process. So the mitochondria within animal cells create energy not only from food and other nutrients but also from photons absorbed by water within the body. Thus we experience increased energy when we are exposed to natural light and remain sufficiently hydrated (by drinking plenty of water). Consuming green leafy vegetables (especially when they are juiced, as chlorophyll cells are carried within water to the body's cells), turmeric, and coconut water further enhances the ability of our cells to absorb and transduce light energy, as does walking barefoot on the negatively charged earth, which is grounding (Pollack 2016).

THE TYPES OF SUGARS (CARBOHYDRATES)
PRESENT IN PLANTS

CARBON ATOMS	CHEMICAL FORMULATION	CARBOHYDRATE
six carbon atoms	$C_6H_{12}O_6$	hexose sugar (glucose, galactose, fructose)
five carbon atoms	$C_5H_{10}O_5$	pentose sugar (ribose, deoxyribose)
three carbon atoms	$C_3H_6O_3$	triose sugar (aldotriose, ketotriose) *important in cellular respiration*
TYPES OF SUGARS		
sugar molecules in isolation	monosaccharides	pentose, hexose *found in proteins (RNA and DNA) and glucose*
sugar molecules formed in pairs	disaccharides	sucrose (glucose + fructose) *found in fruits* lactose (glucose + galactose) *found in milk* maltose (glucose + glucose) *found in germinating grains and root vegetables*
sugar molecules formed in chains	polysaccharides	glycogen and starch *found in roots and root vegetables, rice and leguminous plants*

Nonrenewable Energy

Basically, nonrenewable energy is transformed solar light energy—decomposing organic land and sea plants that lived millions of years ago in an environment that no longer exists. These were buried, along with their store of chemical energy, then compressed and subjected to immense heat and sustained pressure. They eventually transformed or metamorphosed into coal. Similarly, marine phytoplankton, which is also converted and stored chemical energy as a result of photosynthesis, were buried and compacted over millions of years in depressions deep within the ocean bed, eventually converting into crude oil. Natural gas, a hydrocarbon mixture consisting mostly of methane, was similarly created from the decomposition of organic matter and is stored in deep, underground rock formations.

THE PRODUCTS OF PLANT METABOLISM

To reiterate, there are two types of metabolic processes that occur within plants: primary (initiated during the light phase of photosynthesis) and secondary (initiated during the light-independent or dark phase of synthesis). Both processes are interconnected, as one depends on the other, so there is not always a clear distinction between them, yet each phase of metabolism serves a particular purpose. For example, primary metabolism is concerned with the synthesis and utilization of chemicals necessary for the survival and health of the organism. These chemicals also support and sustain animal life. Primary metabolites include:

+ amino acids
+ chlorophyll
+ fatty acids
+ nucleic acids
+ sugars

Secondary metabolism produces chemicals that are not vital to the organism but play an important role in enabling the organism to interact and adapt to conditions in its environment. These use a different production pathway. Secondary metabolites also provide characteristics such as color, scent, and defense of the plant. Secondary metabolites include:

+ alkaloids
+ bitters
+ flavonoids
+ glycosides
+ gums
+ phenols
+ saponins
+ steroids
+ terpenes (essential oils or plant volatiles)

While not present in all plants, essential oils (also referred to as *volatile organic compounds* or *plant volatiles*) are found in a wide range of botanical species. These include biennial or perennial herbaceous plants and evergreen or deciduous shrubs and trees. Essential oils are mostly comprised of terpenes and terpenoids and green-leaf volatiles. Although a by-product of biosynthesis, few essential oils are involved in plant metabolism. Even so, essential oils provide a significant and purposeful role that extends beyond their originating organism, one that touches and influences the wider existential web of life, as we shall see.

Terpenes and their terpenoid derivatives are one of a group of chemicals produced by plants for protection, as many animals and rodents are repelled by the scent and taste of terpenes. Other groups include alkaloids (the bitter-tasting principle in herbs), flavonoids (antioxidants such as those found in fruits, vegetables, and flowers), and saponins (these froth when the plant is cut and they taste soapy).

Phytohormones are chemical messengers that coordinate cellular activity. They relay signals throughout the plant and are transported via sap from one part of a plant to another. Their main roles are to regulate cellular activities and growth, vegetative and reproductive development, and pattern formation in tissues and to initiate stress responses. Essential oils are responsively stimulated into action by plant hormones.

Essential oils are sometimes referred to as phytohormones, or plant hormones. Indeed, some essential oils appear to have hormonelike or aphrodisiac qualities—for example, fennel, clary sage, geranium, rose, niaouli, and ylang-ylang. Also, some plants and herbs exhibit proven hormonelike actions when consumed. Fennel, for example, is shown to stimulate milk production in lactating mothers, and clary sage regulates menstrual flow. However, the process of these actions is not clear, as the mechanisms that instigate such responses are complex and often interdependent. Also, it cannot be assumed that an essential oil in isolation from a plant will exhibit or carry forward the same properties and qualities as those expressed by the whole plant. Essential oils are hormonelike in that they appear to relay messages. However, once removed from a plant, an essential oil is no longer part of the plant's infrastructure. It is highly concentrated and comprised of a unique array, or synergy, of the plant's most volatile chemicals. Therefore it is not representative of the whole plant, nor does it represent the version of the essential oil that was present in the plant before extraction (as you will discover in the following chapters).

Which Part of the Plant?

Essential oils are generally extracted from a specific part of a plant, such as the leaf, stem, flower, fruit, root, or bark. The phytochemicals present in a given part of the plant will vary according to the role it plays; for example, the chemicals found in a flower will differ from those found in the leaf or the roots of the same plant. Furthermore, the chemical composition and predominance of essential oil in a particular part of a plant varies according to the plant's age, stage of development, and health, as well as the environmental context in which it grows, the time of year, and the stage of its reproductive cycle. Some suggest that essential oils carry a vibrational imprint of the energy of the *whole* plant, but this is very difficult to prove or qualify, as there are far too many variables and intangible elements at play.

As a plant matures, the composition of its essential oil alters. Young plants mainly contain terpenic hydrocarbons and simple molecules, and their reproductive organs tend to contain molecules that are richer in oxygenated compounds (as described in detail in chapter 4). Also, young plants tend to produce more essential oil than old plants, while old plants surrender more resinous, darker essential oils due to gradual build-up of the heavier components that are left behind as a result of the continuous evaporation of the lighter, more volatile components.

The strongest-scented plants tend to be found in tropical regions, where solar light energy is most abundant.

The Role of Essential Oils in Plants

Defense and Protection

Most essential oils are antimicrobial and capable of inhibiting the proliferation of invasive bacteria, viruses, and fungi. Leaf, wood, and root oils protect against attack and predation, repelling certain insects and herbivores. Essential oils also attract insects and birds that eat or destroy plant-eating moths, caterpillars, insects, and aphids. They support tissue repair and regeneration. Resinous material (for example, the oleo gum resins of frankincense, myrrh, and galbanum and the resins found in pine, fir, spruce, juniper, cypress, and cedar), which is laced with essential oil, exudes at the site of damage when the trunk of the tree, stem of a plant, or root is injured or damaged; this prevents the loss of sap and/or provides a protective anti-microbial seal against parasites and disease organisms.

Reproduction

Scent exuding from essential oils in flowers and blossoms attracts pol-linating insects and seed-dispersing birds and animals, mainly by creating an odor trail to food (nectar and pollen). Many chemicals found in essen-tial oils are also found in the scent glands of insects (pheromones). Most insects, including honeybees and bumblebees, butterflies, and flower bee-tles, have excellent olfactory acuity and learn to associate scent with food. Most animal-pollinated flowers are typically highly scented, while the least scented are mainly bird-pollinated flowers. The release of essential oil often oscillates in sync with daily environmental rhythms—for example, increas-ing when pollinators are most active, whether during the day or at night, as some pollinating animals are nocturnal, such as moths and bats.

Prevention

Some plants deliberately release essential oils into the atmosphere around them to influence the condition of their immediate environment. This cre-ates an enveloping vapor haze that protects against adversely hot or dry climatic conditions, optimizing temperature control and stomatal closure to prevent water loss. Essential oil vapors also instigate intraspecies communi-cation to warn of predators or to signal changes in the environment.

STORAGE OF ESSENTIAL OILS IN A PLANT

Essential oils tend to remain in their secretory structure or are excreted into intercellular cavities or canals or on the surface of the plant in response to conditions in the environment. Secretory structures are found either on the surface of a plant or within the plant's tissues. The type of secretory structure depends on the type of plant, the role the essential oil plays in a given area (protective, reproductive, etc.), and which parts of the plant the oil is found in.

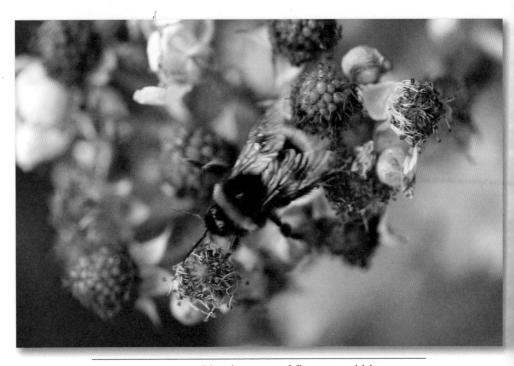

Bees are attracted by the scent of flowers and blossoms
and aid pollination and reproduction.

WHERE THE ESSENTIAL OILS ARE FOUND

STRUCTURE	DESCRIPTION	EXAMPLES OF WHERE THE SECRETORY STRUCTURE IS FOUND
Single secretion-containing cell	Found scattered among other cells, in different plant tissues, single secretory cells are similar in structure to adjacent nonsecretory cells. They may sometimes be larger than other cells or have a thick, cuticularized lining. Often the only distinguishing feature between a secretory cell and surrounding nonsecretory cells is its essential oil content.	**leaf** parenchyma of *Cymbopogon citratus* (lemongrass), *Pimenta racemosa* (bay), *Cymbopogon nardus* (citronella), *Pogostemon cablin* (patchouli) **seed coat** of *Elettaria cardamomum* (cardamom) **rhizome** of *Zingiber officinale* (ginger), *Curcuma longa* (turmeric) **fruit wall** of *Piper nigrum* (black pepper) **perisperm** and **embryo** of *Myristica fragrans* (nutmeg) **bark** of *Cinnamomum zeylanicum* (cinnamon) **root** of *Valeriana fauriei* (valerian)

STRUCTURE	DESCRIPTION	EXAMPLES OF WHERE THE SECRETORY STRUCTURE IS FOUND
Osmophores	Also known as *floral fragrance glands* and found distributed and concentrated in certain regions of floral organs, such as the sapels (mesophyll) and across the surface of petals (epithelium), osmophores are perfectly situated to allure potential pollinators. They differ structurally from adjacent cells and can have different shapes, sizes, and colors.	**isodiametric cells** in orchids
Secretory cavities	These tend to be ovular or spherical in shape and thin-walled, with dense protoplasm. They have two modes of behavior: parenchyma cells separate and leave intercellular spaces (lumina or lacuna); or the cell itself disintegrates, leaving a cavity within the tissue. The spaces created are lined with secretory epithelial cells, which produce essential oils. High-yielding plants generate several layers of secretory cells.	**leaves** and **fruits** of the citrus family, for example, *Citrus bergamia* (bergamot), *Citrus aurantifolia* (lime), *Citrus x aurantium* (sour orange), *Citrus limonum* (lemon), *Citrus x paradisi* (grapefruit) **flower buds** of *Syzygium aromaticum* (clove) **fruit walls** of *Pimenta dioica* (allspice) **bark** of *Commiphora myrrha* (myrrh), *Boswellia sacra* (frankincense)
Secretory ducts	These are elongated cavities that can often branch to create a network extending from roots through to the leaves, flowers, and fruits. As the cells divide they expand the space or cavity. Some of the cells forming the wall of the cavity change into secretory epithelial cells.	**roots, stems, leaves, flowers,** and **fruits** found in all the Umbelliferae family, including *Pimpinella anisum* (anise), *Foeniculum vulgare* (fennel), *Coriandrum sativum* (coriander), *Anethum graveolens* (dill)

WHERE THE ESSENTIAL OILS ARE FOUND (continued)

STRUCTURE	DESCRIPTION	EXAMPLES OF WHERE THE SECRETORY STRUCTURE IS FOUND
Glandular trichomes	Found in modified epidermal hairs— secretory cells that are attached by a single stem or basal cell in the epidermis. The outer surface of the cell is heavily cutinized. Essential oils accumulate in subcuticular spaces, diffusing outward through the cuticle. Epidermal hairs can be found covering leaves, stems, and parts of the flowers in many plants within the Lamiaceae family.	**leaves, stems,** and parts of the **flowers** of many plants in the Lamiaceae family, including *Ocimum basilicum* (basil), *Lavandula angustifolia* (lavender), *Origanum majorana* (marjoram), *Mentha* x *piperita* (peppermint), *Thymus vulgaris* (thyme)
Epidermal cells	Conical epidermal cells form a layer that covers the leaves, flowers, roots, and stems of plants. Essential oil–containing epidermal cells are found mostly within and on the surface of flower petals, where their scent attracts pollinating bees and other insects. The yield of essential oil from these cells is usually very low.	**petals** and **buds** of *Jasminum grandiflorum* (jasmine), *Rosa centifolia* (rose), *Cananga odorata* (ylang-ylang)

Source: Information derived from Tölke et al. 2018 and from Svoboda 2000

THE VARIOUS PARTS OF PLANTS
AND THE ESSENTIAL OILS THEY YIELD

PLANT PART	ESSENTIAL OIL
Bark	cinnamon
Berries	chaste tree/vitex (*Vitex agnus-castus*), juniper
Blossoms	orange blossom/neroli, rose, ylang-ylang
Flowers	calendula, chamomile (German and Roman), clove bud, helichrysum, jasmine
Flowering tops (herbs)	clary sage, hyssop, lavender, lemon balm/melissa, marjoram, peppermint, rosemary, thyme
Fruits	black pepper, may chang, star anise
Grass	citronella, lemongrass, palmarosa
Leaves	basil, cajeput, cassia, cinnamon, chaste tree/vitex, clary sage, eucalyptus, hyssop, lavender, lemon balm/melissa, myrtle, niaouli, patchouli, peppermint, petitgrain, rosemary, sage, tea tree, thyme
Needles	cypress, pine
Resins	frankincense, galbanum, myrrh
Rind	bergamot, bitter orange, grapefruit, lemon, lime, mandarin
Roots and rhizomes	ginger, spikenard, valerian, vetivert
Seeds	bitter fennel, caraway, cardamom, carrot seed, coriander, fennel, nutmeg
Twigs	cajeput, cassia, cinnamon, cypress, eucalyptus, myrtle, niaouli
Branches	petitgrain, tea tree
Whole plant (above the ground)	bitter fennel, geranium, rosemary (poor quality), yarrow
Wood (stumps, trunk, heartwood, sawdust)	cedarwood, rosewood, sandalwood

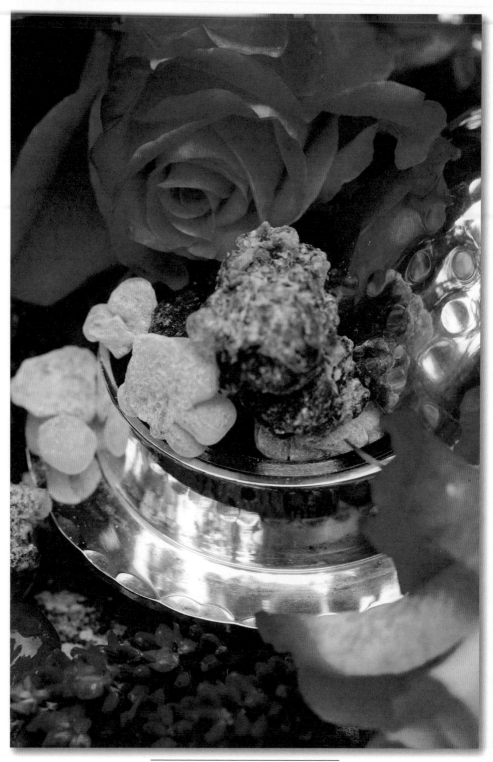

Frankincense and myrrh resin

Types of Essential Oil Molecules Found in Various Parts of a Plant and Their Predominant Role

Flowers

Flowers tend to contain the largest quantity of the most volatile essential oil components, and also the most intensely scented ones, as these need to be far-reaching in order to attract pollinators from a distance. Flowers produce different complex mixtures of essential oil compounds designed to target specific pollinators; thus each species of flower has a unique scent profile. Rose flowers, for example, contain over three hundred volatile compounds that work together to attract butterflies, bees, and hummingbirds, as well as insects that eat pests like aphids. Linalool and beta-caryophyllene are examples of compounds that act defensively in flowers to ward off predators (Cseke et al. 2007).

Leaves and Stems

Green-leaf volatiles include alcohols, aldehydes, and esters, with their characteristically green smell of freshly cut grass. These mostly behave defensively and are released into the immediate environment when a plant is attacked by a pathogen or an herbivore (Scala et al. 2013).

Roots

Roots contain high levels of monoterpenes and sesquiterpenes that attract protective bacteria, which in turn support the balance of the roots' environmental microbiome, aiding nutrient absorption. Examples include angelica, ginger, turmeric, and vetivert roots (Acimovic et al. 2017).

Fruits

Fruits contain a high proportion of esters that attract fruit-eating herbivores, thus aiding seed dispersal.

Seeds

Seeds contain terpinic compounds and phenylprotanoids (cinnamic acids) that defend against microbes and herbivores and also prevent the growth of other plants (allelopathy) when dispersed. Examples include coriander, fennel, caraway, and carrot seeds.

Bark and Wood

Essential oil compounds are found in sticky resins, which protect a tree from insect and pathogenic invasion when its bark is damaged. This type of resin mainly contains terpenes such as alpha-pinene, beta-pinene, delta-3-carene, and sabinene, as well as limonene and terpinene. Some also contain high levels of resin acids, such as cedarwood, frankincense, and myrrh resin.

Plants produce chemical compounds during the process of metabolic activity. As well as water, plants absorb minerals and other elemental nutrients (such as nitrogen, phosphorus, potassium, and magnesium) from the surrounding soil and microbiome through their root systems; some have deep roots, some superficial roots, and some aerial roots. Xylem (tubular woody tissue) conducts and transports water and minerals from the roots up to the rest of the plant, while phloem (tubular plant tissue present within the body of the plant) transports soluble sucrose and other organic nutrients, which are produced by the leaves during photosynthetic reaction, around the plant and back to the roots.

Green plants provide most of Earth's molecular oxygen and form the basis of the most of Earth's ecologies; they also produce about one-fifth of Earth's atmospheric CO_2, which is fixed by land plants, then released back into the air each day as plant volatiles.

A plant's potential for healthy growth, development, and chemical synthesis is influenced and affected by the condition and quality of the soil it grows in and draws vital minerals, ions, and other nutrients from, as well as the gaseous balance and quality of the surrounding atmosphere. For example, to support photosynthesis, a plant requires:

+ **carbon,** from carbon dioxide in the surrounding air;
+ **hydrogen,** from water contained in the soil; and
+ **oxygen,** from both carbon dioxide and water.

To support and maintain healthy development, a plant requires:

+ **mineral salts,** in the form of ions dissolved in water within the soil, which are drawn in by the root hairs and xylem of the plant;
+ **nitrates,** which contain nitrogen, essential for protein formation;

+ **iron** and **magnesium salts,** for the formation of chlorophyll;
+ **phosphorus** as **phosphates,** for the formation of cell nuclei; and
+ **potassium,** for the control of cell division.

Insufficient availability and quantities of any of these ions and nutrients causes deficient plant growth, which also results in a poor or inferior essential-oil yield and quality. Atmospheric pollution and contamination of the soil also have a detrimental effect on the condition and health of plants. Continued growth of the same crop year after year depletes the nutrient content of the soil, hence the practice of crop rotation, allowing fields or growing areas to remain fallow for a season (Williams 2006).

The growth and development of plants and the composition of their essential oils are affected by various environmental conditions:

+ geographical location of growth
+ soil (type and condition), as above
+ altitude
+ climate
+ atmospheric condition
+ exposure to solar light energy
+ time of day
+ time of harvest (time of day and season)
+ use of fertilizers and pesticides
+ genetics
+ age of plant
+ health of plant

Transportation of an essential oil from one part of a plant to another and/or increased expression or prevalence in a particular area of a plant (most essential oils remain in or around the areas they are stored within) is influenced by pollination (reproduction) and response to predation and tissue injury (protection), as well as by the stage of maturity of a plant or flower. The atmospheric conditions and pressure, time of day, and season are also influencing factors, as plants are responsive to atmospheric changes (pressure, light, and temperature).

These are all factors, among others, that play a part in determining the optimum moment to harvest plants for their essential oils. For example, Senatore (1996) found the best time to harvest *Thymus pulegioides* (Italian thyme) to maximize its essential oil yield is immediately before or during full bloom of the flowering plant. Rohloff et al. (2005) similarly found that the essential oil yield from *Mentha* x *piperita* (peppermint) increased from early to full bloom, and maximized at late bloom. Ahmad et al. (1998) found that while the time of day of harvest does not affect the quantity of essential oil yielded from *Jasminum multiflorum* (jasmine), it does influence its chemical composition. For example, the researchers observed that the concentrations of indole and cis-jasmone compounds that characterize jasmine oil's scent are higher in jasmine obtained from morning-harvested flowers compared to evening-harvested flowers. Morning-harvested jasmine also contains higher concentrations of benzyl alcohol, linalool, and benzyl acetate compared to evening-harvested flowers. Thus, the researchers concluded that jasmine flowers should be harvested in the morning to optimize the quality of the essential oil extracted.

Sharma and Kumar (2018) found that the essential oil content of damask rose (*Rosa* x *damascena*) differs according to maturation of the bloom, noting, for example, the higher content of cis-rose oxide, citronellol, nerol, and geraniol and lower content of nonadecane when the petal whorl began to open, compared to other stages (budding or full opening of the bloom). They also observed that distillation time significantly influences an oil's chemical content. For example, linalool, phenyl ethyl alcohol, citronellol + nerol, and trans-geraniol concentration increased for up to five hours from commencement of distillation, but decreased thereafter. In another study, Younis et al. (2009) observed that early morning is the optimum time to harvest rose blossoms to maximize quantity and quality of their essential oil yield.

Many essential oils are found in herbs and edible plants that have been consumed as food and medicine for thousands of years. However, not all plants produce essential oils that are suitable or safe for use in isolation from the plant.

Essential oils represent only 1 to 10 percent of the complex chemical mixture (which also includes volatile, nonvolatile, organic, and

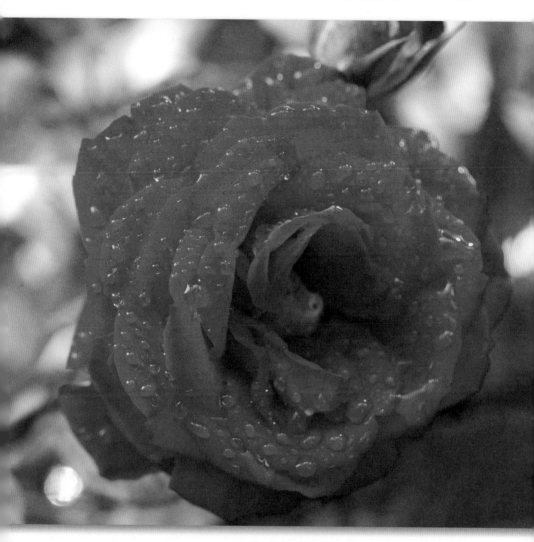

nonorganic components) found within a plant. This means that the amount of essential oil surrendered and isolated from an individual plant is consequently very small. However, when collectively isolated from many plants during the process of extraction, the concentration of essential oil surrendered, along with the removal of other nondistillable and perhaps counterbalancing components left behind during extraction, renders the resulting oil up to fifty to a hundred times more potent than when present in the context of a single whole plant or herb.

It Takes a Lot to Make a Little!

It takes 35 pounds (16 kg) of lavender flowers to produce just 300 drops (15 ml) of essential oil, and 5,500 to 8,800 pounds (2,500 to 4,000 kg) of rose petals to produce just 2 pounds (1 kg, or 1,000 ml) of rose essence. However, this small amount is highly concentrated; just one drop of an essential oil is equivalent to fifteen to forty cups of medicinal tea or up to ten teaspoons of tincture (depending on the type of plant, the amount of oil present in a plant, and whether the plant was dry or fresh when the essential oil was extracted).

The nonvolatile and nondistillable chemical components left behind during extraction often act to counterbalance the potentially irritating or toxic effects of some of the more reactive components found in essential oils when present together in the whole plant.

As identified earlier, some essential oils are found throughout a plant, for example, the whole plant above ground (leaves, flowers, and stalks) of *Pelargonium graveolens* (geranium). Other essential oils are mainly concentrated in one part of a plant, for example, the blossoms of *Rosa centifolia* or *Rosa* x *damascena* (rose species) or *Citrus* x *aurantium* var. *amara* (neroli) during flowering, or the roots of *Vetiveria zizanioides* (vetivert), which is the only grass cultivated solely for its root essential oil (which is used extensively in perfumes and cosmetics). Interestingly, Del Giudice et al. (2008) found that bacteria present in the microbiome surrounding the roots of vetivert may perform a significant role in the biosynthsis of essential oil, their presence significantly influencing the amount of oil present and its chemical composition.

Citrus trees yield three types of essential oil that differ in chemical composition depending on the part of the plant where the oil is found and its predominant role: the twigs and leaves, the blossoms, and the fruit. These differences influence the chemical composition and scent profile of the respective essential oils, as demonstrated below, and also have a bearing on other factors, such as an oil's capacity for irritancy or toxicity.

THREE ESSENTIAL OILS PRODUCED
FROM *CITRUS AURANTIUM* VAR. *AMARA*

ESSENTIAL OIL	PART OF PLANT	MAIN CHEMICAL COMPONENTS	ESSENTIAL OIL APPEARANCE AND ODOR PROFILE
orange, bitter	fruit rind	monoterpenes (90%)	clear to pale orange, with a fresh orange fragrance
neroli	blossom	monoterpenes (35%) alcohols (40%) esters (15%)	pale yellow to amber, with a characteristically sweet, fresh, orange-blossom fragrance
petitgrain	leaves and twigs	esters (55%) alcohols (35%) monoterpenes (10%)	clear to pale yellow to yellow to amber, with fresh, floral (similar to neroli), woody, citrusy fragrance with dry, herbaceous undertones

While *Citrus aurantium* var. *amara* yields three relatively safe essential oils, this cannot be assumed to be the case for all plants. For example, cinnamon bark essential oil contains 40% to 76% cinnamaldehyde (an aldehyde) and 2% to 14% eugenol (a phenol), whereas cinnamon leaf essential oil contains 74% to 96% eugenol and 0.5% to 3% cinnamaldehyde. Cinnamaldehyde is a strong dermal sensitizer, and moderate to large amounts of this component can render an essential oil unsuitable for skin use (Tisserand and Young 2014, 531). Therefore, cinnamon bark essential oil is usually not recommended for topical use (although it may be useful in an antimicrobial blend used in an environmental diffuser). On the other hand, eugenol, although a mild irritant, is considered safe in up to 10% dilution (i.e., 1 to 2 drops of essential oil in 5 ml vegetable oil or other base medium) and is cited by a number of sources as being safe for topical aromatherapeutic use, with the caveat that it be used with caution, in limited amounts (NHR Organic Oils Certificate of Analysis 2021, Tisserand and Young 2014, Good Scents Company 2021).

Basil is a culinary herb considered safe to consume in its whole plant form. There are numerous species of basil and various types of basil essential oil, the majority of which contain estragole, a phenolic ether; phenolic ethers are more powerful than phenols and are neurotoxic in large amounts (Clarke 2002, 61). Basil (*Ocimum basilicum*) ct. estragole for example, contains 70% to 90% estragole; "hairy" basil (*Ocimum americanum*) 0.3% to 0.5%; holy basil (*Ocimum tenuiflorum*) 9% to 14%; basil (*Ocimum basilicum*) ct. linalool up to 1%; basil Madagascar (*Ocimum gratissimum*) 40% to 50%; basil methyl cinnamate (*Ocimum basilicum*) up to 1%; and basil pungent (*Ocimum gratissimum*) up to 2%. Of these varieties, basil ct. linalool is the safest to use due to its low estragole content and high linalool content (linalool, a monoterpene alcohol, counterbalances the irritating effect of estragole, which is a phenol—see chapter 4).

These examples demonstrate how important it is to examine the botanical source, including the Latin name, and the properties and qualities of individual essential oils before using them.

Distilled Essential Oil versus Absolute Oil

Oils can be obtained using different methods (as we'll discover in chapter 3). Two common methods are steam distillation and solvent extraction. Solvent-extracted oils produce what we call *absolute oils*.

Basically, in steam distillation the plant material is placed in a still. Water is added, heat is applied, and as the water heats, the plant material releases its essential oil, which rises with steam droplets that are funneled into a cooling pipe, at which point the oil and oil-infused water (hydrosol) are separated. In solvent extraction, a solvent is combined with the plant material. The solvent then draws the oil out of the plant material and the solvent and oil are then carefully separated; this produces an absolute.

Essential oils and absolutes from the same plant can have characteristics and chemical makeups that can vary a little or vary a lot. Steam distillation produces volatile essential oils comprised of smaller molecules that can dissipate quickly when exposed to air. Solvent extraction produces oils with heavier molecules, which is why many absolutes are often thicker than essential oils. Certain plant materials are better suited for solvent extraction, such as flower petals, because steam distillation can be detrimental to delicate flowers and result in an oil with an undesirable aroma or an oil of lesser quality. In some cases, solvent extractions also produce more oil than other methods of extraction do.

Essential Oils to Avoid in Aromatherapy

The safety of any essential oil largely depends on the knowledge of the person using it. When applied appropriately, most essential oils are safe to use; however, some oils can contribute to skin irritation, respiratory symptoms, and even hormone-related symptoms. Some essential oils can act as endocrine disruptors; some can bring on allergy symptoms (itchy, watery eyes; hives; redness of skin); some oils are photosensitive and if used in the sun can cause skin burning; some oils should not be used directly on the skin in high concentration; and there are possible drug interactions with certain essential oils and pharmaceutical drugs. Inhalation via aromatherapy is perhaps one of the safest ways to use essential oils, but diffusing them should be done with caution and not overdone. For more information on safety, see "Essential Oil Safety" in chapter 5 as well as notes found in the compendium of essential oils in chapter 6.

Avoid using the following oils in aromatherapy:

almond, bitter (unrectified)	mustard
armoise	parsley
basil (high estragole)	pennyroyal
birch (sweet, tar)	*Ravensara anisata*
boldo	sage (Dalmatian)
buchu	sassafras
cade (unrectified)	snakeroot
calamus	tansy
camphor (brown, yellow)	tarragon
cassia	tea (black)
cinnamon bark	tea tree (black river)
costus	thuja
elecampane	verbena
fig leaf	wintergreen
horseradish	wormseed
lanyana	wormwood

A Brief Review

Essential oils develop in plants as a by-product of photosynthesis and secondary metabolism and exist within a plant to protect its health through their antimicrobial and tissue-healing properties. They also aid fertilization and propagation. Minute droplets of essential oil diffuse through the walls of glands or other secretory structures to spread over the superficial surface of a plant, from where they evaporate into the surrounding environment. Thus essential oils repel predators and attract seed- and pollen-distributing insects and animals as well as birds and insects that eat pests. Essential oils also control a plant's immediate environment by exuding vapors that control ambient temperature and humidity. In short, they support a plant's ability to survive and continue to thrive as a species. Animals have a symbiotic and mutualistic relationship with plants and share similar cell structures.

A very simple example of this relationship is seen in the oxygen and carbon dioxide exchange: plants release oxygen required by animals to instigate cellular activity (to convert food into energy, among other things), and carbon dioxide released by animals in turn similarly supports plants to fuel their metabolic processes. Mutualistically, animals assist pollination and propagation of seeds, and plants in turn provide a source of nourishment and medicine. Furthermore, essential oils aid both plants and human microbiomes and immune systems to stave off infection and repair and regenerate damaged tissue. Used appropriately, essential oils work in harmony with our microbiome rather than waging war on it (as with pharmaceutical drugs). In this way we have a mutualistic and symbiotic relationship with our internal and external microbiome. And so in this way these interconnected relationships unfold in the web of life.

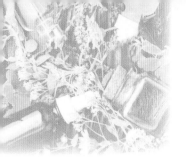

2

Biodiversity, Botany, and Essential Oils

A Deep Dive into the Plant World

*B*iodiversity is a term used to describe the totality of the richness of life on Earth, the total web of all living things and ecosystems, from dolphins to doves, from forests to coral reefs, including the genetic varieties within a species as well as between species. Biologists refer to biodiversity as the complete sphere of life in a region and identify four separate yet unified, interdependent levels of biological activity:

Genes: These are the basic physical and functional units of heredity. Each cell in the human body contains 25,000 to 35,000 genes; by comparison, tree cells have up to 45,000 genes, almost twice as many as humans.

Species: This refers to a group of living organisms consisting of similar individuals capable of exchanging genes or interbreeding.

Ecosystems: These are biological communities of interacting organisms and their physical environments.

Molecules: These are groups of atoms bonded together, representing the smallest fundamental units of a chemical compound that can take part in a chemical reaction. Biomolecules, for example, are carbohydrates, lipids, nucleic acids, and proteins.

This interactive and interconnected (symbiotic and mutualistic) web of life regulates and supports the chemistry and motion of a plant's surrounding atmosphere and its environment, the water supply, and the quality of Earth's topsoil and its microbiome (where minerals and nutrients are recycled, water is purified, and the soil is fertilized to nourish and sustain growth and reproduction).

Life on Earth is not evenly distributed across the planet and varies according to the atmospheric conditions of a given area or climate region. For example, very little life is found at the polar extremes, yet life is extremely rich and diverse in the regions north and south of the equator, areas where the sun is closest to Earth.

THE EIGHT CLIMATE BIOMES

The world is divided into three primary climate zones: tropical, temperate, and polar. These zones are further divided to incorporate eight broad climatic regions, or biomes, each one manifesting a particular weather pattern that influences the natural environment and habitat therein, which includes varieties of species of plants, insects, and animals. Many of these species have adapted and acclimatized over millions of years. Factors that affect regional biodiversity include the altitude (height above sea level), temperature, amount of solar light, precipitation (atmospheric water content and rainfall), and quality and content of soil.

It is impossible to count or measure the existence of *all* life on Earth. However, studies have been (and continue to be) made of regional areas, on land and in the oceans, to identify, ascertain, and catalog varieties of species that are present in a given biome or ecological region. The following table lists the eight climate biomes and their habitats and describes the essential oil–bearing plants in each biome.

CLIMATE BIOMES AND
ESSENTIAL OIL–BEARING PLANTS

CLIMATE REGION	DESCRIPTION	HABITAT	EXAMPLES OF ESSENTIAL OIL–BEARING PLANTS
Tundra/Polar Regions	Treeless polar areas bordering the Arctic and Antarctic are cold, dry, and usually frozen, with long, dark winters and short summers lasting fifty to sixty days. Temperatures rise above freezing for just a few months of the year, when the top layer of soil thaws, creating vast marshes.	**plants:** compact, wind-resistant plants, lichens, and mosses; no deep-rooting plants due to the layer of permafrost **animals:** polar bears, lemmings, reindeer (Arctic), penguins (Antarctic)	no essential oil-producing plants, shrubs, or trees
Mountains	Many high peaks are always covered in snow. Temperatures decrease with altitude and usually drop well below freezing after dark. Wetter and windier conditions prevail. Examples include the extreme northern hemisphere—northern Canada, Greenland, Iceland, Scandinavia, and northern Russia.	**plants:** no trees in higher mountain regions; some vegetation and habitat around rivers draining from mountains in sheltered valleys (e.g., birch, alders, and poplars); growing season lasts 180 days **animals:** mainly birds	no essential oil-producing plants, shrubs, or trees
Northern (Boreal or Taiga) Forests	Forests of conifers spread over a large area, with very cold, long winters and short summers. Temperatures fall to below freezing for four to six months of the year. Examples include the areas lying south of the tundra, stretching across most of northern Canada, Scandinavia, and Russia; also northern Europe, south-central Europe, central-west and eastern Russia, northern Canada, and the northern United States.	**plants:** cone-bearing, needle-leaved evergreen trees such as spruce, pine, larch, and fir **animals:** bears, beavers, squirrels, red deer	pine, spruce

CLIMATE BIOMES AND
ESSENTIAL OIL–BEARING PLANTS (continued)

CLIMATE REGION	DESCRIPTION	HABITAT	EXAMPLES OF ESSENTIAL OIL–BEARING PLANTS
Temperate Forests, Woodlands, and Grasslands	Moderate areas where the weather is seldom very cold or very hot, with warm summers and cool winters, and rain year-round include most of Europe, Russia, western Asia (including China), southern east-west Australia, and the central to western United States.	**plants:** evergreen (pine, fir, juniper, spruce, cedarwood) and broad-leaved deciduous trees (oak, ash, beech, sycamore, chestnut, maple), woody plants, grass, and herbs **animals:** horses, deer, sheep, goats, cattle, various birds	cedarwood, chamomile(s), juniper berry, lavender(s), patchouli, pine, spikenard
Mediterranean or Scrub Regions	Also referred to as shrubland, heathland, or chaparral, these have long, hot, dry summers and short, warm, wet winters. Evergreen scrub prevails. This land used to be covered with trees but has been cleared in many areas to grow crops and graze animals. The main areas include countries bordering the Mediterranean Sea, Australia, California, southern Europe, northern Africa, the Middle East, central and southwest Australia, southern Africa, central South America (e.g., Chile), and the southwestern U.S.	**plants:** from forests to woodlands, savannas, shrublands, and grasslands; olive, vines, pine, cypress, juniper, cedar, citrus, tea tree, oakmoss, frankincense, and myrrh trees; rose bushes, herbs (including lavender), and various shrubs **animals:** goats, sheep, horses, cattle	cajeput, carrot seed, cedarwood, clary sage, frankincense galbanum, geranium, jasmine, juniper berry, lavender, mandarin and other citruses, myrrh, neroli, oakmoss, orange, petitgrain, rose, tea tree, thyme, verbena

CLIMATE REGION	DESCRIPTION	HABITAT	EXAMPLES OF ESSENTIAL OIL–BEARING PLANTS
Deserts	Areas of bare mountains, rocky wastes, and sand dunes, often located in the center of continents, far from the sea, with very high temperatures all year round, although with distinctly hot summers and cooler winters, and scant rainfall of less than 10 inches (250 mm) per year. It may not rain in some areas for several years. Temperatures range from 95 to 104°F in summer, and 68 to 86°F in winter. Examples include northern Africa, the Middle East, central Australia, the southwestern U.S., and the western extreme of South America (e.g., Chile).	**plants:** sparse vegetation—wiry grass, thorny bushes, cacti, succulents **animals:** lizards, camels, rattlesnakes, some birds, black widow spiders, scorpions, jackrabbits, rats	no essential oil–producing plants, trees, or shrubs
Grasslands and Savannas	Dry grasslands are found in the center of continents where temperature variations are extreme. Hot summers, cold winters, and little rainfall prevail. Very few trees grow here. Tropical grasslands or savannas lie near the equator, between deserts and tropical rain forests, where it's hot all year round, with distinctly dry (or drought) and wet seasons (short rainy seasons). Areas of tall, thick-stemmed grasses and flat-topped, or canopied, thorny trees are found, primarily in the southern hemisphere—western (middle to southern) Africa, northern and southwestern Australia, Mexico, and northern (Colombia, Venezuela) and mideastern South America (Brazil).	**plants:** various grasses (with deep, massive, anchoring root systems) such as vetivert, lemon, and eucalyptus trees, mimosa, sunflowers, clovers, and cacti **animals:** giraffes, zebras, elephants, rhinoceroses, lions, leopards, cheetahs, buffalo, crocodiles, flamingos, tree ducks, lizards, anaconda	citriodora, eucalyptus, lemongrass, mimosa, vetivert

CLIMATE BIOMES AND
ESSENTIAL OIL–BEARING PLANTS (continued)

CLIMATE REGION	DESCRIPTION	HABITAT	EXAMPLES OF ESSENTIAL OIL–BEARING PLANTS
Tropical Forests	Found at latitudes within 15 degrees north and south of the equator, these jungles are continuously very hot, humid, and wet (at least 60 mm of rainfall every month), with no real winter or summer. There are five layers of plants in a rain forest: the high trees, the tree canopy, the open canopy, shrubs, and ground plants. Examples include Mexico, South America (Brazil), central-western Africa, southeastern Asia, India, China, Thailand, Burma, Cambodia, Indonesia, Bali, Solomon Islands, Fiji, Puerto Rico, and Hawaii.	**plants:** trees with thick foliage, epiphytes (plants that live on other plants), and climbing plants, e.g., orchids, palms, bamboos, mahogany, rosewood, eucalyptus, cinnamon, cabreuva, and guaiacwood **animals:** tigers, monkeys, tropical birds	benzoin, cabreuva, cardamom, cinnamon, eucalyptus, guaiacwood, palo santo, ravensara, rosewood

The Evolution of Plants

By observing plant impressions preserved in fossils found in lowland or marine sediments, botanists estimate that green photosynthetic land plants appeared around 450 million years ago (and some even suggest one thousand million years ago). Mosses and vascular-type plants, which evolved from algae, began to inhabit water edges, and over time these simple living organisms developed roots, leaves, and secondary woods, with spores and seeds that easily dispersed inland, thus propagating the spread of land plants across continents. Plants evolved as they adapted in accord with the landscape, atmosphere, and prevailing weather conditions. Seed plants that do not rely or depend on available water for the movement of sperm or the development of free-living gametophytes were able to survive and reproduce in extremely arid conditions. Vast forests of tall trees populated land masses. Grasses developed approximately ten million years ago, and flowering plants developed approximately two hundred million years ago.

Humans have cultivated grains, fruits, and nut- and seed-bearing plants and vegetables for thousands of years, ensuring a basic source of energy and vital nutrients (vitamins, minerals, amino acids, trace elements, and fiber). However, the remedial use of medicinal herbs and plants dates back to before records even began, and in many parts of the world plant medicine is still the a primary source of medicine—in fact, 70 to 80 percent of the world's population relies on natural plant remedies for their health-care needs. Some common pharmaceutical medicines that have been around for some time include plant constituents. For example, morphine and codeine, isolated from poppy seeds (*Papaver somniferum*), are used to relieve pain; the pharmaceutical drug digoxin, isolated from foxglove (*Digitalis purpurea*), are used to treat various heart conditions; and isolates such as quinine (chloroquine), from the cinchona tree (*Cinchona officinalis*), is used to treat malaria.

CLASSIFYING LIFE ON EARTH

Life on Earth is divided into two biological domains based on cellular structure and differences: eukaryotes and prokaryotes.

Eukaryote cells contain a nucleus and other structures, known as *organelles,* enclosed within their own membranes. Organelles are centrosomes, rough and smooth endoplasmic reticula, golgi apparatuses, lysosomes (vesicles), mitochondria, ribosomes, and vacuoles. Plant eukaryote cells have additional plastids, such as chloroplasts (responsible for photosynthesis), leucoplasts (responsible for starch storage and found in root and storage organ cells), and chromoplasts (organelles responsible for pigment synthesis and storage in roots, fruits, and flowers).

Prokaryote cells are unicellular organisms (archaea and bacteria) that do not contain a membrane-bound nucleus; all intracellular water-soluble components (DNA, proteins, and metabolites) are located together within the enclosed cell membrane.

Notice in the following diagrams the similarities between a human and a plant cell and the difference between these and the prokaryote cell.

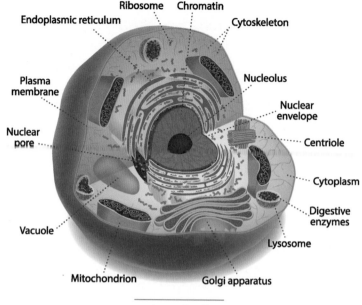

Animal cell

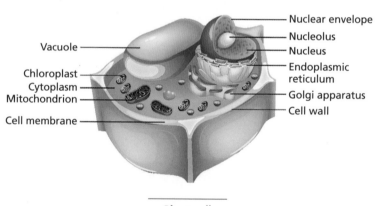

Plant cell

Although plant cells and animal cells are similar in structure, plant cells contain additional plastids—highly specialized membrane-bound structures—and their cell walls are composed of cellulose, a complex carbohydrate; hemicellulose, a type of polysaccharide; pectin, another polysaccharide; and in many instances lignin, a complex polymer that binds together the fibers within the cell walls of plants, making them woody and rigid.

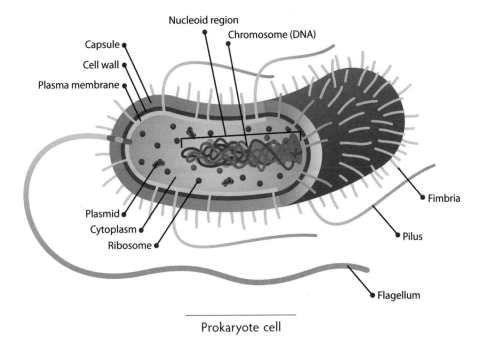

Prokaryote cell

TAXONOMY: IDENTIFYING AND LABELING

Taxonomy is the practice and science of classification and nomenclature. Biological taxonomy encompasses the description, identification, naming, and classification of organisms. Botany is a division of biology and is also known as plant science or plant biology.

Classification of the living world is an ongoing and evolving process that dates back to Aristotle (384–322 BC), who originally categorized plants and animals as separate entities. There were others: Theophrastus (371–287 BC), the "Father of Botany," who succeeded Aristotle and continued his work, as did Dioscorides (40–90 AD), Plinus (23–79 AD), and John Gerard (1545–1612 AD), all of whom made significant contributions to plant taxonomy. However, it was Carl Linnaeus (1707–1778) who further developed Aristotle's classification of the living world by introducing and listing additional subdivisions—class, order, and genus—which differentiated and ranked, or ordered, organisms in terms of their biological characteristics, similarities, variances, and their developmental relationship to one another and to the environment.

Since Linnaeus introduced his ranking system, microbiologists have added more categories. Nevertheless, different opinions and ongoing debates ensue among researchers, scientists, and biologists in terms of the inclusion and exclusion criteria for a given rank. Ranking is based on subjective dissimilarity. This is a devised system that does not necessarily reflect the true pattern or the whole picture. The evolution of life on Earth is highly complex and spans billions of years, and thus we are in a constant state of discovery. Categorization at least provides a system and identifiable pattern that aids in our understanding, and as such, although a complex and incomplete process, it does provide a basic road map to help us begin to understand the nature of living things.

The living world is generally divided into the following hierarchical categories—see examples of eukaryotes and prokaryotes and their divisions on pages 41–42—the range of inclusion for these groups vastly exceeds capacity to list them all below.

Rank		
Life		
Domain or Empire	Eukaryote	Prokaryote
Kingdom (*regnum*): subregnum	Animalia, Chromista, Fungi, Plantae, Protozoa	Archaea, Bacteria

Division or Phylum
  subdivision
  subphylum
  super division		

Class (*classis*) subclassis		
Order (*ordo*) subordo		
Family (*familia*) subfamilia		
Tribe (*tribus*) subtribus		

Genus
  subgenus
  section
  subsection
  series
  subseries		

Species
  subspecies
  variety (*varietus*)
  subvarietus
  form (*forma*)
  subforma		

Apparently, there exists an estimated three to five million discovered and undiscovered eukaryote species; up to approximately 315,000 of these species are plants, of which up to 290,000 (approximately 92 percent) are seed plants. It is difficult to estimate or even predict the numbers of prokaryote species, but researchers suggest that there exist between tens of thousands to billions. Wow! Clearly it would be impossible to categorize and list them all here; however, the following are some simple explanations and examples.

Examples of Eukaryotes

Animalia: corals, sea anemones, sponges, jellyfish, star fish, fish, amphibians (frogs, toads, newts), birds, reptiles, mammals (including humans), insects, spiders, crabs, snails, clams, and squids

Chromista: single-celled plankton, red and brown algae, and large, multicellular seaweeds

Fungi: yeasts, mushrooms, and molds

Plantae: flowering plants, conifers and other gymnosperms, trees, ferns, club mosses, mosses, hornworts, liverworts, green algae

Protists: flagellates (the most numerous soil protozoa), ciliates, and amoebas

Examples of Prokaryotes

Archaea: Members of this domain of single-celled, asexual microscopic organisms have no cell nucleus or any other membrane-bound organelles within their cells. They possess genes and several metabolic pathways that relate them more closely to eukaryotes than to bacteria. Identification and classification of species in this group is problematic and very difficult to clearly define.

Bacteria: There are thousands of known strains of bacteria and many more unknown. Some of the more common known beneficial bacteria include *Lactobacillus acidophilus*, *Bacillus subtilis*, *Bifidobacterium animalis*, *Streptococcus thermophilus*, and *Lactobacillus reuteri*. Harmful bacteria include *Streptococcus pyogenes*, *Escherichia coli*, *Vibrio cholera*, *Enteritis salmonella*, and *Salmonella typhi*.

EXAMPLES THAT ILLUSTRATE HOW
SPECIES ARE CLASSIFIED

RANK	FRUIT FLY	HUMAN	LAVENDER	FLY AGARIC	E. COLI
Domain	Eukaryota	Eukaryota	Eukaryota	Eukaryota	Prokaryota
Kingdom	Animalia	Animalia	Plantae	Fungi	Bacteria
Division or phyla	Arthropoda	Chordata	Tracheo-phyta	Basidiomycota	Proteo-bacteria
Subdivision or subphylum	Hexapoda	Vertebrata	Spermato-phytina	Agaricomycotina	
Class	Insecta	Mammalia	Magno-liopsida	Agaricomycetes	Gammapro-teobacteria
Subclass	Pterygota	Theria		Agaricomycetidae	
Order	Diptera	Primates	Lamiales	Agaricales	Entero-bacteriales
Suborder	Brachycera	Haplorrhini		Agaricineae	
Family	Drosophilidae	Hominidae	Lamiaceae	Amanitaceae	Entero-bacteriaceae
Subfamily	Drosophilenae	Homininae			
Genus	Drosophila	Homo	Lavandula	Amanita	Escherichia
Species	D. melanogaster	H. sapiens	L. angustifolia	A. muscaria	E. coli

The example of *Lavandula angustifolia,* the species of lavender shown in the table above, demonstrates how herbs, flowers, and other essential oil–bearing plants fit into this classification scheme. These divisions continue, however, as there can be several varieties within a species, added to which some plant species naturally cross with one another, while others are purposely cultivated. It can seem quite complicated. Each variation is observed and identified, as in the following boxed example on page 43 of lavender's species divisions.

Further Plant Species Divisions

- The term *subspecies* (abbreviated subsp. or ssp.) often denotes a geographical variation. For example, *Lavandula stoechas* subsp. *atlantica* identifies a lavender plant growing, in this case, in regions bordering the Atlantic. This in turn indicates the potential conditions of growth (geographical region, soil content, altitude, climate, and so on), all of which influence a plant's chemical constituents, and therefore the essential oil's constituents, making this information quite useful.
- The term *variety* (var.) indicates a rank between a botanical subspecies and its forma. For example, for *Citrus aurantium* var. *amara,* the term *amara* indicates bitter.
- The term *forma* (f.) denotes trivial botanical differences. For example, for *Lavandula stoechas* f. *leucantha, leucantha* indicates white flowers.
- A cultivar, which is given a name that is not italicized and appears in quotation marks, is a cultivated variety produced from a natural species and maintained by horticultural cultivation—for example, *Lavandula angustifolia* 'Hidcote.'
- A hybrid, represented by an x (which is not italicized in botanical terminology), is a natural or man-made cross between species. For example, *Mentha* x *piperata* is a cross between *Mentha aquatica* and *Mentha spicata.*
- Chemotypes, named by placing ct. after the botanical name, followed by the chemical constituent, are visually identical plants with significantly different chemical constituents, and so they have different therapeutic qualities. For example:

    Thymus vulgaris ct. linalool (anti-infectious)
    Thymus vulgaris ct. geraniol (similar to geranium)
    Thymus vulgaris ct. thujanol-4 (anti-infectious)
    Thymus vulgaris ct. terpenyl acetate (not usually used in aromatherapy)

Recognizing the nomenclature shorthand helps us decipher constituent content more specifically. It's important to be aware of differences, as they influence the scent, chemical properties, and therapeutic value and safety of a plant and its essential oil, among other things.

EXPLORING THE
PLANT (PLANTAE) KINGDOM

The plant kingdom is divided into three groups:

+ Nonvascular
+ Vascular plants with spores
+ Vascular plants with seeds

Nonvascular plants consist of mosses and related species such as horn-worts and liverworts, which are significant foundation plants for forest ecosystems. They are found growing on the ground, on rocks, and on other plants, and they reproduce by spores, not seeds, as they do not have flowers. Oakmoss, which grows on rocks and trees, is an example.

Vascular plants with spores have a vascular system (unlike mosses), but like mosses they reproduce from spores rather than seeds. Ferns form the largest species in this group. Others include club mosses (lycopods), horsetails, and whisk ferns.

Vascular plants with seeds include conifers (gymnosperms), which reproduce using "naked" seeds found on the surface, for example, in the cones of conifers or the fleshy, covered seed produced by the ginkgo tree. However, these external seed-carrying structures are not fruits or flowers. This group consists of nonflowering trees or shrubs that have needle-like leaves. Species include pines, firs, spruces, cedars, junipers, and yew trees, among others. Conifer "allies" include ginkgo (with a single species, the maidenhair tree) and cycads, which are palmlike and herblike plants that bear cones (such as Mormon tea, *Ephedra viridis*). Magnoliophyta, or angiosperms (flowering plants), form the largest and most diverse group of seed- and fruit-bearing plants and include most trees, shrubs, vines, flowers, fruits, vegetables, and legumes. These provide the largest source of staple food and medicine consumed by animals, which includes, of course, humans. They are differentiated from mosses and related species because they produce their seeds inside an ovary that is embedded in a flower or fruit, for example, sunflowers or dandelions, or fruit such as apples or tomatoes. There are 64 orders, 416 families, approximately 13,000 genera, and over 300,000 known species in this group.

Examples of Plant Types within the Plant Kingdom

NONVASCULAR	VASCULAR (SPORES)	VASCULAR (SEEDS)
Anthocerotophyta (hornworts)	Equisetophyta (horsetails)	Magnoliophyta (flowering plants)
Bryophyta (mosses)	Lycopodiophyta (lycopods)	Coniferophyta (conifers)
Chlorophyta (green algae)	Psilophyta (whisk ferns)	Cycadophyta (cycads)
Hepatophyta (liverworts)	Pteridophyta (ferns)	Ginkgophyta (ginkgo)
		Gnetophyta (gnetophytes)

The vascular seed-producing plant groups Magnoliophyta (angiosperms), which comprise monocotyledons (monocots) and dicotyledons (dicots), and Coniferophyta, which comprise cone-bearing seed plants, also include essential oil–bearing plants and are divided into the following classes:

Liliopsida (Monocotyledonae): This class, also known as the *monocots,* contains only the Liliaceae family. Examples include water poppies, duckweeds, rice, tulips, grasses, pond weeds, water lilies, orchids, and cattails.

Magnoliopsida (Dicotyledoneae): This class, also known as the *dicots,* contains other families of flowering plants. Examples include asters, carrots, daisies, pokeweed, hollies, dogwoods, honeysuckles, geranium, blueberries, clovers, maples, witch hazel, laurels, magnolias, roses, and many more.

Coniferophyta (Pinophyta): This class contains cone-bearing trees (conifers). Examples include cedar, spruce, cypress, and juniper, among others.

Monocots and Dicots

Monocots (Monocotyledonae)

Monocots are characterized by trimerous (having parts in three) flowers, a single cotyledon or embryonic leaf, pollen with one pore, usually parallel-veined leaves, and a fibrous root system (web- or threadlike and reaching in many directions). Monocots comprise some of the largest families of angiosperms, such as orchids, with approximately 20,000 species, and grasses, with approximately 15,000 species. They include some of the most economically important species of plants. In addition, numerous other vegetation types are found in grasslands, palm savannas, sedge meadows, and cattail marshes—some 70,000 species, including:

    Amaryllidaceae: garlic, onions

    Arecaeae: coconut, palms

    Musaceae: bananas

    Poaceae: vetivert, true grasses, including grains (rice, wheat, maize, etc.), sugarcanes, and bamboos

    Zingiberaceae: ginger, turmeric

  Families cultivated for their blooms include lilies, daffodils, irises, amaryllis, orchids, cannas, bluebells, and tulips.

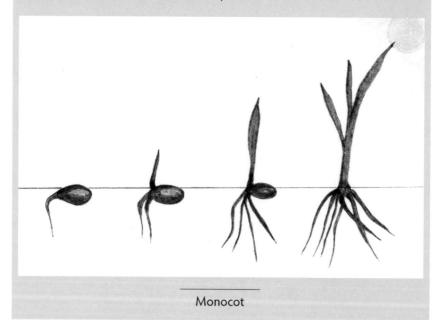

Monocot

Dicots (Dicotyledoneae)

The largest group of flowering plants is characterized by flowers with floral parts in multiples of four or five, and two cotyledons or embryonic leaves in their seeds, netted or spreading veins, and taproots (one main root from which other smaller roots branch off). There are around 200,000 species within this group. They include:

Asteraceae: chamomile, sunflowers, daisies, dandelions

Rosaceae: rose

Rutaceae: bergamot, petitgrain

Lamiaceae: lavender, patchouli, peppermint

Myrtaceae: cajeput, tea tree, eucalyptus

Examples of other plants found in this group include buttercup, sunflower, bean, oak, daisy, dandelion, peanut, cacti, apple, mango, linseed, pea, potato, tomato, and groundnut.

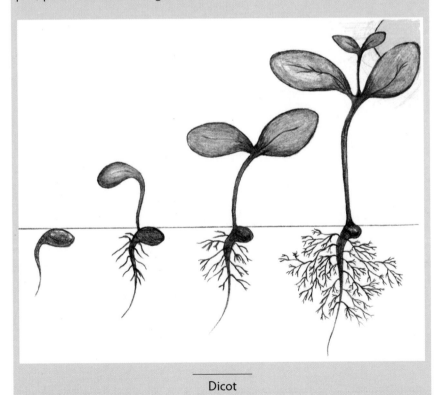

Dicot

PLANT ANATOMY

The following identifies each part of a plant and its fundamental contributing role, including essential oils extracted from secretory glands stored within a plant's structure.

Root System		
PARTS	**GENERAL FUNCTIONS**	**ESSENTIAL OILS**
✦ Primary roots ✦ Lateral roots ✦ Root hairs ✦ Root cap: a thimble-like covering that protects the delicate root tips ✦ Rhizome: a thick, horizontal, underground stem that produces roots and leafy shoots ✦ Tuber: a swollen, rounded, underground stem (for example, a potato) ✦ Bulb: a swollen underground organ that functions as a food store, with overlapping layers of fleshy leaf bases or scales and roots extending from its lower surface	✦ Usually located underground ✦ Anchors the plant in the soil ✦ Absorbs and conducts water and nutrients ✦ Food storage (starch, carbohydrates, amino acids, i.e., energy)	The role of essential oils found in roots: ✦ Deter herbivores and microbial invasion ✦ Act as a food source (for example, sesquiterpenes found in the roots of vetivert) for certain bacteria that prevent colonization of other, potentially pathogenic microorganisms, which in turn also enhances essential-oil biosynthesis in a way that influences the quantity of essential oil and the oil's chemical composition (Del Giudice et al. 2008). Essential oils extracted from roots and rhizomes include: ✦ Angelica (roots and rhizomes) ✦ Garlic (bulb) ✦ Ginger (unpeeled, dried, and ground root) ✦ Spikenard (dried and crushed rhizomes and roots) ✦ Valerian (dried and crushed rhizomes and roots) ✦ Vetivert (dried and chopped roots and rootlets)

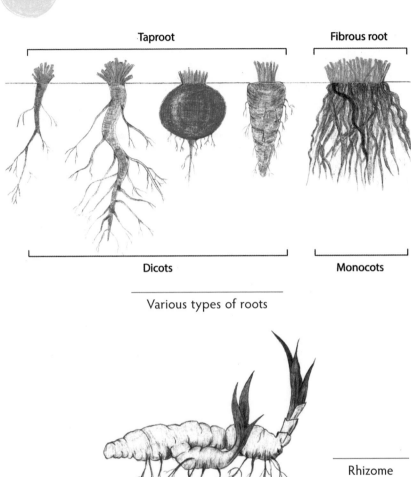

Various types of roots

Rhizome

Tuber

Shoot System

PARTS	GENERAL FUNCTIONS	ESSENTIAL OILS
✦ New growth (sprouts or shoots) formed from a mass of living cells that divide and multiply ✦ Incorporates new stems, leaves, and reproductive organs ✦ Sprouts and shoots can be dormant with the ability to become active when environmental conditions support growth and expansion	✦ Food and water conduction ✦ Reproduction and dispersal ✦ Photosynthesis	The role of essential oils found in shoots—including stems, wood, and bark—and leaves: ✦ Defensive: released locally when plant is attacked by pathogens or herbivores ✦ Act as communication signals within and between plants ✦ Exude characteristic green smell, like freshly cut grass ✦ Bark and wood oils contain a significant amount of resins, secreted when the plant is wounded Essential oils extracted from: ✦ Stems and stalks: galbanum (gum/oleoresin exude), geranium ✦ Grass: citronella, lemongrass, palmarosa ✦ Tree trunk (heartwood): cedarwood, palo santo, rosewood, sandalwood ✦ Bark: birch, cinnamon ✦ Tree resin: frankincense, myrrh ✦ Plant resin: galbanum ✦ Branches, twigs, needles: cajeput, cypress, eucalyptus, myrtle, petitgrain, pine, tea tree ✦ Leaves: cajeput, eucalyptus, geranium, myrtle, petitgrain, tea tree ✦ Flowering herbs (including leaves and stems): clary sage, marjoram, peppermint, oregano, patchouli, tagetes, thyme, yarrow

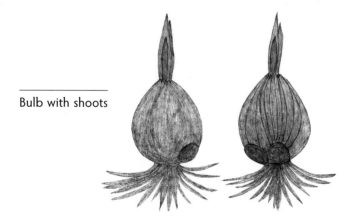

Bulb with shoots

Flowers

PARTS	GENERAL FUNCTIONS	ESSENTIAL OILS
✦ Flowers, blooms, or blossoms (reproductive structures that give rise to fruits or seeds) mostly consist of four structures attached to a stalk, including: • Calyx: outermost whorl of sepals, usually green, which enclose the bud during formation; can be absent or predominant and petal-like • Corolla: the next layer, or whorl, of petals, which are thin, soft, and colored and attractive to insects and birds (as in pollination and reproduction) • Androecium: the inner whorl consisting of stamens, which have two parts, a stalk (filament) topped by an anther, where pollen is produced and dispersed • Gynoecium: innermost whorl consisting of one or more units, called *carpels*, which form a hollow structure called an *ovary*, which produces ovules internally; also known as a *pistil* (comprising the ovary, style, and stigma), the sticky tip (stigma) of which receives pollen. Pollen tubes grow from pollen grains adhering to the stigma.	✦ Attraction (animals and insects) ✦ Fertilization ✦ Reproduction ✦ Provide a mechanism to unite sperm with eggs ✦ Facilitate outcrossing (i.e., fusion of sperm and eggs from different species) or selfing (i.e., fusion of sperm and egg from same flower) ✦ Mediate joining of sperm contained in pollen to the ovules contained in the ovary ✦ Movement of pollen from anthers to stigma (i.e., pollination) ✦ Joining of sperm to ovules (i.e., fertilization) Note: Pollen is normally transported from one plant to another, but many plants are able to self-fertilize	The role of essential oils found in flowers: ✦ To attract pollinators from a distance. During flowering, essential-oil production increases (then decreases once pollination has occurred). Each plant species releases a specific scent to target specific pollinators. ✦ To store and release osmophores from epidermal secretory cells or glands, rather than specific secretory structures ✦ To protect against florivores (insects and ants) Essential oils extracted from: ✦ Buds: clove ✦ Flowers: chamomile, helichrysum, jasmine, lavender, marigold ✦ Blossoms: neroli (orange), rose, ylang-ylang

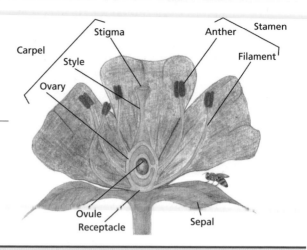

Flower anatomy

Stigma, Anther, Stamen, Carpel, Style, Filament, Ovary, Ovule, Receptacle, Sepal

Fruits and Seeds

PARTS	GENERAL FUNCTIONS	ESSENTIAL OILS
<ul><li>Develop from fertilized ovules</li><li>Pericarp (the wall of a fruit) develops from the ovary wall after fertilization.</li><li>In berries and drupes, the pericarp forms edible tissue around the seeds.</li><li>In accessory fruits (apples, pears), other edible tissue, derived from tissue adjacent to the carpel, develops around the seeds.</li><li>Simple fruits are formed from a single ovary and may contain one to many seeds; they can be either fleshy (berries, drupes, pomegranates) or dry (nuts).</li><li>Aggregate fruits (raspberries, blackberries) are formed from a single compound flower and contain many ovaries.</li><li>Multiple fruits (e.g., pineapple) are formed from the fused ovaries of multiple flowers.</li></ul>	<ul><li>Reproduction</li><li>Food source for insects, birds, other animals</li></ul>	The role of essential oils found in fruits and seeds: <ul><li>Berries, apples, pears, etc., contain low levels of essential oils (mostly nonterpenic esters) and attract fruit-eating herbivores that help disperse seeds. Citrus fruits contain high levels of monoterpene-rich oil, usually stored in single secretory cells. Cardamom and black pepper fruits contain high levels of mono- and sesquiterpenes, alcohols, and aldehydes. Seeds (or dried fruits) contain terpenic compounds and phenylpropanoids (phenols) and defend against invasive microbes and herbivores; they also prevent the growth of other plants (allelopathy).</li></ul>Essential oils extracted from: <ul><li>Fruit, berry: black pepper, juniper, may chang, star anise</li><li>Fruit peel: grapefruit, lemon, lime, mandarin, orange</li><li>Nut: almond, coconut, hazelnut, walnut</li><li>Seed: caraway, cardamom, carrot seed, coriander, cumin, fennel, nutmeg</li></ul>

ESSENTIAL OIL–BEARING PLANTS AND THEIR CHARACTERISTICS

This section lists and briefly describes the characteristics of botanical families that contain essential oil–bearing plants, with examples of essential oils extracted from plants in each family and their general therapeutic traits. The number of genera and species within a botanical family identified below are estimates (because, among other reasons, the adaptation of the ecological landscape in response to climate change inevitably impacts diversity—see "Ecological Sustainability," later in this chapter).

Annonaceae

Class: Dicotyledons

Also known as the custard apple or annona family, these are deciduous or evergreen shrubs, trees, and woody climbers with simple leaves; symmetrical, bisexual, fragrant flowers; and berrylike pulpy fruits that sometimes coalesce into multiple fruits. The bark, leaves, and roots of many species are used traditionally as medicine. There are approximately 130 genera and 2,300 species, and they are found mostly in tropical rain forests in southern Europe, Asia, and Africa and in some temperate regions.

Essential oils: Ylang-ylang; also cananga

Associated therapeutic traits: Sedative and balancing to the nervous system, ease depression and anxiety, support the integumentary and circulatory systems, aphrodisiac

Apiaceae (Umbelliferae)

Class: Dicotyledons

Also known as the parsley family, these are flowering plants that are often aromatic and characterized by hollow stems, alternate featherlike multi-divided leaves, and flat-topped, bisexual flower clusters or umbels that produce ridged fruits that split open upon maturing. Some are very poisonous (due to a high ketone and phenolic ether content, for example, hemlock), some are medicinal, and others are widely used foods such as carrots, celery, fennel, parsnips, and parsley, among others. There are approximately 430 genera and 3,700 species, and they are found throughout the world, mostly in northern temperate regions, particularly the Mediterranean.

Essential oils: Caraway, carrot seed, coriander, fennel, and galbanum; also angelica, aniseed, asafetida, celery seed, cumin, dill, khella, lovage

Associated therapeutic traits: Aid elimination and secretion, support the digestive, respiratory, endocrine, and integumentary (tissue-regenerating) systems

Asteraceae (Compositae)
Class: Dicotyledons
Also known as the aster, daisy, or sunflower family, these are a large and widespread family of herbaceous annual or perennial plants, shrubs, and some trees, including sunflowers, lettuce, echinacea, dahlias, and marigold, among others. The flowers are borne in florets surrounded by a whorl of petal-like bracts. The leaves are simple or occasionally compound and arranged oppositely, alternately, or occasionally whorled, along the stem. This comprises the largest family of flowering plants, with approximately 1,620 genera and 23,600 species distributed throughout the world, spanning all continents, altitudes, and climate regions, although originally native to North America.

Essential oils: Chamomile (German, Roman, Maroc, English), helichrysum/immortelle, and yarrow; also calendula, costus, cotton lavender, marigold, tagetes, tarragon

Associated therapeutic traits: Calming and regenerative to body and spirit, soothe inflammation, support the digestive and integumentary systems

Betulaceae (Fagales)
Class: Dicotyledons
This family includes deciduous nut-bearing trees and shrubs with simple, serrate, alternate leaves and pendulus male (long) or female (short) catkin flowers that produce small nuts or a short-winged samara. Species include birches, alders, hornbeams, and hazels, which are a valued source of timber. The oil (betula) obtained from the twigs of the

birch smells similar to wintergreen. There are approximately 6 genera and 150 species, mostly natives of temperate and subarctic areas of the northern hemisphere, although also found in the Andes in South America.

Essential oil: Birch (sweet, white)

Associated therapeutic traits: Analgesic; supports kidney, muscular, urinary, and respiratory systems; eases muscular pain

Burseraceae

Class: Dicotyledons

Also known as dry fire or torchwood—owing to historical use of its fragrant wood, bark, and resin as incense and ritualistic fumigants—this family of resinous trees and shrubs has leaves composed of many leaflets that alternate along the stem, with solitary or clustered flowers and fleshy fruits. Several species of *Boswellia* (frankincense) and *Commiphora* (myrrh) produce fragrant oleo-gum resin, traditionally used as incense and medicine. Resins are also obtained from other species in this family, including *Canarium luzonicum* (elemi), a tree native to the Philippines. There are approximately 19 genera and 540 species that are native to Central America and the Caribbean, with some species occurring in Africa and Asia.

Essential oils: Frankincense and myrrh; also elemi, linaloe, opopanax, palo santo, West Indian birch, West Indian elemi (the last two of which are neither true birch nor elemi)

Associated therapeutic traits: Sedative and fortifying, cooling and drying, anti-inflammatory, support the respiratory and integumentary systems, vulnerary (wound-healing), expectorant

Caprifoliaceae (Valerianaceae)

Class: Dicotyledons

These are herbaceous flowering plants with strongly odiferous (considered unpleasant by some) foliage and roots, with simple compound leaves and small, clustered, bisexual flowers. The morphology between species varies. Valerian has sweetly scented pink and white flowers, whereas spikenard's are pink and bell-shaped, with berrylike fruits. There are approximately 17 genera and 300 species widely distributed from temperate to tropical regions, except in Australia and New Zealand.

Essential oils: Spikenard; also valerian

Associated therapeutic traits: Sedating and calming; support the nervous system, ease anxiety and insomnia

Cistaceae

Class: Dicotyledons

Also known as rock rose, this family produces aromatic, sweet-smelling, flowering shrubs, with yellow, pink, or white flowers that have crumpled petals and numerous stamens, with alternate simple, scalelike leaves. Self-pollinating species do not have flowers. The fruit is a capsule that opens along a number of valves to release its seeds. There are 9 genera and 200 species found in temperate or warm-temperate areas, especially the Mediterranean region, from Europe to North Africa to Central Asia, as well as North and South America.

Essential oils: Cistus, labdanum

Associated therapeutic traits: Sedative and fortifying; support the integumentary and nervous systems, ease depression, anxiety, and stress-related disorders; vulnerary (wound-healing)

Cupressaceae

Class: Coniferae

Also known as the cypress family, this group includes evergreen, ornamental, and timber shrubs and trees with needlelike leaves and cones, such as juniper and redwoods. There are approximately 30 genera and 133 species distributed throughout the world.

Essential oils: Cedarwood, cypress, and juniper; also cade (juniper)

Associated therapeutic traits: Warming and tonic; support the nervous system, the respiratory system (especially the lungs), and the integumentary system; aid nervous tension, stress-related conditions, and insomnia

Dipterocarpaceae

Class: Dicotyledons

These lofty, lowland rain forest trees with green, leathery leaves and aromatic resin have clustered, fragrant flowers with twisted, leathery petals and winged-nut fruits. *Dipterocarpus glandulosa* yields gurjun balsam, which is used in medicines. As well, it is an important source of timber, aromatic oils, balsam, and resin. Borneo camphor (*Dryobalanops aromatica*) is an endangered tree, and although a crystalline resin is still tapped from the tree's trunk, most borneol essential oils are synthetically created from turpentine or camphor oil. There are approximately 17 genera and 695 species found in Malaysian and Southeast Asian forests.

Essential oils: Borneol, gurjun balsam

Associated therapeutic traits: Anti-inflammatory and decongestant; support the integumentary, respiratory, and circulatory systems; ease joint and muscle pain

Fabaceae (Leguminosea)

Class: Dicotyledons

Known commonly as the pea family, this is a very large family of flowering trees, shrubs, vines, and herbs that have compound stipulate, pinnate, feather-like leaves and fruits known as legumes. An important source of agricultural and food plants, species include carob, chickpea, lentil, mimosa, peanut, soya bean, and tamarind. Most woody species are tropical, with herbaceous species occurring mainly in temperate regions. There are approximately 751 genera and 22,000 species found almost worldwide in tropical and temperate regions.

Essential oil: Balsam (copaiba, Peru/Tolu)

Associated therapeutic traits: Warming and sedative to the nervous system, antiseptic, supports the respiratory (sore throat) and circulatory systems, eases anxiety and depression

Geraniaceae

Class: Dicotyledons

This family of flowering plants whose name derives from the geranium consists of herbs or low shrubs with lobed or otherwise divided leaves that are either opposite or alternate, with five-petaled, symmetrical red, pink, purple, blue, or white flowers. Some species have scented leaves. The *Pelargonium* genus provides the essential oil commonly used in aromatherapy. There are approximately 7 genera and 830 species found in temperate, warm-temperate, and some tropical regions.

Essential oils: Geranium, rose geranium

Associated therapeutic traits: Balancing to the nervous system, antiseptic and antiviral, support the organs of the digestive system (liver, kidneys) and the nervous and integumentary systems, ease nervous tension and depression

Hamamelidaceae

Class: Dicotyledons

Also known as the witch hazel family, these shrubs and trees have simple, palmate, alternate leaves and flowers that are usually held within a spike. They bear woody fruit. Some species are grown for their wood and others for their medicinal properties. There are approximately 30 genera and 100 species that are native to both temperate and warm-temperate regions.

Essential oils: Asiatic styrax, Levant styrax, storax (resins used in perfumery and as flavors), witch hazel (a hydrosol)

Associated therapeutic traits: Soothing and grounding; ease depression, anxiety, and stress-related conditions; support the integumentary system

Lamiaceae (Labiatae)

Class: Dicotyledons

Also known as the mint family, this is the largest essential oil–producing family. These herbaceous plants are characterized by square stems, paired and simple leaves, and two-lipped, open, tubular, fragrant flowers that are usually bisexual. Often the whole plant is aromatic. There are approximately 236 genera and 7,000 species distributed almost worldwide, mainly found in temperate and tropical regions, especially Mediterranean regions.

Essential oils: Basil, clary sage, hyssop, lavandin, lavender, marjoram, melissa, oregano, patchouli, peppermint, rosemary, and thyme; also calamintha, mint

Associated therapeutic traits: Stimulating and warming, vitalizing, and medicinal; support metabolism and the digestive and respiratory systems

Lauraceae

Class: Dicotyledons

This economically important family of laurels produces aromatic woods with leathery evergreen leaves that are alternately arranged or whorled, with small green, yellow, or white single-carpel flowers, usually arranged in clusters that produce single-seeded, fleshy berries or drupes. The essential-oil cavities are found in the leaves, wood, and bark. There are approximately 50 genera and 2,500 species distributed throughout tropical and subtropical regions, mostly in southeast Asia and tropical America, especially Brazil.

Essential oils: Cinnamon and may chang; also bay laurel, camphor, ho wood, ravensara, rosewood, sassafras

Associated therapeutic traits: Stimulant and tonic, antimicrobial (fungicidal, bactericidal, and virucidal), support the nervous and circulatory systems, support tissue regeneration, aphrodisiac

Liliaceae

Class: Monocotyledons

Members of this family consist of herbs and shrubs with six-segmented large flowers and three-chambered capsular fruits that are sometimes berries. The leaves are usually clustered at the base of the plant but are sometimes presented alternately along the stem or in whorls. Most species have underground storage structures such as bulbs or rhizomes. There are approximately 16 genera and species native to temperate and subtropical regions.

Essential oils: Hyacinth (absolute), garlic, onion

Associated therapeutic traits: Anti-infectious and detoxifying, support the circulatory system; hyacinth eases depression and anxiety; onion and garlic are highly antiseptic and antimicrobial (garlic and onion essential oils are extremely pungent)

Malvaceae

Class: Dicotyledons

This family of flowering plants has palmately lobed, compound, palmately veined leaves. The stems contain mucous canals and cavities with snowy, five-petaled single flowers with fused bracts below the sapel.

Many species are cultivated as a source of natural fibers, while others are grown as food crops and ornamentals. Species include cacao, cotton, hibiscus, hollyhock, linden, mallow, and okra. There are approximately 243 genera and 4,225 species found mostly in temperate and tropical regions.

Essential oils: Ambrette seed, linden blossom (absolute)

Associated therapeutic traits: Relieve stress-related conditions, anxiety, and depression; ease muscular aches and pains; support the digestive and nervous systems

Monimiaceae

Class: Dicotyledons

This family consists of evergreen trees, shrubs, and, rarely, woody vines (liana) with simple, oppositely arranged leaves and unisexual flowers that are closed and somewhat fig-like, producing fruit that splits open to expose individual small, fleshy fruits with a single seed inside. Essential oils are extracted from the bark, wood, and leaves. Closely related to the Lauraceae and Hernandiaceae families, there are approximately 24 genera and 520 species found mostly in the southern hemisphere, in the tropical and subtropical regions of Central and South America, tropical Africa, Madagascar, Sri Lanka, Australia, and New Zealand.

Essential oil: Boldo leaf

Associated therapeutic traits: Metabolic stimulant, detoxifying, supports the urinary system; mainly used in medicine rather than aromatherapy, as in the latter it is highly toxic

Myristicaceae

Class: Dicotyledons

These family members consist of evergreen trees (which are often large), shrubs, and, rarely, wood vines (lianas) with fragrant wood, leaves, and small, unisexual flowers that produce fleshy, single-seeded fruits. The dark green, glossy leaves are simple and alternately arranged along stems. The trees produce a colored (often red) sap that exudes when the trees are cut. There are approximately 21 genera and 520 species found throughout moist tropical lowland rain forests, mainly in Malaysia.

Essential oils: Nutmeg; also mace

Associated therapeutic traits: Analgesic and aphrodisiac; support the digestive, circulatory, and nervous systems; cephalic (relating to the head) stimulant

Myrtaceae

Class: Dicotyledons

Also known as the myrtle family, these shrubs and trees have leathery, evergreen, opposite or nearly opposite simple leaves that contain oil glands. The flowers have a base number of five petals with conspicuous, brightly colored stamens (referred to as bottle brush). The trees produce timber. There are approximately 150 genera and 3,700 species widely distributed in the tropics, especially Australia (dry-fruited) and Central and South America (berry-fruited). Eucalyptus and corymbia grow in the semiarid to wet coastal zones of Australia, whereas myrtle and some species of eucalyptus (for example, blue gum, red gum, lemon-scented gum, and red ironbark) grow in more temperate regions of both hemispheres, especially in the Mediterranean region and also South Africa.

Essential oils: Cajeput, clove, eucalyptus, myrtle, niaouli, and tea tree; also allspice, turpentine, West Indian bay

Associated therapeutic traits: Stimulant and tonic, strongly antimicrobial and anti-infectious, support the respiratory system and metabolism

Oleaceae

Class: Dicotyledons

Also known as the olive family, this family includes trees, shrubs, and a few lianas (woody vines). Olive trees are of economic significance (both wood and fruit). These family members are cultivated for their beautiful and fragrant four-petaled flowers (especially lilac and jasmine), which are mostly white or yellow and joined at the base to form a tube. The fruits may be fleshy (olives), winged (ash), a woody capsule, or a two-lobed berry (jasmine). There are approximately 24 genera and 615 species found throughout most of the world; they're especially abundant in tropical and temperate Asia (evergreen), although also found in colder zones (deciduous). Some species are native to forested regions.

Essential oil: Jasmine

Associated therapeutic traits: Calming and uplifting; aphrodisiac; supports the nervous system; eases depression, anxiety, and stress-related conditions; highly scented

Parmeliaceae

Class: Fungi, lichen (lecanoromycetes)

The largest family of lichen-forming fungi has a symbiotic relationship with green algae. With a diverse and complex morphology, these plants are found growing on roadside pavements, alpine rocks, tropical rain-forest trees, and subshrubs in the Antarctic tundra. The species *Evennia prunastri* (oakmoss) is pale to dark olive green and appears as a flat, bushy, highly branched vegetative tissue that grows on trees, mainly on the trunk and branches of oaks, as well as on rocks, in temperate mountain woodlands. There are approximately 87 genera and 2,000 species found in the northern hemisphere, including France, Portugal, Spain, North America, and central Europe.

Essential oil: Oakmoss (absolute)

Associated therapeutic traits: Supports the nervous system; balancing and grounding; aphrodisiac; used as a perfume fixative

Pinaceae

Class: Coniferae

Also known as the pine family, these evergreen and resinous trees and, rarely, shrubs, with subopposite or whorled branches and spirally arranged needlelike leaves, bear both male and female reproductive structures on the same plant, with pollen-bearing male cones and female ovule seed-bearing cones. Species include fir, Douglas fir, spruce, larch, cedars, and pines. The trees are economically significant as a source of timber, paper pulp, oils, and resin. There are approximately 11 genera and 220 species native to northern temperate regions.

Essential oils: Cedarwood Atlas and pine; also Canadian balsam, silver fir, spruce

Associated therapeutic traits: strongly antimicrobial and antiseptic; reviving, warming, and tonic; support the respiratory, nervous, and endocrine systems; especially useful for shallow breathing where there is a deficiency of oxygen

Piperaceae

Class: Dicotyledons

Also known as the pepper family, species include trees, shrubs, woody vines, and herbs with pungent, aromatic leaves that grow singly, and numerous flowers that are crowded in dense spikes and lack sapels and petals. Many species are used in medicine and in food as spices and seasoning. *Piper nigrum* (black and white pepper) is a woody climber native to India and Sri Lanka and is cultivated in mostly warm, moist, tropical regions. There are approximately 13 genera and 360 species widely distributed throughout the tropics and subtropics.

Essential oils: Black pepper; also cubeb (also known as java pepper or false pepper)

Associated therapeutic traits: Warming and drying; stimulating and tonic; support the digestive, circulatory, and nervous systems; ease indigestion and muscle pain; grounding

Poaceae (Gramineae)

Class: Monocotyledons

Part of the grass family, the grasses have stems that are hollow except at the nodes, and alternate leaves borne in two ranks. The flowers are characteristically arranged in spikelets, each having one or more florets. A significant food source, the species are among the top five families of flowering plants and range from lawns to staple cereal crops. Species include bamboo, barley, maize, millet, oat grass, pampas grass, rice, rye, vetivert, and wheat. Species that grow in the tropics are grasslike and scented. There are approximately 800 genera and 12,000 species found on all continents throughout the world.

Essential oils: Citronella, lemongrass, palmarosa, vetivert

Associated therapeutic traits: Refreshing and sedative, strongly anti-microbial, support the nervous and immune systems, ease nervous tension and depression

Rosaceae

Class: Dicotyledons

Also known as the rose family, the species also includes important food crops such as apples, almonds, cherries, pears, blackberries, raspberries, and strawberries. Generally woody plants, mostly shrubs, or small to medium-size trees, many are armed with thorns, spines, or prickles to discourage herbivores. Brambles such as blackberry present as tangled, prickly shrubs or scramblers. Most species have alternate leaves and bisexual flowers that vary from small to large, with colors that range from white to yellow, pink, orange, lavender, or red. The flowers are typically flat or shallow, cup-shaped, and radially symmetrical, with petals in multiples of five or four. Nectar-producing and insect-pollinated, they yield a variety of fruits. There are approximately 91 genera and 4,828 species found primarily in the northern temperate zone, and in a wide variety of habitats.

Essential oils: Rose (Damask otto)

Associated therapeutic traits: Uplifting and tonic; aphrodisiac; support the reproductive, integumentary, and nervous systems; ease emotional shock and grief; balancing to the nervous system

Rutaceae

Class: Dicotyledons

The leaves of these woody and aromatic trees and shrubs, and a few herbaceous perennials, have oil glands on the surface, and the colorful flowers contain nectar that is strongly fragrant, with five or four petals with both male and female reproductive organs that are pollinated by bees and small insects. The fruits are various, consisting of capsules, follicles, drupes, and berries (citrus fruit is a modified sectional berry). Orange, lemon, lime, mandarin, and grapefruit are economically significant fruit-bearing trees. West Indian sandalwood, or amyris, is an intensely scented balsam extracted from the trunk of the amyris tree. Note: West Indian sandalwood and West Indian rosewood are synonymous with amyris; they are not true sandalwood or rosewood. There are approximately 160 genera and 2,070 species distributed throughout the world, especially in temperate and warm, tropical regions such as around the Mediterranean and in South Africa, North America

(California, Arizona, Florida), Central America, and Australia.

Essential oils: Bergamot, grapefruit, lemon, lime, mandarin, orange (bitter, sweet), orange blossom (neroli), and petitgrain; also amyris

Associated therapeutic traits: Tonic to the nervous system; flowers are sedative and fruits are refreshing; support the digestive (especially the liver and kidneys), nervous, and integumentary systems; ease inflammation

Santalaceae

Class: Dicotyledons

Also known as the sandalwood family, this group consists of semi-parasitic trees, shrubs, herbs, and climbers. Although their green leaves contain chlorophyll, which allows some independent manufacturing of food, these plants bind to the roots, stems, and trunks of other plants, forming connections to tap into and leech water and nutrients. Most have small, unisexual flowers, either single or clusters, which produce fruits surrounded by brightly colored flesh with a stony seed. The species *Santalum album,* or Indian sandalwood, now endangered as a result of overexploitation, is used to make furniture and perfumes. *Santalum spicatum,* or Australian sandalwood, offers a substitute. There are approximately 43 genera and 2,525 species found in tropical and temperate regions, including India, Pakistan, Nepal, and western Australia. There are also some species in North America.

Essential oil: Sandalwood

Associated therapeutic traits: Grounding and calming; disinfectant; supports the nervous, respiratory, and excretory systems; balancing to the nervous system; eases lung congestion, urinary infections, and stress-related disorders

Schisandraceae

Class: Dicotyledons

This family includes evergreen tropical shrubs, trees, and woody vines with beetle-pollinated flowers. The genus *Illicium* (formerly listed under the now-defunct family Illiciaceae) is comprised of shrubs and trees that have aromatic leaves and bisexual flowers composed of inner petals that gradually change into stamens. The female, ovule-bearing structures consist of carpels usually arranged in a single whorl. At maturity the flowers produce a woody fruit consisting of a ring of several joining, podlike seed follicles. The essential oil of star anise is extracted from the fruit. Schisandraceae comprises approximately 3 genera and 90 species, of which *Illicium* (various species of anisetree) is one, with approximately 42 species. It is native to Australasia, southeastern Asia, and the southeastern United States.

Essential oil: Star anise (Chinese, Japanese)

Associated therapeutic traits: Supports the circulatory, digestive, and respiratory systems

Tiliaceae

Class: Dicotyledons

This family consists of trees, shrubs, and, rarely, herbs with woody, cylindrical, solid and branched stems with simple alternate leaves and bisexual flowers. Some species are used for timber, and some are a source of jute. Tilia species found in the northern hemisphere produce lime trees (or linden) with highly scented linden flowers or blossoms. There are approximately 50 genera and 450 species found in tropical and subtropical regions, and they are especially abundant in southeast Asia and Brazil, as well as in temperate northern regions.

Essential oils: Linden blossom (absolute) from lime trees (sometimes called linden trees)

Associated therapeutic traits: Supports the nervous system; eases insomnia and stress-related conditions

Verbenaceae

Class: Dicotyledons

This family consists mainly of tropical flowering shrubs, herbs, and a few trees, with mostly simple, whorled, or opposite leaves and clusters of small, tubelike, aromatic, bisexual flowers that yield drupe or capsule fruits. This family also includes deciduous timber plants such as teak (*Tectona grandis*). There are approximately 30 genera and 1,100 species, and most are found in tropical and subtropical regions, while some extend into temperate zones.

Essential oil: Lemon verbena

Associated therapeutic traits: Cooling and refreshing; supports the nervous and digestive systems; eases nervousness

Violaceae
Class: Dicotyledons
Also known as the violet family, these plants include trees and a few vines, as well as herbaceous plants (mainly violas and pansies) that have stipulated and toothed leaves, solitary nectary flowers, and capsular three-seamed fruits that explode to expel seeds. The rhizomes and seeds of *Viola odorata* (sweet violet) are poisonous, but the essential oil is often used in scents. There are 23 genera and 800 species found throughout the world, mainly in tropical to warm-temperate zones.
Essential oil: Violet (absolute)
Associated therapeutic traits: Calms the nervous system

Zingiberaceae
Class: Monocotyledons
Also known as the ginger family, this group includes aromatic perennial herbs that grow in moist areas, with creeping horizontal or tuberous forked rhizomes, many of which are large and spicy in all their parts. The flower clusters are brightly colored, spiral, and conelike, resembling an orchid, and nectar is present in the slender flower tubes. The flowering period is very brief. *Curcuma longa,* turmeric roots, and *Zingiber officinale,* ginger roots, are used as spices and medicine. There are approximately 52 genera and 1,300 species found in mostly moist, sometimes dry areas of the tropics and subtropics, especially Africa, Asia, and South and North America (Hawaii).
Essential oils: Cardamom, ginger, turmeric
Associated therapeutic traits: Warming, cleansing, stimulating, and tonic; support the digestive and reproductive systems; ease muscular and joint pain

Zygophyllaceae
Class: Dicotyledons
These shrubs or small trees are often resinous, with opposite or spirally arranged leaves and five-part, nectary flowers that produce capsule,

berry, or drupelike fruits. The wood of the *Guaiacum* species is hard, dense, and durable and is used to make tools. The wood also contains guaiac gum resin, used medicinally and as a perfume for hundreds of years. There are 27 genera and about 250 species found in desert or saline environments of temperate, tropical, and subtropical regions of both hemispheres, including Africa, Asia, and the warm deserts of South and North America.

Essential oil: Guaiacwood

Associated therapeutic traits: Drying and soothing; supports the integumentary system; eases muscular and joint aches and pains

ESSENTIAL OILS BY PLANT TYPE AND BOTANICAL SPECIES: A QUICK REFERENCE GUIDE

FLOWERS	TREES	HERBS	SPICE/SEED
Apiaceae (Umbelliferae)	Burseraceae	Apiaceae (Umbelliferae)	Apiaceae (Umbelliferae)
khella/ toothpickweed	linaloe	dill, fennel, galbanum, khella, lovage	angelica, aniseed, asafetida, caraway, carrot seed, celery seed, coriander, cumin, dill, fennel
Asteraceae (Compositae)	Betulaceae (Fagales)	Labiatae (Lamiaceae)	Lauraceae
calendula, chamomile (German, Roman, Maroc, English), costus, helichrysum/ immortelle, lavender cotton, tagetes/ marigold, tarragon, yarrow	birch (sweet, white)	basil, calamintha, clary sage, hyssop, marjoram, melissa, mint, oregano, patchouli, peppermint, rosemary, sage, thyme	cinnamon
Violaceae	Cupressaceae	Verbenaceae	Malvaceae
violet	cade juniper, cedarwood, cypress, juniper	lemon verbena	ambrette seed

FLOWERS	TREES	HERBS	SPICE/SEED
	Fabaceae (Leguminoseae)		Myristicaceae
	balsam (copaiba, Peru/Tolu)		mace, nutmeg
	Lauraceae		Myrtaceae
	bay laurel, camphor, cassia, cinnamon, may chang, ravensara, rosewood, sassafras		allspice, clove
	Myrtaceae		Schisandraceae (Illiciaceae)
	allspice, cajeput, eucalyptus, myrtle, niaouli, tea tree, West Indian bay		star anise (Chinese, Japanese)
	Pinaceae		Zingiberaceae
	Canadian balsam, cedarwood Atlas, pine, silver fir tree, spruce, turpentine		cardamom, ginger, turmeric
	Rutaceae		
	amyris, petitgrain (citrus)		
	Santalaceae		
	sandalwood		
	Schisandraceae (Illiciaceae)		
	star anise (Chinese, Japanese)		
	Zygophyllaceae		
	guaiacwood		
FLOWERS/BLOSSOMS	TREES/RESINOUS	GRASS	FRUITS
Annonaceae	Burseraceae	Poaceae (Gramineae)	Piperaceae
cananga, ylang-ylang	elemi, frankincense, myrrh, opopanax, palo santo	citronella, lemongrass, palmarosa	black pepper, cubeba
Liliaceae	Dipterocarpaceae		Rutaceae
hyacinth	borneol, Gurjun balsam		bergamot, grapefruit, lemon, lime, mandarin, orange (bitter, sweet)

ESSENTIAL OILS BY PLANT TYPE AND
BOTANICAL SPECIES: A QUICK REFERENCE GUIDE (continued)

FLOWERS/BLOSSOMS	TREES/RESINOUS	GRASS	FRUITS
Malvaceae	Fabaceae (Leguminoseae)		Schisandraceae (Illiciaceae)
linden blossom	balsam (copaiba, Peru, Tolu)		star anise (Chinese, Japanese)
Oleaceae	Hamamelidaceae		
jasmine	Asiatic styrax, Levant styrax, storax (resins used in perfumery and as flavors)		
Rosaceae			
rose (cabbage, Damask, Maroc)			
Rutaceae			
orange blossom/ neroli			
Tiliaceae			
linden blossom			

FLOWERS/HERBS	TREES/SHRUBS	ROOTS/BULBS	FUNGI/LICHEN
Geraniaceae	Cistaceae	Apiaceae (Umbelliferae)	Parmeliaceae
geranium (Bulgarian, rose)	cistus, labdanum	angelica, lovage	oakmoss
Labiatae (Lamiaceae)	Mimosaceae (Fabales)	Caprifoliaceae (Valerianaceae)	
lavandin, lavender	cassia	spikenard, valerian	
	Monimiaceae	Liliaceae	
	boldo leaf	garlic, onion (pungent)	
		Poaceae (Gramineae)	
		vetivert	
		Zingiberaceae	
		ginger, turmeric	

THE FUTURE OF BIODIVERSITY

The demand for essential oils and the popularity of aromatherapy have increased exponentially over the past decade or so in response to the growing interest in natural healing and the demand for natural products. It is estimated that the market will increase by up to 8 percent over the next six- to seven- year period (that is, between 2020 and 2027) (Market Analysis Report 2020).

The soft-drink industry is the largest consumer of essential oils. They are also used in alcoholic beverages, various types of sweets, some dairy products, fast and processed foods, and pharmaceuticals, perfumes, supplements, herbal products, and animal food. Apart from scent, essential oils are mainly used by these industries for their antimicrobial and flavoring properties. The aromatherapy market mainly uses essential oils in spas and in cosmetics, as well as in therapeutic applications, with the spa sector accounting for over a third of the market (Market Analysis Report 2020).

Global Production of Essential Oils

- The top three crops grown for their essential oils are orange, lemon, and mint.
- Essential oils produced for industrial purposes include citronella, cornmint, eucalyptus, lemon, orange, and peppermint.
- Essential oils produced for domestic purposes include chamomile, eucalyptus, frankincense, geranium, jasmine, lavender, lemon, orange, rosemary, and sandalwood.
- Essential oils produced on small farms or from plant material collected wild from forests include citronella, clove leaf, eucalyptus, geranium, lavender, nutmeg, patchouli, spikenard, vetivert, and ylang-ylang.
- The major producers of essential oils across the world are China and India, followed by Indonesia, Sri Lanka, and Vietnam.
- African essential oil–producing countries include Algeria, Egypt, Morocco, Tunisia, and to a lesser extent Ethiopia, Ghana, the Ivory Coast, Kenya, South Africa, Tanzania, and Uganda.
- Essential oil–producing countries in the Americas include the United

> States, Canada, Mexico, and to a lesser extent Argentina, Guatemala, Haiti, Paraguay, and Uraguay.
> • Other, less prominent essential oil–producing countries include France, Germany, Jamaica, Japan, the Taiwan Region, and the Philippines.
>
> Source: Market Analysis Report 2020

In addition, around 65 percent of the world's production of essential oils takes place in developing countries, a practice mainly supported by small farmers and foragers who depend on wildcrafting as a means of earning a living and supporting their local communities. Labor is also much cheaper in these countries. Crops are cultivated on a large scale by industrial growers. However, wild-harvested medicinal plants are considered more efficacious than those that are industrially cultivated, mainly due to the biodiversity in natural habitats. Moreover, up to 70 to 80 percent of the world's population continue to rely on medicinal plants for their primary health-care needs (Sheng-Ji 2001).

Many of these plants and/or their essential oils are featured in the pharmacopeias of traditional healing such as Chinese, shamanistic, Tibetan, Ayurveda, Unani, and Siddha medicine, as well as in many types of folk medicine.

Ecological Sustainability

Ecological sustainability is concerned with conserving the productivity of water, soil, and the entire ecosystem in order to maintain a healthy equilibrium for all life on Earth. Physician and educator Zach Bush, MD, a longtime advocate of sustainable agriculture, along with other concerned experts, poignantly warns of our planet's trajectory toward ecological disaster. Humans are on track to become extinct in the next sixty or seventy years unless radical changes are made in the way food is produced and harvested, as modern industrial farming methods (both animal and agriculture) are unsustainable (Farmer's Footprint 2021; Bush 2020, June 16; Soil Health Institute 2020).

The depletion of ancient, biodiverse natural habitats—our wetlands, forests, and wildlands—along with excessive timber harvesting done to make way for industrial animal grazing and monocrops, as well as the extraction of natural gas and oil reserves, is stripping our planet of its nutrient-rich, life- and growth-sustaining topsoil, as what remains after these unsustainable practices is dirt, not soil. The destruction of biodiverse habitats also depletes the available atmospheric oxygen that is so vital to life. The excessive foraging of wild-growing medicinal plants to satisfy ever-increasing commercial demands is part of this problem and contributes to the demise of plant, animal, and microbial species, further diminishing Earth's biodiversity. Add to that the extensive use of water-soluble glyphosates to control weeds and insects, along with the proliferation of genetically modified organisms (GMOs) that chemically control the growth behavior of plants and deliberately (and conveniently for industrial growers) dries out plants prior to harvest, which exacerbates this depletion. GMOs wreak havoc in various ways. Not only do they diminish the nutrient content and value of plants by stripping the topsoil of its life-sustaining microbiome, they also disrupt the balance of the wider ecosystem and contaminate the water. Glyphosates now literally run through our rivers and rain down on us—we drink these poisons and wash in them. Within thirty to fifty years (some estimate in even less time), the natural nutritional growth value of most of the world's topsoil will be depleted (Bush 2021; Bush 2020, June 16)—a sobering and quite scary prospect, to say the least.

The commercial harvesting of plants, wood, and their derivatives can only be sustained with considered management of and respect for our planet's natural resources, wildlife habitats, and topsoil. Despite humankind's assault on its landscape and the consequential loss of species and depletion of fertile soil, the Earth at this moment—remarkably, given the challenges—remains abundant, but this is a very fragile and temporary state. We are at a significant juncture, right on the cusp of extinction. The window of opportunity to reverse the current trajectory is almost closed. Yet despite the dire prognostications, Dr. Zach Bush, with inspiring optimism, believes that we, humankind, are gifted with incredible potential and are being presented with an amazing opportunity to harness and positively manage the inevitable transitions we are currently faced with (no matter the cause). He believes we can pull together to create an even more diverse and richer future for generations to come, but the landscape, he admits, will be very different, and we must adapt to the changes or we will not survive. Overcoming the tremendous obstacles that face us—and the next eight years are pivotal—can only come about through concerted effort, mutual collaboration, and generous sharing of skills, expertise, and resources. The benefit will be the restoration of abundant natural, nutritionally rich food, clean water and air, and more. That said, such a vision does not include draconian "one world" dominance and control by a few over the many for the sake of what some of these puppet masters propose to be "the greater good." Instead, I envisage this shift more as humanity's universal awakening that will result in locally led initiatives that bring about a global, mutually cohabitive recalibration.

Indeed, we exert significant influence through the choices we make every day. Recognizing and honoring our individual responsibility, paying conscious attention to what we purchase and consume and how we choose to live ripples around us; no step is too small or insignificant. An ocean, after all, is made up of uncountable billions of tiny drops of water. Respecting and honoring the sovereignty of nature, valuing and treasuring its abundant gifts (by the grace of which go we), and recognizing ourselves as sovereign beings cohabiting with all living beings on Earth sets the foundation for a healthy, thriving interdependency. We are, after all, custodians, not owners and controllers of Earth.

Sourcing Ethically

What does sustainability mean when it comes to essential oils?

The molecular content and energy of an essential oil depend on the condition of the plant it develops within and the environment in which that plant grows. Glyphosates inhibit enzyme synthesis involved in the biosynthesis of aromatic compounds, among other things, and have a direct impact on the condition and content of a plant's essential oil. Topsoil depleted of vital nutrients (nitrogen, phosphorus, potassium, and magnesium) that are necessary for growth and development, in turn, impacts the metabolism and products of plants and their microbiome. For example, potassium helps form and move starches, sugar, and oils in a plant; magnesium and manganese are vital for photosynthesis; calcium is essential for root health and the growth of new shoots and leaves. Even organic farmers and growers are susceptible to industrial fallout and pollution (transposition via wind, rain, and water) from industrial growing operations. Nevertheless, purchasing essential oils from sustainable organic growers and suppliers goes at least some way toward ensuring the integrity of the source and ultimately the authenticity and quality of the essential oil, and adds to the movement toward sustainable production.

Reputable suppliers will provide evidence of the authenticity, chemical content, integrity, and purity of their essential oils in the form of certificates of analysis, soil association certificates, and organic grower certificates, among other means of verifying that their oils are obtained from sustainable regenerative sources.

In developing a consciousness of biodiversity, we must become aware of essential oil–producing plants that are endangered, threatened, or vulnerable. These include, among others, certain plants listed in chapter 6: East Indian sandalwood (*Santalum album*), rosewood (*Aniba rosaeodora*), frankincense (*Boswellia carteri, B. sacra*), galbanum (*Ferula gummosa*), cedarwood Atlas (*Cedrus atlantica*), Scotch pine (*Pinus sylvestris*), and spikenard (*Aralia* spp. and *Nardostachys* spp.). It is possible to obtain these essential oils from sustainable and ethical sources, although they may not always be available or may be very expensive due to limited supply. The good news is that there are always alternatives, as the dynamic qualities of essential oils mean that most oils can be substituted with others, either a similar single oil or a blend of oils. You can use the information presented in chapter 6 of this book to select viable alternatives to threatened and/or costly plants. Spikenard, a threatened species, can be substituted with vetivert or valerian; Indian sandalwood (*Santalum album*) with Australian (plantation grown) sandalwood (*Santalum spicatum*); frankincense (*Boswellia carteri*) with myrrh. Eucalyptus trees grow in other countries apart from Australia—in Portugal, for example—and although the chemistry of the oil will differ accordingly (wildfires and drought destroy habitats around the world, which affects trees and the availability of their yields), it still has appropriate therapeutic value. Purchase your oils wisely. Buy small amounts as needed rather than purchasing in bulk. Buy and use fewer varieties of oils and create your own small, all-around kit, the contents of which you can change from time to time, rotating certain useful oils. And when possible, try to purchase from local farmers, growers, distillers, and suppliers; do your homework and seek out ethical sources.

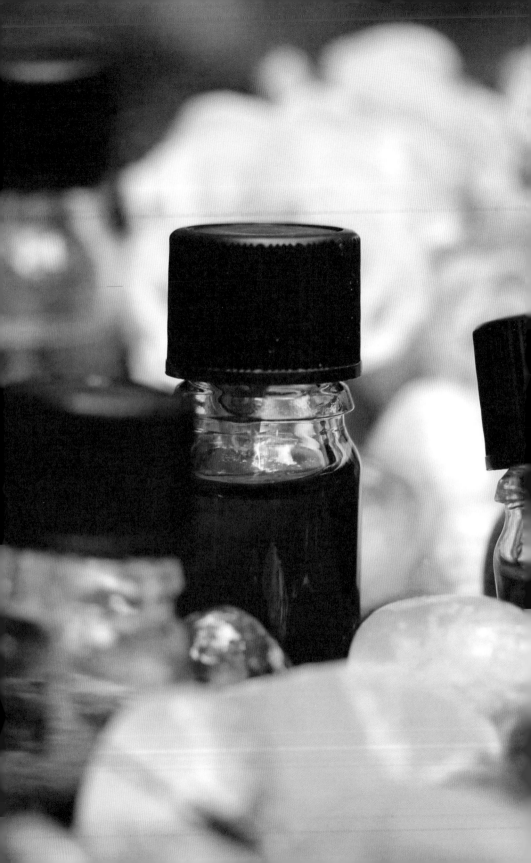

3

Methods of Extraction

From Plant to Bottle

As we know from the previous chapter, essential oils are stored in various parts of a plant, from the delicate petals of flowers and blossoms to the heartwood deep within the trunk of a tree. Most essential oils are released and separated from the plant material by steam distillation, which involves intense heat and pressure. However, some plants require gentler methods due to their delicate structure. For example, the petals of flower blossoms dissolve or disintegrate in the presence of extreme heat. Less aggressive methods of extraction include the infusion of plant material in warm vegetable oil, water, or another solvent to gently coax or soak out the volatile components. Some volatile components are destroyed or chemically altered by heat, particularly terpenes, the aromatic chemical compounds responsible for the medicinal effects of essential oils, so distillation is not a desirable option for plants containing terpene-rich essential oils such as are found in citrus fruits, which contain high quantities of monoterpenes. Instead, the peel of citrus fruits is crushed to erupt or burst the essential oil–containing cavities found there, a process known as *expression*. Fibrous materials such as hardwoods require breaking down into smaller parts or sawdust, and seeds require crushing to expose volatile oils and to ease their extraction.

In this chapter we will describe the various methods of extracting essential oils and how they are evaluated to determine their medicinal qualities, potency, and safe use.

Types of Plant Materials That Contain Essential Oil

SOFT PLANT MATERIAL

flowering heads (e.g., fresh lavender)

flowers (e.g., dried chamomile)

grass (e.g., fresh, partially dried lemongrass)

leaves (e.g., fresh cajeput)

needles (e.g., cypress)

whole plant (e.g., geranium)

delicate flowers (e.g., rose, jasmine, melissa), which must be distilled
   immediately after harvest

resin (e.g., dried frankincense, myrrh, and other oleo gums)

FIBROUS PLANT MATERIAL (CUT-UP, CRUSHED, OR GRATED)

bark (e.g., cinnamon)

roots and rhizomes (e.g., ginger)

seeds (e.g., carrot seed)

twigs and branches (e.g., petitgrain)

wood stumps, trunks, heartwood, sawdust (e.g., cedarwood)

SUPERFICIAL SECRETORY CAVITIES

fruit rind (e.g., mandarin)

FRAGRANT PETALS

blossoms (e.g., rose, jasmine, ylang-ylang)

DISTILLATION

Distillation is the most cost-effective and frequently used method of extracting essential oils from plant material. In general, a distillation apparatus includes the following:

+ heat source
+ water container
+ holding vat (which acts like a pressure cooker)
+ cooling condenser
+ vat to collect the essential oil–impregnated water
+ container to collect the siphoned essential oil

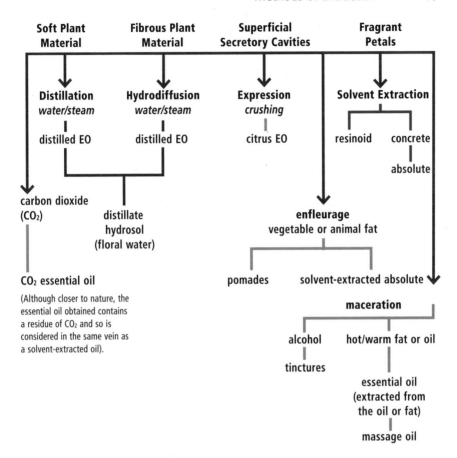

There are three methods of distillation used to extract essential oils from plants: hydrodistillation, water and steam distillation, and hydrodiffusion.

Hydrodistillation

In hydrodistillation, the plant material is completely immersed in water that is contained in a holding vat, which is placed over a source of heat (often an open fire, brick oven, or propane-fueled heater) and brought to boiling point (212°F or 100°C) for a specified period of time, depending on the nature of the plant material. The intense temperature and pressure created by the heat causes the secretory cells within the plant material to either burst open or surrender the essential oil it contains through osmosis (through the cell walls). So at high temperature, the essential oil contained in the secretory cells disperses into water within the cells, and this watery mixture is then able to permeate the water-saturated cell membranes in the swollen plant tissue and pass into the surrounding water and steam contained in the vat.

As the essential oil–infused steam rises, it is funneled into a condenser, where it cools down and returns to a liquid state, or distillate. The distillate is left to stand to allow the essential oil to separate from the mixture and either settle at the top or to sink to the bottom of the vat. The essential oil is then siphoned off. Sometimes essential oils are continuously siphoned off slowly while distillation proceeds.

Hydrodistillation is often employed by small producers, especially when it is imperative that distillation occurs immediately after harvest to prevent enzymes in the plant cells from breaking down the essential oils; examples include fresh flowers such as ylang-ylang, rose, and jasmine. Hydrodistillation is also employed for dense woods and tree bark (such as sandalwood and cinnamon); the wood is broken down into small parts and soaked in water before distillation takes place to macerate the material, thus allowing the essential oil to "wash out" with ease.

It is difficult to maintain a constant, even temperature using this method. There is also increased chance, unless the vat is continually monitored, that the water will dry out and the plant material will burn. Also, the duration of distillation can be inconsistent, which means the chemical composition of the oil extracted can vary. Essential oil molecules are released from the plant material at different rates depending on their volatility, so temperature and distillation time are significant in terms of the ultimate chemical content and quality of the scent of the resulting essential oil.

Water and Steam Distillation

Water and steam distillation involves a similar process as hydrodistillation. A grid is placed above the water on which the plant material is placed, which keeps it separate from the water (reducing the chance the material will burn should the water level reduce). The water is brought to boiling point. The rising steam passes through the grid and plant material, causing the secretory cells to either erupt or saturate (osmosis) and surrender their essential oils. Just as in hydrodistillation, the essential oil–infused steam is funneled through a pipe into a cooling condenser (usually filled with cold water) that returns the vapor to water, at which point the essential oil is siphoned off into a separate container. This method is preferred in the field in the case of delicate plants or flowers that require immediate extraction to avoid degradation of the essential oil.

Some small steam-distillation apparatuses include a separate basket-like holding container that fits into a larger holding vat. This basket-like container is filled with plant material (freshly harvested lavender, for example); the external walls of the main holding vat act as a sleeve. Steam is created in an adjacent container and piped with some force into the vat, permeating through the plant material (something like a steamer pan used to steam vegetables). The essential oil–impregnated steam is funneled, cooled, and siphoned off as previously described.

Industrial steam distillation employs similar methods but on a much larger scale. Steam is produced in a separate water boiler, then channeled under pressure through pipes into the base of an adjacent vat containing the plant material. Larger-scale operations tend to enable more efficient and consistent control of temperature and pressure.

Hydrodiffusion

Hydrodiffusion, developed in the 1990s, is similar to steam distillation in principle. It employs the force of gravity and atmospheric pressure to assist percolation (in the same way a coffee percolator extracts coffee essence from ground coffee beans). Steam percolates down with force from jets situated above the plant material, rupturing essential oil–containing secretory cells as it passes through. Steam infused with essential oils is channeled (this time from the bottom rather than the top of the vat), condensed, and siphoned off in the same manner as in steam distillation. This method uses less water, takes less time to perform, uses less energy, and is less harsh, while the essential oils maintain more of their original chemical components and aroma. However, even though the color and aroma are reported as being darker and stronger, it is not clear whether hydrodiffused essential oils are actually therapeutically superior.

Hydrodiffusion is most useful for fibrous material such as wood and bark, which benefits from the force of the pressurized steam. It is an expensive method of distillation and so is not widely used.

Terpenes are the first components to be released from the secretory cells, followed at varying rates and intervals by others (depending on their volatility). Terpenes are also the most vulnerable components and are easily destroyed if the pressure and temperature are too great. The larger, more viscous molecules take the longest time to release from the plant material. In this method, esters react with water to form acids and alcohols (for a further discussion of essential oil chemistry, see chapter 4).

Sometimes (for the sake of increasing profits) distillation time is deliberately reduced to accommodate a quick turnaround, which means some of the slow-releasing molecules are consequently not extracted at all. Some of the more volatile chemical components are unavoidably destroyed by the intensity of the pressure and heat applied, and some components are lost through diffusion into the water, while others are changed.

Soft plant material (leaves and flowers, for example) do not require pretreatment with this method. However, fibrous material (bark, wood, roots, and seeds) must be broken down before being distilled—either cut up, crushed, or grated—to assist the release of essential oil from the secretory cells, particularly those that lie deep within the denser parts of

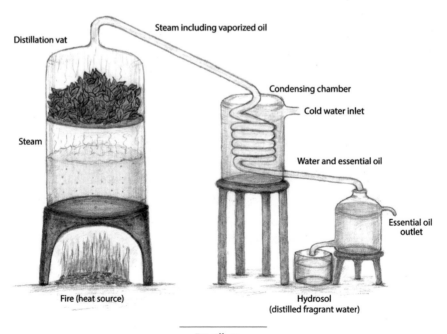

Distillation

the plant's fiber or within the heartwood of trees such as sandalwood, cedarwood, and pine. As noted earlier, some delicate flowers such as rose or jasmine require immediate extraction following harvest to prevent the enzymes in the plant cell from breaking the essential oil down. For others, such as calendula, the process of distillation is too harsh and will destroy much of the flowers' delicate, volatile, active components. Less fragile flowers like chamomile are dried before distillation. Patchouli is another example; it is dried and left to ferment before being distilled.

Is Essential Oil Really Oil?

The term *essential oil* can be misleading. Essential oils appear to behave like oil as they coalesce and tend to remain separate from water. However, essential oil molecules do not readily bond with water molecules. They are mostly lighter (less dense) than water molecules, so they tend to float on the surface, although some are heavier and will sink to the bottom of the distillation vat. Some hydrophilic (water-loving) molecules bond with oxygen molecules in the water, thus dissolving into the distillate. Once the essential oils are siphoned off, the remaining distilled water impregnated with plant chemicals is known as a hydrosol or hydrolate (for example, witch hazel, rose, and other floral waters are hydrosols).

Rectification, Fractionation, Folding

Redistilling (either in steam or in a vacuum) to remove chemical compounds or unwanted impurities from a distillate is known as *rectification*. Bergamot essential oil is rectified, for example, to remove the phototoxic furanocoumarins (the result is labeled *bergamot FCF,* i.e., bergamot that is furanocoumarin-free). Some essential oils such as peppermint and clove are rectified to standardize their chemical consistency, a common practice in the drug and food industries. The essential oils of eucalyptus and cajeput are rectified to remove impurities such as resinous matter and plant dust, while other essential oils may be rectified to remove terpenes or water carried over from distillation. As Valnet (1990) and Gattefossé (1937, 1995) affirm, deterpenated essential oils last longer and are more soluble in alcohol, a trait preferred in perfumery. While removal of terpenes will influence the scent profile and the oil's chemical mixture, the therapeutic properties are not necessarily diminished; in fact, in many cases these are even improved as the remaining constituents are less volatile and therefore more consistent/stable.

Essential oils such as ylang-ylang are richly fragrant and are able to tolerate redistillation or *fractional distillation,* a term that describes the separation of volatile oil into different fractions or portions at various boiling points. During this process, distillation is deliberately stopped at specified times (or fractions) or when a specific density is reached; in the case of ylang-ylang, this occurs four or five times and at each stage of fractionation the essential oil is siphoned off. This process produces different grades of oil. Ylang-ylang "extra," for example, refers to the first extraction, which is usually collected in the first hour or so and contains the lightest volatiles. The next three fractions, called ylang-ylang 1, 2, and 3, are collected over 12 to 20 hours of distillation; these are regarded as low grades and tend not to be used in aromatherapy. However, when all four fractions are combined or folded together, the resulting mixture, known as ylang-ylang complete, is considered a therapeutic-grade oil due to the resultant chemical structure being very close to the plant's original oil. Fractionation is undertaken in order to procure or squeeze out as much of the available essential oil as possible from the freshly picked flowers. Fractionated distillates are also used to bulk out expensive essential oils to increase profit. Carried out appropriately, fractional distillation, like rectification, can actually enhance rather than diminish the properties of the resultant essential oil or isolated component (Perini et al. 2017). Of course, this process steps away from the definition of a *pure* essential oil—that is, *nothing added, nothing taken away* from the original distillate. However, removal of impurities or unwanted toxic elements is sometimes necessary. Fractional distillation of essential oils is applied in the food, flavor, cosmetic, and pharmaceutical industries to control the oils' chemical content—that is, to intensify or enhance a particular property or characteristic or to isolate individual components. For example, rosemary essential oil is fractionated to islolate verbenone, linalool, and geraniol (Silvestre et al. 2019); verbenone has a champhoraceous menthol-celery-like odor and is applied as an ingredient in perfumery, in herbal teas and remedies, and in insecticides.

Lavender, a very popular essential oil, provides an example wherein distillates from different batches and crops of the same or similar botanical species may be mixed, or *folded* together. (Note that a label that states "pure lavender essential oil" does not give this information.) Lavender 40/42 (i.e., 40% linalool to 42% linalyl acetate) consists of blended, or folded, oils from various lavenders harvested from different crops and different species of lavender, which are deliberately combined to create an essential oil with a consistent chemical and odor profile, a process preferred in perfumery.

The process of separating an essential oil from the plant alters its chemistry. Some molecules are changed, and other molecules are newly created by the distillation process—for example, matricin, which converts to form the blue-colored chamazulene in German chamomile, and linalyl acetate, a monoterpene acetate found in lavender, bergamot, and clary sage, which partially converts to linalool (a monoterpene ester). Also, molecules continue to change post-distillation (extraction) as a result of reactions instigated by light, heat, and oxygen (see chapter 4).

Hydrosols

Essential oils are a mixture of hundreds of organic chemical components. Some are water-loving (hydrophilic) and some are fat-loving (lipophilic). When the secretory cells are disrupted through distillation, the essential oil mixture disperses and breaks down into component parts as each evaporates. Water-loving components bond with oxygen molecules in the atmosphere or in the water in which the plant is suspended.

Examples of Common Hydrosols

chamomile	peppermint
cypress	rosemary
geranium	rose otto
helichrysum/immortelle	tea tree
jasmine	thyme
lavender	verbena
lemon balm/melissa	witch hazel
orange blossom/neroli	

The fat-loving, oil-like components tend to remain separate when suspended in water, floating to the surface or sinking to the bottom of the containing vat. The distilled water left behind, after the essential oil has been removed, contains traces of water-loving essential oil molecules as well as nonvolatile or less volatile chemical components and plant acids, and this is known as a *hydrosol*. Synonymous terms are *aqueous solution, colloidal suspension, hydrolate, floral water,* and *essence water*.

Hydrosols can be reused for subsequent distillations, bottled for other uses, or discarded, depending on the plant material distilled. Fresh hydrosols are used in medicine as herbal distillates and also in cosmetics and skin-care preparations as well as food flavorings. In some instances, hydrosols are produced primarily for this purpose only— for example, witch hazel, from *Hamamelis* spp., which is used for its astringent properties. Some retailers suggest that hydrosols are a weaker version of the distilled essential oil and possess similar but gentler therapeutic properties. Some also suggest that hydrosols contain the vibrational qualities of both the plant and its essential oil. Clearly, hydrosols do contain *some* of the plant's chemical properties and traces of its scent profile, and they may also retain some aspect of the plant's energetic imprint, a phenomenon postulated by French immunologist Jacques Benveniste (Benveniste 1988). But synergistically, hydrosols are *not* representative of the whole herb or plant, or even the extracted essential oil. Hydrosols mainly contain hydrophilic (water-loving) molecules and as such exhibit their own unique, dynamic qualities. Rosewater (*Rosa* x *damascena*) is a classic example of a hydrosol used variously (in perfume and in skin-care and food preparations) since ancient times, in China, India, Assyria, Egypt, Greece, and Rome. Indeed, the Mycenaeans and Persians developed a lucrative trade exporting rosewater to China and countries throughout the Islamic world more than three thousand years ago. Orange blossom water is another such example with an ancient history of use.

The high temperatures required for distillation and the slightly acidic pH balance of the resulting hydrosol will initially prevent bacterial growth. However, this is a temporary state, as hydrosols are not sterile; when stagnant, water rapidly becomes contaminated by bacterial growth. This means hydrosols bottled for cosmetic, flavoring,

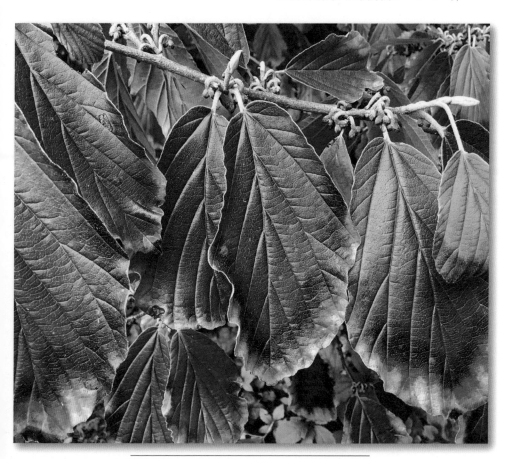

Witch hazel leaves touched by autumn

or medicinal purposes have a very limited shelf life and, like fresh produce, must be kept cool and discarded after a limited period of time, especially after opening a sealed bottle. Considering this, it is imperative that hydrosols are regarded as perishable and that appropriate caution should be observed when purchasing and storing them. Factors such as freshness, authenticity, plant source, place and date of production, sell-by/use-by date, and adherence to appropriate methods of storage (in a cool, dark place, such as a fridge, and containment in UV-protecting dark blue or brown glass bottles with tightly secured lids, just like essential oils) must be considered before using a hydrosol, especially if it is to be used internally as a food ingredient or medicine.

Distillation Review

- Distillation in its various forms is the most common method of extraction employed.
- Plant material is heated with either water or pressurized steam.
- The heat and pressure rupture plant cells, releasing essential oils into steam vapor.
- Essential oil molecules are carried with the steam, then cooled and separated from the condensed water.
- Some of the water-loving (hydrophilic), more volatile and heavier molecules are left behind in the water or residual plant material or are lost during the process.
- Some molecules convert to new or altered molecules during the process of distillation and after distillation.
- The distilled essential oil is not the same as the essential oil present in the plant before extraction.
- Hydrosols (hydrolates) are derived from the water used to distill the essential oil, and although a by-product of distillation, they are also produced in their own right for various purposes.
- Hydrosols have a short shelf life.
- The first distillation usually produces the best-quality essential oil.
- Redistillation is known as *rectification*.
- Some rectification is necessary to remove unwanted plant residue such as dust and resinous matter that gets extracted with the essential oil.
- The second and subsequent distillations produce a cheaper oil (generally unsuitable for aromatherapy); these are sometime used to "bulk out" the oils originally extracted.

EXPRESSION

Expression involves applying pressure, squeezing, or compressing the fresh plant material to force the essential oils from their secretory cells. Historically, most essential oils were produced using this method. Today, expression is generally reserved for the extraction of essential oil from citrus fruits (bergamot, orange, lemon, lime, mandarin). Secretory cells in citrus fruits are present in abundance in the rind, where the flavor and aroma of the fruit is contained in concentrated form. Citrus essential oils are rich in terpenes, which are highly volatile. Expression, sometimes referred to as *cold pressing,* preserves the integrity of terpenes and these days tends to be carried out using machinery to mechanically crush the peel. The peel is scraped (scarification) or abraded to break open the surface secretory glands before or during the crushing process to improve extraction efficiency.

Citrus fruits are easy to grow and harvest, and the large quantities of essential oil in the fruit peel means that citrus essential oils remain relatively cheap to produce. Lemon and sweet orange essential oils are mainly obtained as a by-product of the food and manufacturing industries. The peel is sometimes distilled after expression to extract residual oil. However, most of the terpene molecules that are left in the peel after expression are lost during distillation due to the extreme heat applied, and consequently an inferior essential oil is produced. Steam-distilled citrus essential oils are colorless, while expressed citrus oils retain flavonoids and other nondistillable compounds and are consequently richly colored (from green to deep orange and red); these are preferred in aromatherapy. Bigarade orange essential oil is produced from the outer part of the peel of bitter Seville oranges and is richly colored and odiferous. Terpeneless (rectified) citrus essential oils are favored by the perfume and food industries, as they provide less volatile, more stable ingredients.

Expression Review

- This method is reserved for citrus oils, which have a high content of terpenes that are lost or destroyed when heated.
- Essential oil is found in small sacs under the surface of the fruit rind.
- Mechanical crushing machines are used to squeeze oil from the plant material.
- Expression is a by-product of the fruit industry; the resulting essential oils are often adulterated with subsequent extractions, which are of lesser quality, to increase bulk.
- Distilled fruits rinds produce an inferior essential oil.

SOLVENT EXTRACTION

Solvent extraction involves the use of organic (i.e., carbon-based), oil-soluble solvents such as acetone, hexane, toluene, petroleum ether, methanol (methyl alcohol), and ethanol (ethyl alcohol) to extract essential oils. Benzene is no longer used because it is carcinogenic, so toluene, which has similar solvent activity, is used as a safer alternative. The process is similar to steam or water distillation in that the volatile components of essential oil are encouraged or "soaked out." This process is less heat-intensive, thus preserving the more volatile, delicate components found in essential oils. Solvent-extracted oils, known as *absolutes,* are preferred by the perfume industry and are generally not used in aromatherapy.

In this method, aromatic plant material is placed into a vat and immersed within the solvent, for example, hexane (see "About Hexane," at right). The vat is agitated to assist even dispersal of the solvent throughout the plant material; sometimes rotating blades are used to disperse the plant material to achieve thorough saturation. As with distillation, plant material such as bark, wood, and other fibrous material may require more thorough breaking down prior to immersion. As well as volatile odiferous compounds, chlorophyll and other pigments, natural waxes, and resinous material are also surrendered to the solvent. The residual plant material may be washed a few more times with fresh solvent to maximize its yield. The liquid solvent solution is then channeled into a receiving vessel, where under reduced pressure it is kept at a gentle heat to allow the vaporous components of the solvent to evaporate. The remaining concentrated extract is channeled off and cooled to become a solid, waxy mass known as a *concrete.* The concrete is washed in a strong alcohol solution (for example, ethanol) to remove as much of the wax and any remaining solvent as possible (wax may comprise up to 50% of the concrete). The resulting alcohol solution is then filtered to remove impurities. The alcohol is removed by vacuum distillation, a process known as *dissolving,* leaving behind a heavy, sticky resinoid: this is the *absolute* (see as well "Distilled Essential Oil versus Absolute Oil" in chapter 1).

Next, alcohol is used to dissolve out or separate gums and unwanted resins from dried, solid, resinous exudes, or soft oleoresins, such as from frankincense, myrrh, and galbanum, and is also used to soak out or macerate extracts from dry material to produce tinctures. The final absolute will contain traces of the alcohol used to wash out the concrete and dissolve alcohol-soluble molecules from the plant material and other constituents of low volatility not usually found in essential oils (such as benzenoid compounds). As well, this is used to wash out traces of the extracting solvent initially used, which may be present in amounts between 1 to 5 parts per million. This means that although an absolute does contain extracted essential oils, it is not regarded as a pure essential oil.

About Hexane

Hexane, a constituent of gasoline (petroleum), is toxic and an irritant and sensitizer, especially in cases of prolonged or long-term exposure. Some of the symptoms that may be caused or exacerbated by traces of hexane found in absolutes include acne, anxiety, asthma, breathing difficulties, burning, eczema, headaches, hives, itching, redness, and skin rashes. There are several types of hexane used in solvent extraction, and the level of sensitization will depend on which type is used, in what quantity, and in which context; for example, n-hexane is used by perfume industry as well as in food manufacturing (where, for example, it is used to extract vegetable oils from crops such as soybeans). Author Robert Tisserand, one of the world's leading authorities on aromatherapy, suggests that hexane used to extract essential oils is generally mildly to negligibly toxic or irritating (Tisserand and Young 2014, 9). Even so, it is advisable to consider this potential because not all absolutes or essential oils are equal when it comes to quality and integrity.

The production of absolutes tends to be reserved for blossoms and flowers such as rose, lily, and jasmine, which are too delicate to endure the high temperatures involved in distillation or which contain few distillable odorous molecules. Absolutes tend to produce scents that are closer to the plant's natural perfume, scents that are stronger and more intense than distilled essential oils. This occurs because at a low temperature, the solvent draws out more of the plant's nonvolatile, less volatile, and trace components, as well as other organic and inorganic matter that is either not distillable or is destroyed by the heat and pressure used during distillation. Most absolutes, consequently, tend to be richly colored compared to a distillate from the same plant. For example, rose absolute presents with a rich, reddish color, while rose distillate is clear to opaque, as seen at right.

Why a Rose Is a Rose Is a Rose

Rose owes its distinctive odor to the presence of minute amounts of beta-damasconone, beta-damascone, beta-ionone, and rose oxide, which make up just 1% of the chemical constituents but contribute 90% of the scent profile (due to their low odor detection thresholds). These constituents are also found in other exotic absolutes and essential oils, like neroli and jasmine. This phenomenon is true for many essential oils. For example, dextro-limonene, a chemical present in orange essential oil in amounts up to 95%, actually contributes very little to the distinctive scent and flavor characteristics associated with this oil; instead, it is the remaining 5%, which consists of many other chemicals, some present in barely detectable amounts, that act together to produce the lovely, fresh, citrusy scent we are so familiar with. Conversely, the major effect of a relatively small amount of a molecule can be detrimental too. For example, the furanocoumarin bergapten in bergamot essential oil is phototoxic; phototoxic constituents often constitute only 1% of an essential oil yet have dramatic effects (for example, burning, blistering, drying, and reddening of skin and alteration in pigmentation that produces brown patches) in the presence of UV light (Tisserand et al. 2021, 25).

Be aware that exotic or rare oils are often adulterated due their high market value. Fortunately (or unfortunately), because of the complex chemical mixture and the minute, or in some instances barely traceable, constituents found in many floral blossoms, their scents are rendered impossible to truly mimic synthetically. This does not deter their adulteration, however. Maude Grieve (1858–1941), the renowned English herbalist, wrote about this nearly a century ago in her comprehensive classic, *A Modern Herbal,* published in 1931:

> Geraniol and citronellol are the chief ingredients of rose oil as regards percentage, though not the most characteristic as regards odour. Citronellol, a fragrant, oily liquid, forms about 35% of the oil.

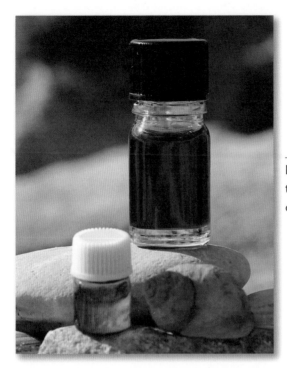

Distilled rose otto on
the left, rose absolute
on the right

Geraniol, which may be present to the amount of 75%, is a colorless liquid, with a sweet, rose-like odour. It is also found in palmarosa or Turkish geranium oil and in oils of citronella, lavender, neroli, petitgrain, ylang-ylang, lemongrass and some eucalyptus oils. It is largely obtained industrially from the oils of palmarosa and citronella and is much used to adulterate Otto of roses. The temptation to adulterate so expensive an oil is great and it is widely practised. (Grieve 1931, 686)

According to Grieve, "It takes 30 roses to make 1 drop of [rose] Otto and 60,000 roses (about 180 lb. of flowers) to make 1 oz. of Otto" (Grieve 1931, 687). *Rosa damascena* contains about 0.015% to 0.02% of essential oil per blossom, producing a distilled average yield of around 2.2 pounds of essential oil per 8,818 pounds of petals compared to 10 pounds of concrete per 10,000 pounds of rose blossoms. Rose essential oil thus remains costly to produce due to the low essential oil yield of its blossoms, and it is thus very expensive (0.30 ounces, or 10 milliters, can cost between $137 to $550 at today's exchange rate as of this writing). For this reason, adulteration remains an option for those wishing to bulk out rose essential oil to increase profit or to sell competitively. Absolutes are a less costly alternative, as they produce a higher yield of essential oil. In addition, the scent profile of rose absolute is much more intense than that of the distillate, while the pure distillate has a round, soft, sweet, smooth scent, with gentle, pleasant, subtle tenacity.

Generally, absolutes are less volatile and therefore more tenacious than distilled essential oils. They are used in perfumery as fixatives to prolong a fragrance and provide stable residual base notes. This is why absolutes are preferred (along with terpeneless essential oils, which are rendered less volatile) by the cosmetics and perfume industries.

Solvent Extraction Review

- Solvent extraction does not yield a pure essential oil.
- Organic (i.e., carbon-based) solvents are used, such as hexane, acetone, ethanol, methanol, toluene, and petroleum ether.
- Traces of the solvent used remain in the concrete and sometimes the final absolute.
- Dissolved materials include other substances such as natural waxes, resinous materials, chlorophyll, and other pigments.
- The first waxy substance produced is called a *concrete*.
- The concrete is further washed in alcohol to dissolve out waxes and solvent residue to produce an absolute.
- The odor and color of an absolute is stronger and more intense than the pure essential oil produced by distillation.
- Frankincense, myrrh, and galbanum may be produced by solvent extraction but are also distilled from their crude resin exudes to produce a pure essential oil.
- Benzoin is produced by solvent extraction and is thus not technically an essential oil.
- Solvent extraction is employed for exotic blossoms and flowers such as rose, jasmine, neroli, and champaca.
- Absolutes are more tenacious than pure essential oils and are used as fixatives in perfumes.
- Absolutes (along with terpeneless oils) are preferred by the perfume and cosmetics industries and are generally not used in aromatherapy.

Benzoin is insufficiently volatile to distill and is produced as an absolute by solvent extraction to provide a resinoid, so benzoin is not a true essential oil, even though it is listed as one. Frankincense, myrrh, and galbanum, like rose, can be prepared in the form of both resinoids (concretes and absolutes) and as distilled essential oils.

Although absolutes such as rose are not recommended in aromatherapy, they do provide potent hedonistic qualities and make significant contributions to aesthetic perfumes. Besides rose, absolutes produced by solvent extraction used in perfumery include benzoin, carnation, champaca, hyacinth, immortelle, jasmine, lotus, marigold, melissa, mimosa, narcissus, neroli, oakmoss, sandalwood, tonka, tuberose, vanilla, and violet leaf.

CARBON DIOXIDE EXTRACTION

Carbon dioxide extraction is similar to distillation, but with carbon dioxide replacing water as the extracting medium. Carbon dioxide comprises two oxygen atoms and one carbon atom and is abbreviated CO_2. It is a gas at standard atmospheric temperature and pressure and exists as a trace gas within Earth's atmosphere. Carbon dioxide behaves differently than water. The boiling point of water is 212°F (or 100°C); note that boiling points depend on liquid density and atmospheric pressure. The boiling point of CO_2 is 134°F (57°C)—much lower than that of water (by comparison, the boiling point of the solvent hexane is between 122°F and 158°F, or 50°C and 70°C).

The boiling point is the stage at which a liquid transforms into a gaseous state, known as the *critical point.* Pressure reduces the boiling point of a liquid, which is also true of CO_2. Under pressure, the boiling point of CO_2 is further reduced, reaching a supercritical point at 88°F (31.1°C) and just above. At this supercritical pressure, CO_2 adopts the properties of both gas *and* liquid, expanding like gas to fill the contained space, but with the density of water. It has the added advantage of being less destructive due to the reduced temperature compared to water.

In CO_2 extraction, which is instigated at 87°F to 98.6°F (31°C to 37°C), pressurized carbon dioxide is pumped into a vat containing organic plant material, and like a solvent, it draws out pigments, chlorophyll, and other matter, along with essential oil. Compare this to steam distillation, activated at a temperature of 140°F to 212°F (60°C to 100°C), or solvent extraction, which occurs between 122°F and 158°F (50°C and 70°C). Heat potentiates chemical changes, and so controlling the temperature range and pressure means there is a greater chance of managing the chemical reactions that can be instigated. CO_2 extraction draws out chemical constituents other than volatile odorous components, and there are some advantages to extracting essential oils this way. Let's take German chamomile (*Matricaria recutita*) as an example. During distillation, matricin, a sesquiterpene found in German chamomile, transforms into the aromatic chemical compound chamazulene in reaction to the presence of heat. Chamazulene is what's responsible for the dark blue color of distilled German chamomile (it is also present in distilled yarrow after transformation of proazulene). However, due to the comparatively low temperature, matricin remains unchanged, so CO_2-extracted German chamomile is green; its scent is also softer and closer to that of the flower; the anti-inflammatory properties of matricin are superior to those of chamazulene. Compared to organic solvent extraction, CO_2 surrenders oils with more volatile components, or top notes (notes, in perfumery, are descriptors of scent, and top notes are those immediately perceived), as well as a higher proportion of esters and some larger molecules, but fewer terpenes due to their lower solubility in the carbon dioxide.

Another advantage is that CO_2-extracted oils are closer to those found naturally in the original plant, according to some sources. Certain sources say that because traces of CO_2 remain and because the acidic quality of CO_2 alters the chemical structure of the resultant essential oil, it is not a true essential oil—nor an absolute. Tisserand and Young (2014, 6, 11, 22) refer to CO_2 *extracts* when discussing oils obtained by this method. CO_2 extracts are more prone to degradation than essential oils. Certainly CO_2 extraction produces oils with a different odor profile compared to distilled essential oils. It is also a very expensive process, so it is not widely used to produce essential oils and is used primarily for producing oils for the food and pharmaceutical industries. For example, coffee is decaffeinated using this process, and cannabis oil is also refined using this method. However, there are some essential oils extracted this way: agarwood, ambrette seed, angelica root, calendula, caraway, cardamom, champaca, cinnamon bark, coriander seed, frankincense, ginger, jasmine, juniper berry, orris root, patchouli, and vanilla.

In reality, all methods of extraction, whether involving exposure to oxygen, heat, or solvents, are responsible for denaturing the original essential oil and altering its odor profile to varying degrees as it separates from the raw plant material. However, distilled essential oils contain no additional chemicals or substances after extraction and therefore represent the purest version, especially when considering their use in aromatherapy.

Carbon Dioxide Extraction Review

- Carbon dioxide (CO_2) is used as a solvent and is considered by some to produce absolute-type oils.
- This method creates a supercritical fluid at low temperature, 86°F (30°C), therefore preserving more chemical components in the essential oils extracted. It is therefore potentially closer to the original plant chemistry, with more top notes, esters, and larger molecules, which may be lost or left behind in steam or water distillation, but with fewer terpenes.
- Carbon dioxide is an acidic gas and therefore is considered by some to be detrimental to essential oils.
- CO_2 extraction is a very expensive method to employ at present.
- CO_2 extraction is primarily used in the food and pharmaceutical industries and in perfumery.

MACERATION

Maceration, which dates back to the ancient Egyptians, is the process by which fresh or dried plant material, when steeped and saturated in an appropriate liquid, becomes soft, breaks up, and surrenders its soluble (miscible) constituents to the liquid (for example, tea leaves left to stand in a teapot macerate in the boiling water). Also known as *liquid-liquid extraction* and similar in principle to solvent extraction, maceration is reserved for plant material containing volatile chemical derivatives that are otherwise destroyed by the intense heat and pressure of distillation, or valuable nondistillable derivatives such as natural waxes or pigments, which may contribute desirable qualities such as flavonoids, which are water-soluble plant pigments that are responsible for most of the red, pink, purple, blue, and especially yellow colors (*flavus* means "yellow" in Latin) found in vascular plants. Flavonoids are responsible for the rich color of macerated oils, as in the deep reddish-orange of carrot oil, the rich orange of calendula oil, and the bright red of St. John's wort oil. Flavonoids are anti-allergic, anti-inflammatory, antioxidant, antifungal, and antiviral.

Macerated oils are mostly used for their skin-healing properties (often without additional essential oils). Maceration (along with expression) was historically the main method used to separate out essential oils and other plant components, until the discovery of distillation. These days, maceration is rarely used commercially as a method to extract essential oils, but it is used to produce plant-infused vegetable oils. It is also still viable for small batches made at home on the stovetop or by small producers.

Flavonoids: What Gives a Rose Its Color

Flavonoids are among the major nonvolatile plant pigments (along with chlorophyll, carotenoids, and betalains); they provide the colors yellow, red, blue, and purple. They give flower petals their color and are designed to attract pollinators. They are involved in UV filtration and act as chemical messengers, physiological regulators, and cell-cycle inhibitors. Also known as vitamin P, flavonoids are found in virtually all fruits, vegetables, herbs, and spices and are most abundant in the skins of fruits and vegetables. Food sources rich in flavonoids include apples, apricots, blueberries, pears, raspberries, strawberries, black beans, cabbage, onions, parsley, pinto beans, spinach, and tomatoes, as well as green tea, black tea, and dark chocolate. Flavonoids act as antioxidants and are enhanced when combined with vitamin C (each enhances the antioxidant properties of the other). They also help prevent blood vessels from rupture or leakage, prevent excessive inflammation throughout the body, and protect cells from oxygen damage. This is why macerated vegetable oils, such as calendula, are employed as skin-care agents.

In this method, fresh dry or dried plant material (usually flowers or herbs) is steeped in a vat of either hot or cold vegetable oil, which, depending on the plant material used, is agitated daily for a period of several days or weeks. Once the oil is saturated with the plant exudes, the mixture is strained to remove the residue. This process can be repeated a number of times, adding fresh plant material until the oil medium is sufficiently saturated.

An absolute can also be produced from the saturated, macerated oil by "washing out" the oil solution with a strong alcohol such as ethyl alcohol. After a few such washouts, the alcohol and oil mixture is left to stand to allow the alcohol to separate. The essential oil–imbued alcohol is then poured off and left to stand to allow the alcohol to evaporate from the mixture, leaving behind a viscous, richly colored absolute.

Selecting an appropriate vegetable oil to use in this process will enhance the quality and properties of the plant material. Olive, sweet almond, jojoba, and coconut oils are popular choices, as these are less inclined to become rancid (adding vitamin E will slow this process); others include sunflower, safflower, avocado, and castor oil. Calendula is an example of a macerated essential oil that has potent anti-inflammatory properties, which may improve dry skin, eczema, dermatitis, psoriasis,

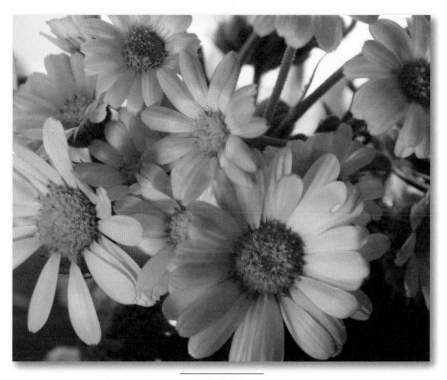

Calendula

and scar tissue, as well as sunburn and inflamed skin conditions. Kept in the refrigerator or a cool place, macerated oils will last for about three weeks to a month.

Examples of macerated, or infused, essential oils used in aromatherapy include arnica, calendula, carrot, champaca, comfrey, daisy, hypericum, jasmine, rose blossom, and St. John's wort.

Maceration Review

ESSENTIAL OIL

- The plant material is soaked in hot oil to draw out the essential oil and other volatile and nonvolatile substances.
- The saturated oil is then washed with alcohol to separate out the plant's essential oil.
- This method is used for essential oils that cannot be extracted by distillation, such as calendula and jasmine, and also hyacinth and tuberose (for perfumery).
- As with other types of solvent-extracted essential oils, the resulting essential oil is not considered a true essential oil because the process leaves traces of the vegetable oil and washout alcohol.

MASSAGE OIL

- The plants are steeped in warm oil. The container is agitated at least once a day for a few days to encourage the release of essential oil and other volatile and nonvolatile substances.
- This method produces a macerated massage oil such as calendula, carrot, and hypericum.
- Due to the inclusion of flavonoids and other waxy, nonvolatile substances along with essential oil, macerated oil is useful for general skin care and for alleviating conditions such as inflammation, eczema, psoriasis, dermatitis, and dry and aging skin.

ENFLEURAGE

Enfleurage is another ancient method historically employed to extract fragrant components from plant material, especially delicate flowers and blossoms. Although rarely employed commercially these days, this method is still used by producers in some remote or small farming areas. Time-consuming and expensive, especially when measured against yield, this process has been superceded by solvent extraction, which by comparison is commercially more viable in terms of cost, time, labor, and yield.

In this method, framed glass plates are coated with layers of cold, odorless fat such as lard or tallow (from pork or beef) or vegetable fat (such as coconut, palm, or jojoba oil and beeswax) that is solid at room temperature. Whole flowers or petals are spread evenly over the fat. The framed plates are then stacked and left to stand for two to three days to allow the plant extracts to permeate the fat. The plant material is removed and replaced with fresh flowers, and the process is repeated until the fat is sufficiently saturated with the exuding fragrant essential oils and other extracts. Hot fat can also be used in this process. The fat is placed in a receptacle with access to an external heat source such as a fire. The flowers are placed in the fat and stirred; the fat is strained to remove the flowers and replaced with more fresh blossoms. This process is repeated until the fat is sufficiently saturated. The fat is then cooled. The resulting pomade can be applied as a perfume or skin salve. As with maceration and solvent extraction, the infused fat can also be soaked and washed in ethyl alcohol to separate out fragrant molecules to produce an absolute-type scent.

Enfleurage Review

- Enfleurage is similar to maceration but uses animal or vegetable fat.
- Framed glass plates are covered in fat onto which plant material such as flowers, blossoms, or petals are evenly distributed.
- The plant material is removed and replaced with a fresh batch every few days until the fat is sufficiently saturated with essential oils and other surrendered exudes.
- For faster results, hot fat or oil can be used, strained, and refreshed, until fully saturated.
- The resulting oil can be used as a perfumed pomade or processed further to create an absolute-type scent.

EVALUATING ESSENTIAL OILS

Each species, variety, cultivar, and so on of a plant consists of a particular array of organic and inorganic components. Essential oils are comprised only of volatile components, and thus the chemical profile of an essential oil may have similarities to that of the whole plant but will actually be quite different. The properties of an essential oil cannot be assumed to be the same as that of the whole plant. Identifying the chemical constituents of essential oil is necessary not just to evaluate their therapeutic properties but also to screen for undesirable components. Each component is measured and identified (as described below), either during extraction or at various stages post-extraction, to evaluate the content and also the condition of the essential oil. This process produces standard profiles. These can be used to compare an essential oil with other essential oils extracted from the same type of plant (allowing for minor natural fluctuations) to reveal the current state, age, and rate of oxidation and transmutation of chemical components present in that oil. Reputable suppliers will be aware of their chain of supply, from grower to consumer, and will be able to provide traceable evidence of the source, quality control, chemical composition, and safety data information in relation to the essential oils they sell.

An essential oil that presents with additional components, fewer components, or components present in quantities outside the expected and acceptable parameters (either too much or too little) must be considered questionable; it usually means the oil is either overoxidized or not authentic. It may be adulterated, inappropriately or rapidly extracted, derived from a plant source of inferior quality or from another species altogether, or comprised of synthetic or other substitute components. The acceptable range of difference in terms of the quantity of a given compound present in an essential oil post-extraction is between 10% and 20%.

Essential oils are easily spoiled by heat, light, water, and exposure to air, and they must be stored in well-sealed, noncorrodible containers. Aluminum containers are generally used to store large quantities of essential oil; small quantites (2 ml to 250 ml) are stored in dark-colored glass bottles. Although aluminum is a poisonous heavy metal that will corrode when in contact with water, when it comes into contact with oxygen a protective layer is created, unlike the case for iron or steel. Aluminum bottles used to store essential oils are sometimes additionally coated with an epoxy phenolic lining. To ensure their integrity, essential oils are constantly monitored along the chain of production and supply (from growth and distillation to consumer), not only for the above reasons, but to also screen for undesirable deterioration and toxicity. While the scent of some essential oils may improve with age and oxidation (rose, patchouli, and sandalwood, for example), other essential oils can become chemically unstable, toxic, and unsafe, and potentially capable of causing skin or mucous-membrane sensitization and/or irritation, especially those essential oils with a very high terpene content such as are found in pine or citrus fruits.

Methods Used to Evaluate Essential Oils

There are various methods used to evaluate the chemical constituents, authenticity, and condition of essential oils. Although appearance is not a completely reliable determinant of the quality of an essential oil, it does provide a useful instant guide that can be used by anyone along the chain of production, from the farmer or grower to the consumer. When observing an essential oil, we compare its qualities to the standard description of that oil. The qualities we look at include color, brilliance, transparency, viscosity, and scent/odor. For example:

+ Expressed essential oils such as lemon, lime, orange, and so on are always strongly colored due to the presence of flavonoids and colored pigment present in the fruit rind, from yellow to orange, red, and green.

+ Good-quality distilled essential oils are transparent or slightly hazy, colorless, or tinted. Bergamot is colorless after distillation to remove the furanocoumarins (expressed bergamot is yellow to green), and German chamomile, yarrow, and blue tansy are naturally dark blue or greenish olive due to the chemical reaction incurred by the intense heat of distillation. German chamomile produced using CO_2 extraction (undertaken at a low critical temperature) remains green.

+ Absolutes are usually a very dark or deep color, often viscous, and frequently hazy, translucent, or opaque due to residues of insoluble natural waxes and in some instances the extracting solvent used.
+ Some essential oils, such as rose, are naturally solid at room temperature.
+ An adulterated or questionable essential oil is likely to present as being more hazy, cloudy, or more viscous than expected for that particular type of essential oil. Oxidation (due to poor storage, water contamination, or age) can render an essential oil more viscous, darker, or altered in color.

As well as visual observation, the scent profile of an essential oil can be tested and compared against that of a sample of the same type and grade of essential oil. Smelling strips, dipped respectively into the sample essential oil and the essential oil being tested, are left to dry out at the same time and under the same conditions. The scent exuding from each strip is observed at specific intervals until the dry-out is complete. Visual observation is also made of any color, tint, stain, or ring mark left behind.

Scent observation is a subjective process and so not a completely reliable indicator alone. But it must be noted that old essential oils lose their fresh scent or develop "off scents" (often due to the formation of carboxylic acids from aldehydes), so odor can be a very useful indicator. And when visual and scent observation are used together, they provide an initial comparative guide that may help us flag any disparity and indicate the need for further evaluation. It's a simple method that anyone can use.

Analytical Testing

Analytical testing is more complicated than the simple methods described above and requires special equipment, so it is usually performed in laboratory-type environments. This type of testing can take various forms.

Specific Gravity

Specific gravity is used to indicate how much heavier or lighter a particular substance is compared to the same volume of pure water at room temperature (or a consistent, controlled ambient temperature, for example, 68°F, or 20°C). Most essential oils are lighter than water; a few are heavier (for example, rose, vetivert, and myrrh). To measure the weight of a particular essential oil, a small bottle is filled with a specific amount of water and weighed; the weight is recorded. Then another bottle of the same size and weight when empty is filled with exactly the same quantity of good-quality essential oil; again the weight is recorded. The difference between the weight of the water and the weight of the essential oil is noted and provides a standard against which to compare other samples. Significant deviation from this standard indicates the need for further evaluation.

Refraction

Refraction measures the speed of light when passing through air into a denser medium, such as water. As the beam of light passes from air into the denser medium, the speed at which the light is traveling reduces, and the beam will appear to bend in the same way a knitting needle or pencil will appear to bend at its point of contact when inserted into water. (Do you remember doing this experiment in school?) The angle of refraction (that is, change in direction) of a beam of light passed through a given essential oil is measured against a standard sample, and deviation from the anticipated standard range of refraction indicates possible adulteration or compromised quality and the need for further evaluation.

Optical Rotation

Polarized light waves are passed at speed through the essential oil to measure changes in polarization or the angle of rotation (for example, clockwise or counterclockwise). Twists of the angle of the light beam as it passes through the essential oil are measured and identified—for example, clockwise, or dextrorotatory (the name of the compound identified is prefixed with *dextro-* or the letter *d-*), and counterclockwise, or laevorotatory (the name of the compound is prefixed with the word *laevo-* or the letter *l-*).

The molecules causing this rotation are isomers, which are molecular variants that contain exactly the same constituent atoms, but which are arranged in a different order or shape. Optical isomers are molecules that contain exactly the same atoms arranged in opposite formation, like a mirror image, that will cause the beam of polarized light to change direction to either the left or right. Different or reversed orientation of the same constituent atoms will significantly alter the molecule's behavior, including its scent profile. For example, the scent of *laevo*-linalool is fresh, floral, woody and lavender-like, while *dextro*-linalool has a sweet, floral, petitgrain-like, lavender like scent, and *dextro*-carvone, found in caraway essential oil, actually smells of caraway, with spicy, minty, breadlike tones, yet *laevo*-carvone smells sweet, minty, and herbal and is found in spearmint (Good Scents Company 2021; Williams 2006, 135–39; Tisserand and Balacs 1995, 14).

Again, the optical activity is measured against a standard reading for the given essential oil, a significant deviation from which indicates adulteration or compromised quality.

Acid Value

Because essential oils are volatile, their molecules will alter, degrade, or deteriorate, particularly in the catalytic presence of heat and solar or ultraviolet (UV) light. Consequently, essential oils can rapidly deteriorate when inappropriately stored or if they are old and exceed their recommended shelf life. Oxidation causes the most volatile components within an essential oil, especially terpene molecules, to evaporate, and others, especially aldehydes and esters, to transmute, causing the content of free acids to increase in many essential oils. Measurement of the acid value of an essential oil compared to the standard acid value for that particular essential oil will reveal such anomalies if they are present.

An acid test determines the condition, age, level, and rate of deterioration and will indicate whether or not the essential oil is safe to use, and if it is safe, for how long it should continue to be stored before and after being opened and used.

Gas Liquid Chromatography

Gas liquid chromatography (GLC), also known as *column chromatography*, determines the presence and amount of different chemical constituents within an essential oil. GLC involves injecting a droplet of essential oil using a micro syringe into a cylindrical tube within a small, very hot injector oven that rapidly heats (known as *flash evaporation*) the essential oil. The vaporized essential oil is mixed with an inert gas and channeled into a coiled column (approximately 1 mm in diameter and 30 to 100 meters long), which is contained within a larger, cooler, temperature-controlled oven.

The heat in this oven is strategically adjusted to prevent the molecules from being destroyed while being suspended in a gaseous state long enough to be detected and registered. This condition allows molecules to break free from the essential oil substance according to their individual boiling point, while being sustained in a gaseous state, thus making detection easier. As each molecule is released, it is registered. A pen attached to detecting instruments continuously records this release as peaks and depressions on a chart, which indicates the quantity of each chemical present and the time and order of its release up to detection. These graphic records are compared to a standard reading to verify authenticity.

Mass Spectrometry

Mass spectrometry (MS) is used to determine the specific chemical identity of molecules that have been detected by the GLC instruments (not just their quantity and rate of release). MS instruments are usually attached to the GLC detector equipment. A very small sample from a given group of molecules passing through the detector oven is channeled into a vacuum and bombarded with a stream of electrons that causes the molecules to form positively charged ions, which are detected by recording instruments. The fragmentation pattern of the ions enables identification of the molecular structure and identification of individual chemicals. Measured against a standard, this readout will also reveal the level of oxidation and toxicity of a given compound.

Chemical Abstracts Services (CAS)

The Chemical Abstracts Services, or CAS, governs a system of labeling and identification devised by the American Chemical Society. The acronym CAS, or CAS RNs, with "RNs" referring to registry numbers, appears with a unique number or code assigned to every known

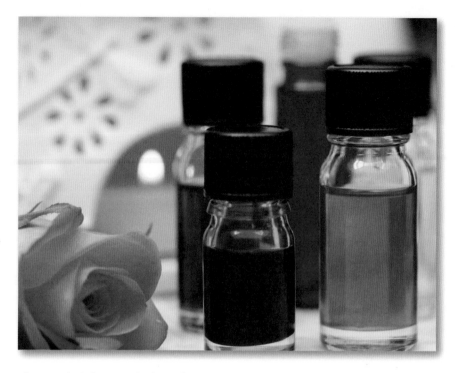

chemical. This includes elements, isotopes, organic and inorganic compounds, ions, organometallics, metals, and materials of unknown, variable composition or biological origin, including nonstructurable materials—for example, ethanol, which is a volatile, flammable colorless liquid. The numbers of each chemical are assigned for the purpose of listing and cataloging only; they have no other significance.

Every essential oil as well as each chemical component in an essential oil is assigned a unique identifying CAS number, which is recorded on all accompanying documents. For example:

German chamomile (*Matricaria recutita*)   CAS No. 8002-66-2
patchouli *(Pogostemon cablin)*   CAS No. 8014-09-3
rose (*Rosa damascena*)   CAS No. 8007-01-0
tea tree (*Melaleuca alternifolia*)   CAS No. 68647-73-4

Knowing the chemical composition of an essential oil goes a long way toward determining its appropriate use. That is the subject of the next chapter.

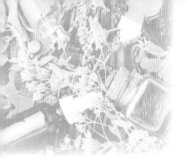

4

Essential Oil Chemistry

A Brief Introduction to the Science of Plant Constituents

Organic chemistry is a vast, complex, and fascinating subject merely touched upon here. Stepping along the shoreline, so to speak, this chapter takes a look at the various chemical constituents that comprise essential oils so that we may best use them in therapeutic applications.

Essential oils are typically made up of up to 250, and sometimes more, individual molecules. Each constituent molecule presents its own chemical, scent, and therapeutic profile. The scent that exudes so delightfully from an essential oil does so by virtue of these volatile molecules, which evaporate at different rates and lend dynamic depth, layers, and contours to the quality of an essential oil's odor. An essential oil's therapeutic profile is also determined by the presence and arrangement of these molecules.

Beginning with a look at the building blocks from which molecules evolve, this chapter identifies the various chemical components that contribute to and influence the characteristic qualities of essential oils, including their scent profiles and therapeutic values.

FORMS OF MATTER

All matter is made up of atoms and molecules, which, although invisible to the naked eye, form the basic building blocks of everything that physically exists. In its simplest state, matter is defined as anything that has mass and occupies space.

Matter is observed in four discernable states: solid, liquid, gas, and plasma (plasma forms a major component of the sun and is found mainly in space). To illustrate quite simply, water solidifies into ice as it freezes; heat then melts ice into its liquid state, water; and intense heat transforms water into steam or vapor (gas) and condenses back into water as it cools. The different manifestations of matter can be observed in various states in everything around us—in the clouds, snow, air, rocks, sand, metal, wood, rivers, and so on. Heat and light energy interacts with the atoms and molecules that comprise matter, influencing a reaction that transforms its state to create different manifestations, qualities, and substances, as when heat energy causes ice to melt or water to evaporate, or when light energy instigates a chemical reaction in plants through photosynthesis.

Atoms

Atoms are the basic building blocks of chemistry and the smallest units of matter that participate in chemical reactions. They cannot be naturally broken down without the release of electrically charged particles, and they cannot be subdivided without destroying their identity.

Invisible to the naked eye, atoms measure approximately one hundred millionth of a centimeter in diameter. The nucleus of an atom is very dense and extremely small compared to its outer sphere; in fact, atoms are mainly empty space. The nucleus of an atom is made up of particles known as *protons,* which are positively charged (+), and *neutrons,* which are electrically neutral (neutrons do not affect the chemical properties of an atom but act to prevent the positive (+) proton charges from repelling one another). *Electrons,* which are negatively charged (−), orbit the protons (+) and neutrons in a cloud surrounding the nucleus. This electron cloud has a radius ten thousand times greater than that of the nucleus. The number of protons (+) in the nucleus equals the number of orbiting electrons (−), and thus the atom remains electrically neutral. Protons, neutrons, and electrons are made up of even smaller particles, known as *quarks.* Atoms do not exist in isolation from one another (with the exception of helium and neon) but bond with other atoms comprising the same atomic construct to form *elements.*

Protons and neutrons have approximately the same mass, and they are denser and heavier than electrons; a proton is nearly two thousand times the size, or mass, of an electron. Atoms always have an equal number of protons and electrons, and the number of neutrons is usually the same but sometimes varies. Adding a proton to an atom makes a new element. Adding a neutron makes an isotope, which is a heavier version of that atom.

The number of protons (+) gives the *atomic number* of each element; this, along with the number of neutrons and electrons (–), determines the atom's and ultimately the element's unique quality and identity. For example, atoms within the element helium have 2 protons, 2 neutrons, and 2 electrons, and atoms within the element carbon have 6 protons, 6 neutrons, and 6 electrons. However, hydrogen, which is the simplest chemical element and present in almost all carbon compounds and in all animal and vegetable tissue, has 1 proton and 1 electron, which affects the element's bonding properties.

If an atom has a different number of electrons (more or less) than protons, it is known as an *ion*. Ions are created when an atom either loses or gains electrons. If an atom gains electrons, it has a net negative charge and is known as an *anion;* if an atom loses electrons, it has a net positive charge and is known as a *cation*. If an atom possesses the same numbers of electrons as protons, its electrical charge is neutral. Cations and anions attract each other and combine to form *ionic compounds* (for example, salts are ionic compounds). Conversely, cations repel one another, and so do anions.

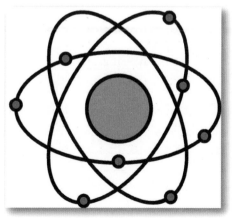

An atom and its orbitals

Elements

Elements are pure chemical substances consisting of one type of atom, identified by the number of protons (atomic number), neutrons, and electrons present. Elements form the simplest substances that cannot be further broken down by chemical reactions. There are ninety-two naturally occurring elements (and twenty or so additional, less stable elements created through nuclear physics). Elements form the basic substances from which all others derive; substances are built by chemical bonding, that is, by atoms joining with one another.

The periodic table, an icon of chemistry, used in chemistry, physics, and other sciences, is a useful visual construct that groups and orders the elements in a grid according to their atomic number. Working across the table, each element, which is abbreviated according to the Latin, Greek, Arabic, or other common name of the element, increases by one proton (neutron and electron) to form another basic substance. For example, platinum's atomic number is 78, gold's is 79, mercury's is 80, and so on. The vertical rows in the grid are known as *groups,* and the horizontal rows are known as *periods.*

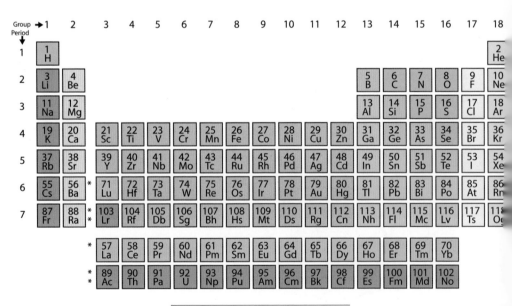

The modern periodic table

Molecules

A molecule is the simplest unit of a chemical compound or element that can exist in a free state, and it consists of two or more atoms held together by chemical bonds. There are two types of molecules: *homonuclear molecules,* which consist of atoms of a single chemical element, for example, molecular oxygen (O_2); and *heteronuclear molecules,* which consist of more than one element, for example, oxygen and hydrogen, as found in water (H_2O).

COMPOUNDS

A compound is a chemical substance consisting of two or more different elements chemically bonded together, which can only be separated into simpler chemical substances by means of chemical reactions. When elements are joined to form a compound, the atoms they are comprised of lose their individual properties, and the compound formed maintains its own unique and defined chemical structure. Examples of compounds include:

+ Table salt ($NaCl$), which comprises one sodium (Na) atom, an alkali metal, and one chlorine (Cl) atom, a nonmetal from the halogen group
+ Carbon dioxide (CO_2), which comprises one carbon (C) atom, a nonmetal, and two oxygen (O) atoms, another nonmetal
+ Water (H_2O), which comprises two hydrogen (H) atoms and one oxygen (O) atom, both of which are nonmetals
+ Ethanol (alcohol) (C_2H_5OH), which comprises two carbon (C) atoms, six hydrogen (H) atoms, and one oxygen (O) atom, all of which are nonmetals
+ Terpenes (C_5H_8), which are comprised of five carbon (C) atoms and eight hydrogen (H) atoms, and with their derivatives, terpenoids, form the main chemical structures of essential oils

MIXTURES

Mixtures are made up of two or more substances that are not chemically bonded and do retain their individual identities or characteristics. The components of a mixture can be separated from one another. For example, seawater is a mixture of salt (sodium chloride, NaCl) and water (H_2O). The salt is dissolved in the water. When heated, the water evaporates as steam and then condenses purely as water, leaving behind solid salt crystals.

Mixtures can have any number and amount of ingredients and may take the form of solutions, suspensions, and colloids. There are two types of mixtures: *homogeneous* and *heterogeneous.* In a homogeneous mixture, all components are evenly distributed, and every part of the solution has the same properties; for example, salt or sugar dissolves in water to create a homogeneous mixture or solution. In a heterogeneous mixture, the ingredients remain discernibly separate—for example, sand and water, or water and oil.

Essential oils are fluids that are made up of a complex mixture of volatile organic terpene and terpenoid compounds. All molecules comprising essential oils contain oxygen and hydrogen atoms in varying proportions; a few also contain sulfur constituents, and fewer still, nitrogen. Some of these constituents are present in such minute quantities that they are barely detectable. All molecules present contribute (with varying degrees of potency) to the essential oil's qualities. However, essential oils are not stable (that is, they are volatile), and this means their characteristics will change over time.

ESSENTIAL OIL CONSTITUENTS

Essential oils are comprised of hydrocarbons (terpenes), such as monoterpenes, sesquiterpenes, and diterpenes, and their oxygenated derivatives (terpenoids). Terpenoids include alcohols, aldehydes, ketones, esters, oxides, phenols, ethers, furans, lactones, and acids. The charts in this chapter list these components and identify the essential oils they are found in. Identifying these components provides some indication of the general therapeutic properties of an oil and which oils can be blended together to enhance certain therapeutic actions or, conversely, to quench or counterbalance potential irritating or otherwise less desirable components.

The individual essential oil profiles found in chapter 6 provide a complete overview of the properties of fifty-eight essential oils. You can cross-reference these with the information in this chapter to guide you so you can hone your use of an essential oil.

Terpenes

Terpenes are the aromatic, bioactive chemical compounds found in many plants that give plants their distinctive odor and endow certain protective qualities to the plant. In the case of essential oils, they also impart certain health benefits, such as antiviral, antibacterial, anti-inflammatory, antiseptic, analgesic, stimulant, sedative, and decongestant activities, among many others.

Terpenes are a class of hydrocarbons, which are naturally occurring organic chemical compounds composed solely of the elements carbon (C) and hydrogen (H). Carbon atoms join together to form a framework, and the hydrogen atoms attach to them in many configurations. A hydrocarbon is a five-carbon unit, known as *isoprene* (C_5H_8). Isoprenes combine to form *isoprenoids*. Terpenes are derivatives of isoprene units. The smallest terpene molecule contains ten carbon atoms, or two isoprene units, and is called a *monoterpene* ($C_{10}H_{16}$). Monoterpenes are mostly volatile and fragrant. Terpenes develop in structure by the addition of one isoprene unit (five carbon atoms) at a time, with each additional unit rendering the terpene less volatile and more stable. A terpene consisting of fifteen carbon atoms (three isoprene units) is called a *sesquiterpene* ($C_{15}H_{24}$), with *sesqui* meaning "one and a half." A terpene consisting of twenty carbon atoms (four isoprene units) is called a *diterpene* ($C_{20}H_{32}$), a terpene consisting of three terpene units or six isoprene units is a *triterpene* ($C_{30}H_{48}$), and a terpene consising of eight isoprene units is a *tetraterpene* ($C_{40}H_{64}$). Essential oils are comprised mostly of monoterpenes, some sesquiterpenes, and very few diterpenes.

Essential oils that have a large proportion of monoterpene molecules include citrus oils such as lemon, orange, and grapefruit, as well as cypress, frankincense, galbanum, juniper berry, and pine. Sesquiterpene molecules are found in abundance in essential oils such as carrot seed, cedarwood, chamomile, black pepper, patchouli, and ginger. Diterpene molecules are rarely found in essential oils, although small amounts are found in clary sage.

Below are listed 1) the three types of terpene hydrocarbons

(monoterpenes, sesquiterpenes, and diterpenes) and their associated chemical components; 2) the essential oils these components are found in; and 3) the associated scent and therapeutic profile attributed to each group. The percentages attributed to the chemical components in a particular essential oil are based on averages and are included as a general guide. Remember, an essential oil is influenced by all molecules present in its mixture; however, knowing the predominant functional group present offers an initial guide when selecting oils. Always follow this up by checking out an essential oil's complete profile, as found in chapter 6.

Monoterpenes ($C_{10}H_{16}$)

Among the most volatile group of constituents, monoterpenes readily combine with oxygen in the air and transmute over time into peroxides, then epoxides and alcohols. These are usually the first molecules to evaporate from an essential oil and the first molecules surrendered during extraction.

Examples of individual chemical components found in monoterpenes have names ending in *–ene:* Camphene, delta-3-carene, para-cymene, dextro-limonene and laevo-limonene (dipentene), beta-myrcene, beta-ocimene, alpha-phellandrene, alpha-pinene and beta-pinene, sabinene, alpha-terpinene and gamma-terpinene, terpinene, terpinolene, thujene

Examples of essential oils containing some of these components: Bergamot (52%), bitter orange (90%), black pepper (60%), caraway seed (40%), carrot seed (22%), cypress (70%), dill (40%), *Eucalyptus dives* (30%), fennel (24%), fir needle (90%), frankincense (75%), galbanum (84%), ginger (20%), grapefruit (98%), hyssop (28%), immortelle/helichrysum (28%), juniper berry (80%), lemon (87%), lime (72%), mandarin (90%), sweet marjoram (40%), myrtle (60%), neroli (35%), nutmeg (75%), pine needle (84%), red thyme (35%), rose (20%), rosemary (19%), sage (20%), Scotch pine (70%), summer savory (34%), Spanish marjoram (9%), sweet orange (96%), tagetes (35%), tea tree (41%), yarrow (28%)

Associated scent profiles: Woody, piney, resinous; citrusy, fresh, light; camphoraceous; sweet, light, balsamic; scent that rapidly diminishes

Associated therapeutic properties: Analgesic (mild), antifungal, antiseptic (especially for airborne pathogens), antiviral, bactericidal, expectorant/decongestant, diuretic, insecticidal, stimulating

Sesquiterpenes ($C_{15}H_{24}$)

Sesquiterpenes are not as volatile as monoterpenes and slightly more viscous (eventually forming long-chain resins); they are not soluble in water, and they react in the presence of heat and light and transmute to form epoxides and alcohols, and eventually resins. Old and oxidized oils with a high sesquiterpene content, such as patchouli, sandalwood, myrrh, and vetivert, can become thick and sticky as a result.

Examples of individual chemical components have names ending in *-ene:* Aromadendrene, beta-bergamotene, beta-bisabolene, alpha-bulnesene, alpha-cadinene, beta-calarene, beta-caryophyllene, alpha-cedrene, copaene, alpha-curcumene, daucene, beta-elemene, alpha-farnesene, germacrene, 6,9-guaiadiene, guaiene, beta-gurgunene, alpha-himachalene, beta-himachalene, gamma-himachalene, alpha-humulene, italicene, alpha-muurolene, patchoulene, alpha-santolene, beta-santolene, selinene, seychellene, vetivenene, viridiflorene, alpha-zingiberene and beta-zingiberene, chamazulene (a by-product of distillation)

Examples of essential oils containing some of these components: Black pepper (30%), carrot seed (64%), cedarwood (60%), German chamomile (35%), ginger (55%), immortelle/helichrysum (33%), melissa (20%), myrrh (40%), patchouli (60%), sandalwood (10%), spikenard (35%), vetivert (up to 3%), yarrow (45%), ylang-ylang (40%)

Associated scent profiles: Warm, woody, spicy, dry, deep sweetness, cedar-like, camphoraceous

Associated therapeutic properties: Analgesic, anti-inflammatory, antispasmodic, antiviral, bactericidal, balancing, calming, hypotensive, sedative

Diterpenes ($C_{20}H_{32}$)

Diterpenes are rarely found in essential oils. The molecules are heavy and do not readily distill. They transmute to form diterpenols.

Examples of individual chemical components have names ending in *-ene:* Camphorene; diterpenols have names ending in *-ol:* salviol, sclareol

Examples of essential oils containing these components: Clary sage
(2%)

Associated scent profile: Light, faint sweet balsam, amber, woody,
weedy

Associated therapeutic properties: Mildly antifungal, anti-
inflammatory, antioxidant, antiviral, bactericidal, detoxifying, expectorant, immunostimulatory

Terpenoids

Terpenoids derive from terpenes as a result of oxidation—as terpene molecules gain oxygen atoms, their structure and behavior alter. So whereas
terpenes are hydrocarbons (meaning the only elements present are hydrogen and oxygen), terpenoids have been denatured by oxidation (drying
and curing flowers, for example) or chemically modified (as in distillation). Terpenoids are categorized according to the functional group present within their molecule. These functional groups are substituent atoms
(i.e., an atom or group that replaces another atom or group in a molecule)
that form a very small part of the molecule. They have valency, which
means they readily attract and combine with other atoms and ions, and
thus they are volatile, unstable, and reactive and easily transmute from one
state to another to form new molecular structures. Primary alcohols, for
example, can oxidize to aldehydes (examples include geraniol, citronellol,
and myrtenol); secondary alcohols can oxidize to ketones (examples
include menthol, isoplegol, borneol, and verbenol); tertiary alcohols
cannot oxidize and so do not form aldehydes or ketones (examples of
tertiary alcohols include linalool, terpinen-4-ol, and alpha-terpineol)
(Tisserand et al. 2021). To add to the obvious complexity, each molecule
possesses a different mechanism of action, which is widely shared by other
molecules belonging to different functional groups, so isolating specific
actions and attributing these to specific molecules is not exact; there is
still much to discover about these properties. Even though they form a
very small part of a molecule, functional groups tend to determine that
molecule's general characteristics and properties.

As before, below are listed 1) the main related functional groups—
for example, alcohols, aldehydes, ketones, and so on—and their
associated chemical components; 2) the essential oils these components

are found in; and 3) the associated scent and therapeutic profile attributed to each group. Again, the percentages attributed to the chemical components in a particular essential oil are based on averages and are included as a general guide; they may be greater or less than the amount shown (+/– %). Some of the essential oils listed below are not covered in chapter 6 but are included to provide a useful reference.

Alcohols

Chemical profile: Based on monoterpenes and, rarely, sesquiterpenes; can oxidize to form aldehydes and acids or resins; relatively nontoxic and nonmutagenic (not causing change in an organism's genes); low irritancy and allerginicity

Examples of individual chemical components (names ending in -*ol*):

Monoterpene alcohols: Benzyl alcohol, borneol, careol, cinnamyl alcohol, beta-citronellol, beta-eudesmol, dihydrocarveol, fenchyl alcohol, geraniol, isoborneol, isopulegol, lavandulol, dextra-linalool, laveolinalool, menthol, myrtenol, nerol, perillyl alcohol, 2-phenylethanol, phenylethyl alcohol, phytol, trans-pinocarveol, alpha-terpineol, delta-terpineol, terpinen-4-ol, (S)-*cis*-verbenol

Sesquiterpene alcohols: Atlantol, bergamotol, alpha-bisabolol, cadinoll, carotol, caryophyllene alcohol, alpha-cedrol, daucol, elemol, eudesmol, farnesol, isovalencenol, khusimol, nerolidol, norpatchoulenol, paradisol, patchoulol, pogostol, alpha-santalol, beta-santalol, vetiverol, viridiflorol, zingiberol

Examples of essential oils containing these components (+/– %): Carrot seed (26%), catnip (62%), cedarwood (35%), clary sage (20%), coriander (70%), *Eucalyptus smithii* (17%), geranium (68%), German chamomile (20%), jasmine (24%), lavender English (36%), lavender fine (45%), lavender spike (32%), Spanish marjoram (20%), sweet marjoram (50%), myrrh (40%), neroli (40%), palmarosa (85%), patchouli (33%), peppermint (42%), petitgrain (30%), rose otto (63%), rosewood (90%), sandalwood (80%), spearmint (20%), tea tree (45%), thyme linalool (45%), vetivert (40%), ylang-ylang (20%)

Associated scent profiles: Soft, sweet, flowery, green, herbaceous, or woody; floral, fruity, waxy; roselike; lily of the valley–like; fresh, cool, minty; fragrance generally pleasant

Therapeutic properties: Analgesic, anesthetic, antioxidant, anti-infectious, antibacterial, mildly anti-inflammatory, antiviral, balancing, uplifting, gently stimulating, tonic to the nervous system, sedative, warming

Aldehydes

Chemical profile: Derived from primary alcohols through partial oxidation; very reactive and readily oxidize to corresponding organic acids (can be irritant or sensitizing and cause allergic reactions)

Examples of individual chemical components (names ending in *-al* or *-aldehyde*):

Monoterpene aldehydes: Citral, beta-citronellal, cumin aldehyde, geranial, neral, perillaldehyde

Others: Acetaldehyde, anisaldehyde, benzaldehyde, caproic aldehyde, cinnamaldehyde, 2-decenal, dodecanal, 2-dodecanal, myrtenal, nonanal, phellandral, piperonal, salicylaldehyde, sinensal, teresantal, valeranal, vanillin

Examples of essential oils containing these components (+/– %): Cinnamon bark (72%), citronella (40%), *Eucalyptus citriodora* (80%), lemongrass (80%), may chang (75%), melissa (60%), palmarosa (7%), spikenard (trace amount), vanilla (85%)

Associated scent profiles: Sharp, lemony (citrals), floral to intensely green, cinnamon, spicy, medicinal, soaplike; powerful scent; major constituent in tropical oils

Therapeutic properties: Anti-infectious (not as consistent as alcohols, though), antifungal, anti-inflammatory, antiviral, calming to the nervous system, cooling; can be irritant (citral and cinnamaldehyde are skin allergens)

Ketones

Chemical profile: Derived from secondary alcohols through oxidation; relatively stable but resistant to metabolism by the liver and can cause problems (ketoacidosis); do not readily oxidize further. Some ketones are dangerous or damaging to the central nervous system (neurotoxic) (for example, camphor, thujone, and pinocamphone). Essential oils with high ketone content should be used moderately (for example, caraway seed, dill, and hyssop), while others should be avoided or used with extreme caution (for example, western red cedar, wormwood, thuja, ho leaf, Spanish lavender, Spanish sage, rosemary ct. camphor, Spanish marjoram, pennyroyal—profiles for these oils are not covered in chapter 6).

Examples of individual chemical components (names ending in -*one*):

Monoterpenoid ketones: Alpha-asarone, beta-asarone, camphor, carvone, cryptone, beta-damascenone, trans-beta-damascone, fenchone, alpha-ionone, alpha-irone, beta-irone, cis-jasmone, iso-menthone, menthone, methyl amyl ketone, methyl heptenone, methyl nonyl ketone (2-undecanone), perilla ketone, pinocamphone, iso-pinocamphone, pinocarvone, piperitone, delta-pulegone, santolinenone, alpha-thujone, beta-thujone, thymoquinone, verbenone

Sesquiterpenic ketones: Alpha-atlantone, gamma-atlantone, nootkatone, turmerone, valeranone, alpha-vetivone, beta-vetivone

Others: Acetophenone, methoxy phenyl acetone, 2-nonanone methyl heptyl, 3-octanone, tagetone

Aliphatic ketones: 6-methyl-5-hepten-2-one, italidione (found only in helichrysum/immortelle)

Examples of essential oils containing these components (+/– %): Caraway seed (54%), cedarwood (19%), dill (50%), *Eucalyptus dives* (45%), hyssop (46%), immortelle (6%), lavender spike (10%), may chang (4%), pennyroyal (80%), peppermint (30%), rosemary (25%), sage common (35%), spearmint (55%), rose otto (trace amount), tagetes (50%), thujone (75%), vetivert (8%)

Associated scent profiles: Celery-like (cis-jasmone in jasmine absolute), violet-like (orris absolute and clove); powerful, herbaceous, fresh, camphoraceous, minty; honey-like; vast range of scent types

Therapeutic properties: Analgesic, anticonvulsant, antifungal, anti-inflammatory, antiparasitic, antiviral, calming, expectorant, mucolytic, sedative, stimulant, uplifting, vulnerary (wound-healing)

Esters

Chemical profile: Derived from alcohols and acids; generally quite stable; often have an intensely sweet and fruity odor; highest levels reached upon maturity of fruit or plant or on reaching full bloom of flowers or blossoms; for example, in peppermint (–)-menthol is converted to (–)-menthyl, and in bergamot fruits linalool is converted to linalyl acetate (Tisserand and Young 2014, 19).

Examples of individual chemical components (names ending in -*yl* or -*ate*): Iso-amayl, angelate, benzyl acetate, benzyl benzoate, benzyl cinnamate, benzyl salicylate, bornyl acetate, bornyl isovalerate, butyl angelate, iso-butyl angelate, cinnamyl acetate, beta-citronellyl acetate, citronellyl butyrate, beta-citronellyl formate, dimethyl anthranilate, eugenyl acetate, geranyl acetate, hexyl acetate, lavandulyl acetate, linalyl acetate, linalyl propionate, menthyl acetate, methyl anthranilate, methyl benzoate, methyl butyrate, methyl cinnamate, methyl salicylate, neryl acetate, trans-pinocarveol acetate, propyl angelate, sabinene hydrate, cis-sabinyl acetate, alpha-terpinyl acetate, iso-amyl tiglate, vetiveryl acetate

Examples of essential oils containing these components (+/– %): Benzoin (70%), bergamot (40%), chamomile Roman (75%), clary sage (70%), jasmine (54%), lavandin (27%), lavender English (45%), myrtle (39%), petitgrain (55%), *Thymus vulgaris* (40%), ylang-ylang (15%)

Associated scent profiles: Fruity, richly herbaceous and agrestic (reminiscent of the countryside, i.e., fields, meadows, farmyard, hayloft); sweet, floral, and slightly medicated; jasmine-like; also found as volatile, non-distillable component in fruits such as banana, pineapple, and raspberry

Therapeutic properties: Antifungal, anti-inflammatory, antispasmodic, balancing, calming, cicatrizant (aids formation of scar tissue), relaxant, sedative, uplifting, vulnerary (aids healing of wounds)

Phenols

Chemical profile: Chemical names sometimes confused with alcohols; form esters when reacting with acids; very reactive; can cause skin sensitization and dermatitis; avoid during pregnancy.

Examples of individual chemical components (names ending in -*ol*):

Monoterpenoid phenols: Australol, carvacrol, thymol (carvacrol and thymol are isomers of the same molecule; they are powerful antibacterials but also skin irritants)

Phenylpropanoids: Chavibetol, eugenol, iso-eugenol, guaiacol, methyleugenol, para-cresol (phenylpropanoids protect plants from predation; they contain flavonoids, lignin, coumarins, and many small phenolic molecules, and they are bitter and astringent.)

Examples of essential oils containing these components (+/– %): Basil eugenol (60%), cinnamon leaf (86%), clove bud (90%), fennel sweet (62%), oregano (75%), savory summer (40%), savory winter (50%), tarragon (70%), thyme red (48%)

Associated scent profiles: Medicinal (thymol and carvacrol), pungent and spicy (eugenol), herbaceous, thyme-like; spicy, woody, and camphoraceous (carvacrol); sickeningly sweet and tarry

Therapeutic properties: Analgesic, antiviral, antiseptic, antispasmodic, emmenagogue, immune-supporting, raises blood pressure, stimulating, strongly antibacterial

Ethers

Chemical profile: Derived from phenols and alcohols; generally quite stable.

Examples of individual chemical components (names ending in -ether, -ol, -ole, -cin):

Phenolic ethers: Trans-anethole, beta-asarone, chavicol, cresyl methyl ether, dill apiole, elemicin, estragole (methyl carvicol), eugenol methyl ether, methyl isoeugenol myristicin, parsley apiole, phenyl ethyl methyl ether, safrole, iso-safrole, thymol, thymol methyl ether

Alcohol ethers: phenyl ethanol

Examples of essential oils containing these components (+/– %):

Phenol ethers: Anise (98%), star anise (98%), basil Comoro islands (85%), basil estragole (88%), basil Madagascar (50%), ravensara bark (95%), fennel (92%), myrtle/aniseed (95%), tarragon (60%)

Alcohol ethers: Rose absolute (75%)

Associated scent profiles: Sweet, aniseedy, pungent, medicated (methyl ether); spicy, warm, balsamic, woody, smoky, burnt; sweet-herbaceous

Therapeutic properties: Antispasmodic, analgesic, anti-infectious, antiseptic, antibacterial, immune-boosting, stimulant to nervous system

Oxides

Chemical profile: Derived from alcohols and named after the alcohol with *oxide* included in the name; scarce in essential oils but found in the Myrtaceae botanical family; sometimes classified as phenols or phenolic ethers; can be skin irritants; can decompose into alcohols through oxidation (can become sticky).

Examples of individual chemical components (names ending in *oxide*):

Sesquiterpenoid oxides: Alpha-bisabolene oxide, alpha-bisabolol oxide, beta-caryophyllene oxide

Monoterpene oxides: 1,8-cineole (eucalyptol) is the most commonly occurring oxide; 1,4-cineole, geranyl oxide, linalool oxide, nerol oxide, pinene oxide, (–)-cis-rose oxide

Diterpenoid oxide: Sclareol oxide

Examples of essential oils containing these components (+/– %): *Eucalyptus globulus* (82%), *Eucalyptus smithii* (78%), German chamomile (35%), lavender spike (34%), Spanish marjoram (55%), myrtle (22%), niaouli (60%), ravensara (60%), rosemary (30%), rose otto (trace amount)

Associated scent profiles: Gives essential oils strength of odor, even when present in very small amount (for example, rose oxide); fresh, dry woody, camphoraceous

Therapeutic properties: Anti-infectious (respiratory tract), expectorant, decongestant, mucolytic, respiratory anti-inflammatory, stimulant

Furans

Chemical profile: Found in very few essential oils. Menthofuran occurs in most mint oils.

Examples of individual chemical components (names ending in *-furan* or *-ide*): Alpha-argofuran, butylidine phthalide, 3-butyl phthalide, dihydrobenzionofuran, furanoeudesma-1,3-diene, ligusti-lide, menthofuran

Examples of essential oils containing these components (+/– %): Angelica root (20%), lovage root (2%), myrrh (34%), palo santo (12%), peppermint (9%)

Associated scent profiles: Herbal, lovage, celery; green, vegetable; pungent, nutty, musty, earthy, coffee

Therapeutic properties: Toxic in isolation, especially hepatotoxic; antibacterial, antibiotic

Furanocoumarins

Chemical profile: Found in many citrus oils; usually phototoxic.

Examples of individual chemical components (names ending in *-in, -ol,* or *-en*): Bergamottin, bergapten, bergaptol, citropten, oxypeucedanin, xanthotoxin

Examples of essential oils containing these components (+/– %): Angelica root (1%), bergamot (33%), lime (33%)

Associated scent profiles: Citrusy

Therapeutic properties: Phototoxic, neurotoxic, and carcinogenic in isolation, although potentially anti-cancer in controlled amounts (Sumorek-Wiadro et al. 2020, Ahmed et al. 2020)

Lactones

Chemical profile: Present only in very small amounts in essential oils; coumarin is a form of lactone; resemble ketones, esters, and ethers; monoterpenoid or sesquiterpenoid; do not oxidize readily; do not metabolize easily; can have adverse effects (neurotoxic, skin sensitization, allergies, and blistering); neurotoxic and skin-sensitizing.

Examples of individual chemical components (names in this group are variable and end in *-lactone, -in, -ine, -ide, -en*): Alantolactone, bergapten, *cis*-ambretteolide, costunolide, coumarin, dehydrocostus lactone, massoia lactone, (–)-pentaecanolide, umbelliferone (7-hydroxycoumarin)

Examples of essential oils containing these components (+/– %): Ambrette seed absolute (15%), bergamot (1%), cassia bark and leaf (2.5%), lime (1%), massoia (70%), orange (1%), tonka bean absolute (60%)

Associated scent profiles: Earthy, pungent; sweet, creamy, coconut, herbal; warm, nutty, caramel

Therapeutic properties: Analgesic, anti-inflammatory, expectorant, mucolytic

Acids

Chemical profile: Rarely found in essential oils due to low volatility; those found in essential oils are usually carboxylic acids.

Examples of individual chemical components (names containing *-ic* or *acid*): Anisic acid, benzoic acid, cinnamic acid, citronellic acid, thujic acid, valerenic acid

Examples of essential oils containing these components (+/– %): Benzoin (trace amount), bergamot (trace amount), cinnamon (trace amount), citronella (trace amount), valerian (trace amount), vetiver (trace amount), western red cedarwood (25%), mainly found in floral waters

Associated scent profiles: Balsamic, urine; fatty, waxy, floral, citronella, vegetable, tobacco; woody, aromatic, lime, spicy, coumarin, peppery; cedar, thujonic

Therapeutic properties: Stimulant

Peroxides

Chemical profile: Rarely found in essential oils; decompose easily, especially at high temperature, also with prolonged exposure to air and water; very reactive.

Examples of individual chemical components (rare in essential oils): Ascaridole (toxic)

Examples of essential oils containing these components (+/– %): Wormseed (70%) (never used in aromatherapy)

Associated scent profiles: Eucalyptus-like, camphoraceous

Therapeutic properties: Purgative (toxic)

Sulfur

Chemical profile: Found in very few essential oils used in aromatherapy; major constituent of garlic, leek, onion, shallot essential oil; found in other essential oils but only in trace amounts; pungent; reactive; simple structures; not derived from terpenes.

Examples of individual chemical components (names containing -sulph, -sulf, -thio): Allylimethyl, allyl isothiocyanate, diallyl disulfide, dimethyl sulfide, dipropyl disulfide, methyl disulfide

Examples of essential oils containing these components (+/– %): Garlic (95%), onion (90%)

Associated scent profiles: Very pungent, powerful, diffusive; diallyl disulfide found in garlic essential oil

Therapeutic properties: Antimicrobial, antifungal

Nitrogen

Chemical profile: Essential building block of amino acids; not directly useful to plants or animals until converted to a reduced state for higher plants and animals; very rare in essential oils.

Examples of individual chemical components (rare in essential oils): Indole, methyl anthranilate, methyl N-methyle anthranilate, pyrazines, pyridines

Examples of essential oils containing these components (+/– %): Bergamot (trace amount), black pepper (trace amount), galbanum (trace amount), lemon (trace amount), mandarin (trace amount), orange (trace amount), vetivert (trace amount), and floral absolutes including jasmine (14%)

Associated scent profiles: Penetrating and very strong harsh odor; green and sharp, reminiscent of green peppers or peas in a pod; fruity (grape, orange blossom) and floral; animal, musty, fecal

Therapeutic properties: Makes up approximately 79% of Earth's atmosphere; crucial component to all life on Earth; component of all amino acids; converted for use by plants through process of fixation, which transforms nitrogen from its gaseous state; crucial to all plant growth; absorbed from soil by roots and converted within plant, usually roots, or as a process of decomposition by nitrogen-fixing bacteria, e.g. rhizobia; used in chlorophyll molecules

Common Constituents and Scent Profiles of Essential Oils

Extracted from their plant source, essential oil molecules combine to form a unique substance that presents a dynamic scent and therapeutic profile. Each molecule in an essential oil also has its own chemical fingerprint, and thus an associated scent and therapeutic signature. It is the combined influence of these components, observed in the depths and layers of an essential oil's scent, that creates the therapeutic and odor qualities of the oil as a whole. Many of these components are present in miniscule, almost undetectable amounts. Their odor profiles are therefore negligible, yet their presence can have a significant influence, whether it's through potentiating other molecules and contributing to synergy (see the section later in this chapter on synergy) or simply because they are potent, or a combination of these factors. Isolated compounds can behave quite differently when separate from the whole oil.

The following chart lists a few examples of common constituents, their scent profiles, and a few of the essential oils these constituents are found in to demonstrate the way an essential oil's scent is influenced by the various individual chemical components that make up each mixture.

FUNCTIONAL GROUP	CHEMICAL CONSTITUENT	SCENT PROFILE	ESSENTIAL OILS THE CONSTITUENT IS FOUND IN
Monoterpene	camphene CAS no: 79-92-5	odor strength: medium woody, herbal, fir needle, pine, camphoraceous, cool	cajeput, mints, pine needle, turpentine
	delta-3-carene CAS no: 13466-78-9	odor strength: medium citrus, terpenic, pine, solvent, resinous, cypress, medicinal, woody	frankincense, eucalyptus, juniper, dill, summer savory
	para-cymene CAS no: 99-8-76	odor strength: high chemical, woody, terpenic, citrus, lemon, spicy, cumin, oregano	lemon, grapefruit, mandarin, orange, palo santo, caraway, dill, white camphor
	dextro-limonene CAS no: 5989-27-5	odor strength: medium citrus, orange, fresh, sweet	nutmeg, chaste tree, juniper berry, yarrow, ho leaf/cineole, black pepper
	laevo-limonene CAS no: 5989-54-8	odor strength: medium terpene, pine, herby, peppery	sage, pine, pepper (white), cypress, galbanum, basil
	alpha-pinene CAS no: 80-56-8	odor strength: high fresh, camphoraceous, sweet, pine, earthy, woody	spruce, fir needle, pine, sage, rosemary
	sabinene CAS no: 3387-41-5	odor strength: medium woody, terpenic, citrus, pine, spicy, camphoraceous	thyme, oregano, camphor, cumin, tea tree
	alpha-thujene CAS no: 2867-05-2	odor strength: medium woody, herbal	turpentine, frankincense, ferula, mastic, myrtle, juniper, pine, rosemary, nutmeg, helichrysum, galbanum, carrot seed

FUNCTIONAL GROUP	CHEMICAL CONSTITUENT	SCENT PROFILE	ESSENTIAL OILS THE CONSTITUENT IS FOUND IN
Sesquiterpene	bisabolene CAS no: 495-62-5	odor strength: medium balsamic, citrus, myrrh, opoponax, spicy	chamomile (Moroccan), opoponax
	alpha-cadinene CAS no: 24406-051	odor strength: medium woody, dry	pine (traces), manuka, balsam poplar, cananga, ylang-ylang, German chamomile
	alpha-cedrene CAS no: 469-61-4	odor strength: medium woody, cedar, sweet, fresh	cedarwood, cade
	beta-elemene CAS no: 33880-83-0	odor strength: medium herbal, waxy, fresh	myrrh, copaiba, citronella (Java), turmeric, ginger, basil linalool
	alpha-humulene CAS no: 6753-96-6	odor strength: medium woody, oceanic-watery, spicy-clove	ginger, coriander, clove, cypress, peppermint, sage, turmeric
Alcohol	benzyl alcohol CAS no: 100-51-6	odor strength: medium floral, rose, phenolic, balsamic	Tolu balsam, benzoin, hyacinth absolute, jasmine sambac absolute
	beta-eudesmol CAS no: 473-15-4	odor strength: medium woody, green	cypress, European valerian, amyris, blue tansy, vetiver, *Eucalyptus smithii*
	geraniol CAS no: 106-24-1	odor strength: medium sweet, floral, fruity, rose, waxy	bergamot, palmarosa, lemon thyme, geranium, citronella, damask rose, melissa, lemon basil, lemongrass, neroli, ylang-ylang
	menthol CAS no: 89-78-1	odor strength: medium peppermint, cooling, woody	peppermint, cornmint, lemon basil
	nerol CAS no: 106-25-2	odor strength: medium sweet, natural, neroli, citrus, magnolia, fresh, floral	lemon basil, helichrysum, damask rose, melissa, neroli, geranium, may chang
	alpha-terpineol CAS no: 98-55-5	odor strength: medium pine, terpenic, lilac, citrus, woody, floral	*Eucalyptus radiata*, cedarwood, ho leaf, palo santo, cajeput, sweet marjoram, tea tree, petitgrain, frankincense serrata, neroli

FUNCTIONAL GROUP	CHEMICAL CONSTITUENT	SCENT PROFILE	ESSENTIAL OILS THE CONSTITUENT IS FOUND IN
Aldehyde	cinnamaldehyde CAS no: 104-55-2	odor strength: high sweet, spicy, aldehydic, aromatic, balsamic, cinnamyl, resinous, honey, powdery	cassia leaf and bark, cinnamon bark and leaf
	citral (geranial) CAS no: 5392-40-5	odor strength: medium sharp, lemon, sweet	lemon myrtle, lemongrass, lemon-scented tea tree, may chang, lemon verbena, honey myrtle, melissa, lemon basil, lemon balm, lemon thyme, lemon, orange, palmarosa
	citronellal CAS no: 106-23-0	odor strength: high sweet, dry, floral, herby, waxy, aldehydic, citrus	combava leaf, citronella, melissa, lemon-scented tea tree
	cuminaldehyde CAS no: 122-03-2	odor strength: high spicy, cumin, green, herbal, vegetable-like	cumin, *Eucalyptus polybractea*
	neral (cis-citral) CAS no: 106-26-3	odor strength: medium sweet, citrus, lemon, lemon peel	myrtle, lemongrass, may chang, lemon-scented tea tree, lemon, lemon-scented thyme
	salicylaldehyde CAS no: 90-02-8	odor strength: medium medicinal, spicy, cinnamon, wintergreen, cooling	cassia leaf and bark
Ketone	dextro-camphor CAS no: 464-49-3	odor strength: high camphoraceous, minty, phenolic, herbal, woody, medicinal	ho leaf, Spanish lavender, sage, basil, rosemary, green yarrow, blue tansy, coriander seed, mugwort, wormwood, red spruce
	carvone CAS no: 99-49-0	odor strength: medium minty, licorice	caraway, dill seed
	trans-beta-damascone CAS no: 23726-91-2	odor strength: high fruity, floral, berry, plum, black currant, honey, rose, tobacco	damask rose
	dextro-fenchone CAS no: 4695-62-9	odor strength: medium camphoraceous, herbal, thujonic, cedar, earthy, woody	Spanish lavender, thuja, fennel, Scotch pine, African wild sage, cistus
	dextro-menthone CAS no: 3391-87-5	odor strength: medium mentholic, minty	calamint, peppermint, cornmint, pennyroyal, geranium, spearmint
	laevo-piperitone CAS no: 4573-50-6	odor strength: high pungent, minty, peppermint	*Eucalyptus dives*, calamint, peppermint
	alpha-thujone CAS no: 546-80-5	odor strength: medium cedar, thujonic	western red cedar, thuja, sage, tansy, yarrow
	valeranone CAS no: 106-68-3	odor strength: medium fresh, herbal, lavender, sweet, mushroom	European valerian

FUNCTIONAL GROUP	CHEMICAL CONSTITUENT	SCENT PROFILE	ESSENTIAL OILS THE CONSTITUENT IS FOUND IN
Ester	benzyl acetate CAS no: 140-11-4	odor strength: medium sweet, floral, jasmine, fruity, fresh	jasmine absolute, ylang-ylang, narcissus absolute, hyacinth absolute, orange champaca absolute
	benzyl salicylate CAS no: 118-58-1	odor strength: low balsamic, clean, herbal, oily, sweet	ylang-ylang, carnation absolute, tuberose absolute
	geranyl acetate CAS no: 105-87-3	odor strength: medium floral, rose, lavender, green, waxy	thyme (geranial), ylang-ylang, palmarosa, citronella, damask rose, petitgrain, geranium, neroli, lemon balm, lemongrass, carrot seed, myrtle, lemon-scented thyme
	linalyl acetate CAS no: 115-95-7	odor strength: medium sweet, green, citrus, bergamot, lavender, floral, woody	clary sage, petitgrain, mint (bergamot), lavender, bergamot, sweet marjoram, neroli, cardamom, Spanish sage
	methyl salicylate CAS no: 119-36-8	odor strength: medium wintergreen, minty, camphoraceous	wintergreen, sweet birch, ylang-ylang, tuberose absolute
	neryl acetate CAS no: 141-12-8	odor strength: medium floral, rose, soapy, citrus, dewy pear	helichrysum/immortelle, lemon petitgrain, melissa, neroli, Australian lemon balm, bergamot
	alpha-terpinyl acetate CAS no: 80-26-2	odor strength: medium herbal, bergamot, lavender, lime, citrus, spicy, woody, floral, waxy	cardamom, Spanish sage, petitgrain, cypress, myrtle
Phenol	carvacrol CAS no: 499-75-2	odor strength: medium spicy, wood, camphoraceous, thyme, herbal	oregano, wild marjoram, savory, thyme, ajowan
	thymol CAS no: 89-83-8	odor strength: high herbal, thyme, phenolic, medicinal, camphoraceous	thyme, oregano, ajowan, savory, fir needle, blue tansy
	eugenol CAS no: 97-53-0	odor strength: medium sweet, spicy, clove, woody	clove bud, leaf, and stem; cinnamon leaf and bark; pimento leaf and berry; basil, carnation, jasmine, rose absolute, Java citronella, cistus, damask rose
	methyl eugenol CAS no: 93-15-2	odor strength: medium sweet, fresh, warm, spicy, clove, carnation, cinnamon, waxy	black tea tree, huon pine, pimento berry, estragole basil, laurel leaf, damask rose, pimento leaf, East Indian nutmeg, myrtle, elemi, mace

FUNCTIONAL GROUP	CHEMICAL CONSTITUENT	SCENT PROFILE	ESSENTIAL OILS THE CONSTITUENT IS FOUND IN
Ether	trans-athenole CAS no: 4180-23-8	odor strength: high sweet, anise, licorice, mimosa, medicinal	anise, star anise, myrtle, sweet and bitter fennel
	elemicin CAS no: 487-11-6	odor strength: medium spicy, floral	elemi, East Indian nutmeg, Indian mace
	myristicin CAS no: 607-91-0	odor strength: medium spicy, warm, balsamic, woody	Indian nutmeg, Indian mace
	estragole CAS no: 140-67-0	odor strength: medium sweet, sassafras, anise, spicy, green, herbal, fennel	ravensara bark and leaf, tarragon, basil, marigold, star anise, sweet and bitter fennel, myrtle
	safrole CAS no: 94-59-7	odor strength: medium warm, sweet, spicy, woody, floral, sassafras, anise	camphor, ho leaf, Indian nutmeg, Indian mace, cinnamon leaf and bark, star anise
Oxide	beta-caryophyllene oxide CAS no: 1139-30-6	odor strength: medium sweet, fresh, dry, woody, spicy	melissa, Scotch pine, labdanum, angelica root, hyssop, carrot seed, Italian helichrysum, palmarosa, East Indian lemongrass, frankincense sacra
	1,4-cineole CAS no: 470-67-7	odor strength: high cool, pine, minty, camphoraceous, terpenic, green, eucalyptus	distilled lime, cedarwood
	1,8-cineole CAS no: 470-82-6	odor strength: high eucalyptus, herbal, camphoraceous, medicinal	eucalyptus, cajeput, white sage, niaouli, ho leaf cineole and linalool, Spanish marjoram, rosemary, saro, cardamom, Spanish sage, myrtle, spike lavender, holy basil, tea tree, hyssop, oregano
	linalool oxide CAS no: 1365-19-1	odor strength: medium floral, woody, herby, earthy, green	ho leaf, bergamot mint, rosewood, orange champaca absolute, lemon-scented thyme

Source: Information derived from Good Scents 2020, Tisserand and Young 2014, Williams 2006

SYNERGY

According to the *Oxford English Dictionary,* synergy is "the inter-action or cooperation of two or more organizations, substances, or other agents to produce a combined effect greater than the sum of their separate effects." Mathematically, the phenomenon of synergy is expressed as 2 + 2 = 5. So, using this same principle, when components, whatever they be, come together and share equally, the sum can be represented as 2 + 2 = 4, indicating harmony. And where there is a negative, detracting influence, the sum can be represented as 2 + 2 = 3, indicating negative synergy or antagonism.

The molecules in essential oils appear to act harmoniously or synergistically in various ways, sometimes complementing and/or enhancing the action of one or more compounds, sometimes diluting or quenching the less desirable effects of others. Whole essential oils can also be combined or blended in a way that enhances one or more actions and quells others. For example, one study (Onawunmi et al. 1984) explored the antibacterial actions of three major constituents found in lemongrass: myrcene, neral, and geranial. The researchers observed that although myrcene itself had weak antibacterial actions, when it was combined with either alpha-citral (geranial) or beta-citral (neral), it significantly increased the respective antibacterial actions of these components. This is an example of a synergistic effect. Another study (Bassolé et al. 2010) found synergy between eugenol and linalool or menthol, which resulted in a significant increase in the antimicrobial action of these components. The combination of carvacrol and thymol and of carvacrol, thymol, and eugenol was found to increase synergistic potency in yet another investigation (García-García et al. 2011). Antimicrobial synergy was also found between whole essential oils, for example, coriander and cumin (Bag and Chattopadhyay 2015), oregano and thyme, oregano and cinnamon, oregano and tea tree, oregano and mint, peppermint and tea tree, and thyme and cinnamon (Hossain et al. 2016).

Lemongrass (*Cymbopogon citratus*), which contains up to 85% citral (neral and geranial) (an aldehyde), when blended with grapefruit (*Citrus* x *paradisi*), which contains up to 95% dextro-limonene (a monoterpene), reduces the irritant effect of citral in lemongrass. Citral is also found in lemons, but its irritant effect is quenched or quelled by the presence of limonene and pinene.

In reality, creating truly synergistic blends of essential oils is quite difficult to achieve, although not impossible. In principle, the aim of blending essential oils together is to enhance specific properties to support a desired positive outcome. Even so, in many instances when using essential oils therapeutically, a carefully selected single essential oil can work very well too. It is best to blend no more than two, three, or at most four oils together when creating therapeutic blends to ensure and manage the blend's integrity. Keeping it simple definitely supports the creation of an effective additive blend, that is, 2 + 2 = 4, or harmony; this can even lead to synergy. I find that when working with clients, focusing on one outcome, and initially one signature essential oil, hones the process; it is then easy to add one or two other oils to complement that oil's qualities. On the other hand, having too many objectives at once and blending several oils together in one blend increases the chance of overdiluting or canceling out any beneficial effects.

Of course, this doesn't mean that blends that include several essential oils will not be successful, especially when creating perfume. Blending oils with similar antimicrobial or antiviral properties can potentiate an action. However, blending does require careful consideration and practice, and the more oils included in a blend, the greater the chance of missing or cancelling out the intended outcome. But not to worry, as there are many essential oils (and also perfumes) that are singularly potent antimicrobials and antivirals that can be used alone with good effect; tea tree, lavender, and geranium are just a few examples of single oils that each possess strong antimicrobial qualities and are also relatively safe oils to use singly.

Some of the most powerful antimicrobials and antivirals, though, are also strong irritants and potential sensitizers, and this is where blending can be particularly useful. By selectively adding other essential oils, it is possible to create a blend that balances out, quells, and calms these irritating effects (but remember, essential oils should always be added to an emollient, such as a vegetable oil or organic, scent-free lotion or cream, before using them on the body).

Potent Antimicrobial/Antiviral Blends

Some of my favorite antimicrobial/antiviral blends, which I use in an environmental diffuser, are comprised of up to seven components. These blends ease breathing and support the respiratory tract to ward off infection by many types of microbes, bacterial, viral, and fungal. Use only one drop of each essential oil in the following blends:

- cinnamon leaf, clove bud, lavender, peppermint, pine, rosemary, and thyme
- cinnamon leaf, clove bud, geranium, grapefruit, and nutmeg
- cinnamon leaf, clove bud, eucalyptus, lemon, rosemary, and tea tree
- cinnamon leaf, clove bud, lavender, patchouli, peppermint, rosemary, and orange bitter
- cinnamon leaf, clove bud, and bergamot or bitter orange

Antimicrobial/antiviral blends can also be used with a nasal inhaler. Use two drops of each oil in each of the following blends, because the amount of essential oil consumed with each inhalation is small. When using steam inhalation, use one drop of oil in each of the following blends, as more essential oil is consumed with this method:

- eucalyptus, geranium, and peppermint
- eucalyptus, lavender, peppermint, rosemary, tea tree, and thyme
- clary sage, bitter orange, patchouli, and peppermint
- geranium, lavender, and tea tree
- eucalyptus, lemon, and tea tree
- clove bud, bitter orange, and patchouli
- grapefruit, lavender, and thyme

You may have noticed that some of the oils listed in this chapter have a high eugenol (phenol) content, such as clove bud and cinnamon leaf, or a high cineole (oxide) content, such as eucalyptus and rosemary. Both constituents are very strong antimicrobials and antivirals, but they are also irritants to the skin, mucous membranes, and respiratory tract. However, in the blends listed above, these components are balanced and complemented by oils rich in alcohols like linalool, geraniol, and citronellol and esters like linalyl acetate, such as lavender and geranium; others are rich

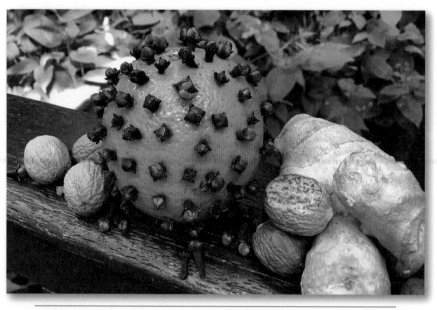

Antimicrobial and antiviral: clove, orange, ginger, and nutmeg

in monoterpenes like limonene and alpha- and beta-pinene, such as grape-fruit, lemon, orange, and pine. All of these oils are antimicrobial (among other qualities) and may support the body's immune system to stave or prevent infection (see chapter 5 for other complementary methods to support the immune system). These are examples of additive blends, which may also be rendered synergistically.

The following chemical components found in the above-mentioned essential oils are also shown to disrupt the cell membranes of bacteria microbes, or cells hijacked by viruses, causing leakage of the cells' ions and inactivation, or cell death, of microbes (Langeveld et al. 2013).

carvacrol	gamma-terpinene
cinnamaldehyde	rho-cymene
cinnamic acid	thymol
eugenol	

Other whole essential oils shown to similarly disrupt cell integrity and provide antibacterial and anitviral protection (Chouhan et al. 2017) include:

African basil (estragole, camphor, limonene)
black pepper (limonene)
fennel (estragole, limonene)
garlic (diallyl trisulfide, diallyl disulfide)
ginger (zingerberene, curcumene)
horse mint (menthol, menthone)
may chang (geranial, neral, limonene)
oregano (carvacrol, thymol)
turmeric leaf and root (alpha-phellandrene, camphor)

Other antimicrobial/antiviral combinations could have a refreshing citral theme. For example, using lemongrass or may chang as signature oils rich in aldehydes such as geranial or neral, to which are added complementary monoterpene-rich oils such as grapefruit or orange bitter, along with other antimicrobial/antiviral middle and base-note oils to further quell any irritancy, can balance the scent and add tenacity to the blend. Experimenting with different essential oil combinations will inspire your creative spirit and aid you in familiarizing yourself with their individual characteristic qualities and personalities.*

Other essential oils that have strong to moderate antimicrobial/antiviral properties include the following:

bergamot	myrtle
carrot seed	palmarosa
cassia (strong)	pine
citronella	rose
fennel (sweet and bitter)	sandalwood (Australian)
frankincense	thyme, red (strong)
melissa/lemon balm	vetivert

Always remember to check out the individual profile and safety criteria of an essential oil before using it.

---

*My previous book, *Essential Oils for the Whole Body,* provides more details about the practical process of assessing the scent of essential oils and creating blends.

Antimicrobial/Antiviral Room Fumigation

The aforementioned room-diffusing quantities provide good background preventive support against pathogenic bacteria and viruses. However, to fumigate an environment efficiently, a higher quantity of essential oil is required—at least 30 drops in total, although this will depend on the size of a room. For fumigation to be effective, all doors and windows must be closed to contain the essential oil vapors during diffusion, which should continue for thirty minutes; any longer and the antimicrobial impact diminishes. Of course, no one should be in the room during this process to avoid irritation of the airways and eyes. Once fumigation is complete, doors and windows should be opened to allow the inflow of fresh air to clear residue vapors.

If you wish, fresh herbs such as sage, rosemary, and juniper can also be used as fumigants instead of essential oils (use either one or the other method at a time). These are usually smoked or smudged—smoldered rather than burned—to cleanse the environment.

Making Your Own Hand Sanitizer

Add from fifteen to twenty drops of essential oil to nonperfumed liquid soap dispensers. Rinse your hands thoroughly after lathering with the essential oil–infused soap. Do not add essential oils to antibacterial sanitizers or scented sanitizers; it is not necessary and may cause an irritant reaction.

Note that it is possible to overuse essential oils and create microbial resistance to their molecules (although that is less likely than with pharmaceutical antibiotics), so it's better not to oversanitize, to change the oil or combination of oils regularly, and to take breaks from using essential oils. Remember, soap itself is antibacterial—soap and water, and careful handwashing and drying, is usually quite effective to sanitize.

Creating Synergy and Optimal Blends: Key Points

These principles apply whether you are creating therapeutic blends or aesthetic perfumes.

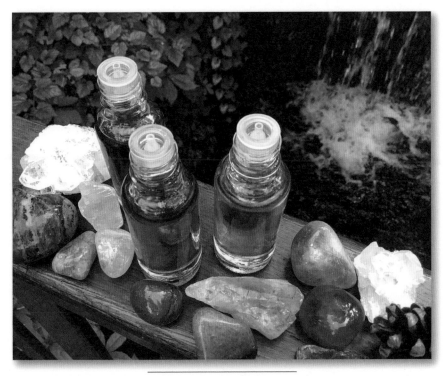

Blending essential oils

Basic Principles

+ Synergy cannot automatically be assumed to be present in a blend or in a single essential oil. The ratio and quantity of essential oils used will significantly influence the outcome. The integrity of an oil—its age and stage of oxidition, appropriate storage, the condition of the plant the oil was extracted from, and so on—also influences its potency.
+ Antagonism, or negative synergy, is a possible outcome.
+ Blending a number of essential oils together can actually negate the intended response instead of enhancing it by overdiluting the dose of active components or canceling their actions out by mixing oils with opposite properties.

Factors That Influence the Effectiveness of a Blend

+ The number of drops of each essential oil and their ratio
+ The number of different essential oils

+ The predominant therapeutic actions of individual essential oils (e.g., stimulating, sedating, invigorating, relaxing)
+ The actions of the individual chemical components present in an essential oil and the collective actions of these when essential oils are blended together, for example, enhancing/synergy, additive, quenching, diluting, negating/antisynergy
+ The strength of character of the individual essential oils and their components
+ The scent of individual essential oils and their constituents, including their dry-out scents, which is significant when creating perfumes or therapeutic blends that are used in products such as ointments, creams, lotions, and carrier oils, which are intended to last over a period of time—days, weeks, or months

Ways to Enhance the Potential for Achieving Synergy

+ Limit the number of essential oils blended together to between two and seven to decrease the possibility of diluting out, antisynergy, or saturation.
+ Blend essential oils from the same species or botanical family.
+ Blend essential oils with similar or supporting chemical constituents.
+ Blend essential oils with similar or supporting therapeutic actions.
+ Focus on one specific outcome rather than many.
+ Avoid blending predominantly stimulating essential oils with predominantly sedating essential oils.
+ Use good-quality essential oils that are fresh and appropriately stored.
+ Blend essential oils into appropriate base mediums—vegetable oils, creams, or lotions—to ensure that the medium selected complements the essential oils' actions and desired therapeutic outcome. For example, vegetable oil is more effective than mineral oil when blending essential oils for their antimicrobial activity, and aqueous bases support essential oil activity more than petroleum- or oil-based ointments.
+ Make sure the working environment, instruments, and materials you use are clean and free from contamination (Harris 2002).

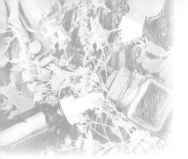

5

Using Essential Oils

Optimizing Our Body-Mind-Spirit

Essential oils have a multitude of uses, from ethereal and cosmetic to psycho-emotional and medicinal. Essential oils are protective and rejuvenating and also act preventively. Most significant of all, though, essential oils are team players (just as they are within the plant), supporting and complementing most body systems. Their qualities also work well with other therapeutic, well-being, beauty, and aesthetic modalities.

Health and wellness are maintained best by acknowledging the cornerstones of well-being:

+ Eating a fresh, nutritious, balanced diet and remaining sufficiently hydrated (drinking fresh water and eating fresh vegetables and fruits, which also contain water)
+ Exercise, movement, and mobility
+ Meditation and relaxation
+ Love, joy, friendship, and community

This chapter looks at the immune-supporting and psycho-emotional qualities of essential oils, their safe use and measurement, and their use on children.

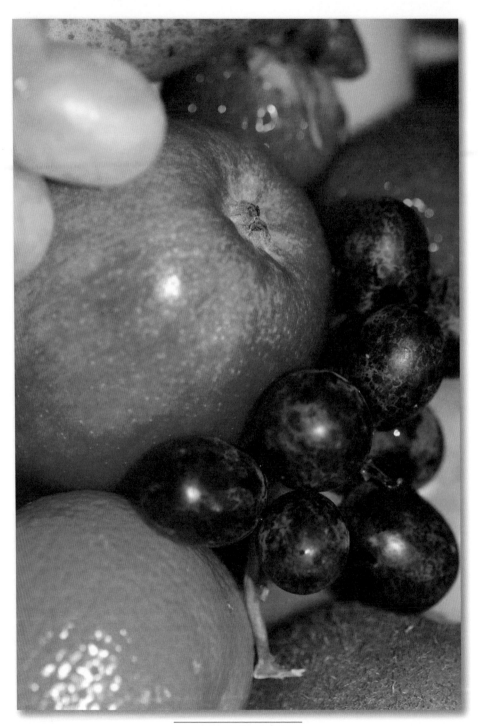

Fruits of the earth

ESSENTIAL OILS AND IMMUNITY:
HOW WE CAN HELP OURSELVES

We are, quite literally, not alone in our bodies. This is not as spooky as it may sound, though it is, in fact, a well-designed feature of our physical existence, a beautiful, collaborative and natural phenomenon.

Supporting the Microbiome

The human microbiome, just like a plant's microbiome, consists of trillions of microbes, including viruses, bacteria, and fungi that live symbiotically in and on the body—on the skin, in the gut, and in cavities such as the mouth, ears, and vagina, all within an auralike cloud surrounding the body. The microbiome plays a significant role in protecting and maintaining immunity and aids a number of vital bodily functions, such as, for example, assisting the breakdown and synthesis of nutrients in the gut and aiding their appropriate absorption, and providing a protective barrier against invasion or proliferation of harmful microbes and pathogens. We coexist with microorganisms—our body houses, feeds, and depends on their presence to maintain its functional equilibrium. Poor diet, refined and sugary foods, overuse of antibiotics and pharmaceutical drugs, stress, and illness, among other factors, can disrupt the harmonious balance of the microbiome and consequently increase our susceptibility to pathogenic invasion, disease, and dysfunction.

Viruses and Exosomes

Viruses are many times smaller than bacteria. They are highly complex and very difficult to accurately detect, let alone analyze. Viruses are not alive; they are apparently parasitic, infiltrating and hijacking the processes of living cells to evolve and replicate. Some suggest otherwise—for example, that viruses are functional exudes or "downloads" of the natural process of cellular detoxification or cell death and, like exosomes, convey vital information from one cell to another, from one environment to another (Bush 2020, June 16; Virgin 2013; Rohwer et al. 2009). Viruses are comprised of biologically active DNA or messenger RNA protein strands and lipids and are very similar in structure and behavior to exosomes.

Exosomes are naturally ocurring particles produced and secreted by all living cells and are also comprised of RNA and DNA protein strands. They are much smaller than viruses and a thousand times smaller than cells. Exosomes aid toxin removal from cells, but more significantly they carry messages from cell to cell via body fluids (extracellular and brain fluid, blood, saliva, and urine, as well as amniotic fluid and breast milk) and instigate processes such as wound-healing, tissue-regeneration, and anti-inflammatory responses. They also aid and boost the immune system.

Exosomes exist in plants, too, and perform similar functions. For example, they carry cell wall–building enzymes that may be involved in plant growth and development, pathogen defense proteins that are delivered to sites of infection, and RNAs that interfere with pathogen genes in a way that inhibits fungal growth. There is speculation that plant exosomes find their way into animal/human gut tissue during plant digestion (Keener 2019). Knowing this, I wonder if essential oil molecules, which are also transported throughout the organism via body fluids, somehow instigate cellular responses via exosome messeging. For example, essential oils are also shown to aid wound-healing, tissue regeneration, and anti-inflammatory and antimicrobial responses and support the immune system and the balance the body's microbiome.

So, our first line of protection and defense when considering immunity and well-being is to observe the four cornerstones of health mentioned above and support our microbiome's equilibrium (and thus also our health and vitality) through optimum nourishment and resistance to pathogenic microbial invasion. Eating nutritionally rich, fresh, seasonal, unrefined, organic whole foods, especially green leafy vegetables, fruits, nuts, lentils, and peas and other legumes, along with fermented foods; drinking plenty of water to hydrate and oxygenate our cells and flush out waste material from our system; getting plenty of fresh air and sunlight to support cellular photosynthesis and photochemical formation of vitamin D; movement and gentle exercise to stimulate peristalsis in the gut and the circulatory and lymphatic systems in order to remove waste products efficiently from our body—all these practices support optimal health. A plant's microbiome can also feed ours, hence

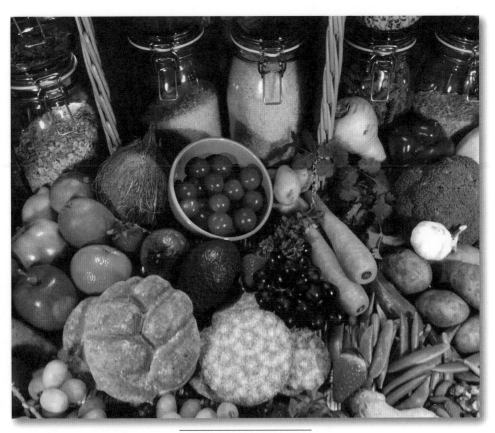

Eating the rainbow

the advisability of leaving the skin on (not peeling) organic vegetables and fruits and eating them raw or just lightly cooked.

Honoring Our State of Being

The boundaries between body, mind, and spirit overlap. Indeed, feeling happy, relaxed and calm, positive and optimistic, demonstrably influences physical function—heart rate, blood pressure, cortisol levels, endorphin release, digestion, and so on. Therefore, our second line of defense in terms of a healthy immune system is our overall state of being. Are we "being in stress" or "being in equanimity"? Are we "being in fear" or "being in peace"? We are often reminded that unconditional love is an optimal state of being. Our state of being influences our state of body, and vice versa. Essential oils instigate psycho-emotional responses that can instill a sense of peace and calm, upliftment and groundedness—states that also support efficient function of the immune system.

Hygiene

Good hygiene, of course, is another practical line of protection and defense. Here we are speaking of cleanliness—soap and water—not some form of obsessive sterilization. We are swimming in a sea of microbobes of all kinds, and so microbial coexistence is our basic human reality. Far from being harmful, we actually thrive by coming in contact with microbes, as this is how we develop immunity. And the health of our microbiome plays a significant role in fighting invading pathogens.

Where Essential Oils Shine

There are times, though, when our defense mechanisms are compromised and our resilience weakens, whether through illness, stress, overwork and inadequate rest, shock, anxiety, feelings of insecurity, poor diet, or lack of sufficient sleep. Complementary interventions are useful preventives that help us manage and maintain our health, wellness, and resilience and support recovery, and this is where essential oils really come into their own. Essential oils work very well preventively, staving off infection and pathogenic invasion. They appear to be especially useful during the early stages of infection, stimulating the immune system into action by promoting the activity of lymphocytes (immune-supporting white blood cells), increasing phagocytosis (the process by which an immune cell uses its plasma membrane to engulf large particles such as viruses or an infected cell), and inducing interferon production (interferons are signaling proteins that "interfere" with viruses to prevent them from multiplying) (Peterfalvi et al. 2019). Thus essential oils support the immune system and support hygiene. They also alleviate symptoms like those associated with colds and flu, such as headache, nasal and sinus congestion, runny nose, cough, and muscle aches, plus all the associated symptoms, including insomnia, depression, and anxiety.

Significantly, unlike conventional antibiotics, essential oils do not disrupt the body's microbiome. This is not to say they are not capable of doing so or that the immune system will not develop resistance to them—the molecular complexity of essential oils means resistance may be delayed through their use but not necessarily prevented, especially if they are repeatedly overused. This is why it is advisable to be moderate in the use of essential oils: use higher amounts for short duration during infection and modest amounts when used as a preventive or when used in skin-care products or for psycho-emotional applications. Always remember that essential oils work very well in very small amounts. And it is advisable to frequently change the essential oil or essential oil blend you use, with periods of abstinence or breaks from using essential oils.

All essential oils possess antimicrobial properties to varying degrees. Essential oils inhibit and slow the growth of bacteria, yeasts, and molds, and their molecules affect the lipid structure of bacterial cell membranes in a way that increases their permeability, causing those cells to lose ions and other cellular components, which leads to cell death. As well, essential oils can act synergistically, potentiating other antiviral or medicinal agents, including biomedical antibiotics (Da Silva et al. 2020, Nazzarro et al. 2013).

Some essential oils possess broad-spectrum bactericidal and antiviral qualities, while others are more specific in their action depending on the chemical composition of the essential oil and the type of microbe or virus. *Broad spectrum* in this context does not mean a single essential oil or blend of essential oils will kill *all* viruses or *all* bacteria, though. Essential oils are generally and variously tissue-regenerating, antiviral, antibacterial, antifungal, anti-inflammatory, mucolytic, and more, and as observed in the previous chapter, considered blending of essential oils with regard to their chemical composition can potentiate their strength, increase their range of action, and quell irritant effects, with certain molecules counterbalancing the less desirable effects of others. In fact, blending essential oils goes a long way toward decreasing the risk of microbial resistance.

COMING TO OUR SENSES: THE PSYCHO-EMOTIONAL INFLUENCE OF ESSENTIAL OILS

A wisp of scent is enough to immediately transport us on a sensory journey—a jasmine kiss on a starlit night; a rose garden in summer;

the earthy-agrestic woodiness of a northern forest in the spring; Mediterranean citrus groves in the winter; a woody-smoky log fire on a cool, dusky evening; spicy, warm fruitcake fresh from the oven; sunshine on the cloudiest day. Tones, colors, and shades, nuances that seamlessly imbue from conjured images, memories, and impressions complex and deep, often experienced beyond words, are all sensually illuminated by the gift of smell. Magical! Yet scent detection is initially instigated by a chemical response.

When we smell and acknowledge the scent of a flower or a fruit, or even the scent of the soft skin of a newborn, we are responding to messages instigated by odor molecules permeating our immediate environment. Scent molecules—terpenes and terpenoids—are detected like a key in a lock by our olfactory receptors, located at the top of each nasal cavity; these in turn relay nerve impulses to the limbic system, located in the brain. Odor receptors are found in other parts of the body, as well, such as in the skin and other organs. However, by grand design it seems, proximity of the master olfactory portal guarantees immediate awareness and an instinctive reflexive response. Initially, we instantly decipher whether something is safe or noxious (do we accept or reject it?). But scent recognition is a complex process.

The limbic system incorporates various functional structures located in the central paleomammalian part of the brain, which includes the amygdala, hippocampus, and hypothalamus, responsible for basic physiological and emotional responses to sensory stimulation. The hypothalamus functionally connects the limbic system to the frontal lobe, where the brain rationalizes and makes sense of information and sensory input, and to the pituitary gland. The pituitary gland, the master endocrine gland, initiates hormone release in response to sensory signals, activating either the sympathetic or parasympathetic nervous system. Depending on the nature of the stimuli, the sympathetic nervous system prepares the body for fight or flight (protection), and the parasympathetic nervous system maintains a state of peace and relaxation (rest and digest) and disengages the sympathetic nervous system from post-alert states, returning the body to its optimal functional resting state.

Initially, our response to an essential oil is reflexive, based on whether we like or dislike its scent—a simple, subjective response, and not an unreasonable indicator of whether the oil is good or bad for us. Essential oils, though, are multidynamic. As well as being antimicrobial and beautifully perfumed, they aid mental alertness and memory and instigate positive psycho-emotional states such as feeling uplifted, calm and grounded, clear-headed, invigorated, and bright and wakeful.

As discussed in chapter 2, essential oils are secondary metabolites, produced as an indirect consequence of photosynthesis in certain plants. Most essential oil–bearing plants are found in areas just north or south of the equator, where the sun is closest to Earth. Thus plants that give us essential oils are intrinsically linked and responsive to the ebb and flow of changing seasons and patterns of available light, as well as to such environmental conditions as temperature, moisture, and atmospheric pressure—just as we humans are.

Essential oils can journey with us through the seasons both actually and metaphorically, protecting and supporting us while we recalibrate and adjust to changing conditions. By harmonizing body, mind, and spirit, essential oils are stabilizing and grounding. For example, frankincense and myrrh have earthy, warming, drying, antimicrobial, and calming qualities. They support the immune system, stave off colds and flu, and serve as a good antidote to the dampness of winter. When combined with bitter orange or another citrusy oil, they also dispel feelings of anxiety and depression. Mandarin and the earthy-smoky scent of vetivert, combined with the sweet, rose-like scent of geranium, express similar uplifting yet grounding qualities. These essential oils can be used to support the transition from autumn to winter and may also aid conditions such as seasonal affective disorder (SAD). Cypress, rose, and lavender aid the transition from spring to summer. Cypress inspires us to metaphorically walk tall and move on as we step out of winter's cave. Rose, the queen of oils, blesses us with a sense of beauty and rejuvenation, while lavender gifts us with its calming, uplifting, and protective qualities. Try it and see for yourself! Indeed, there are so many essential oils to choose from, and it just takes a few carefully selected oils to create your own scent pharmacopeia. Your sense of smell will guide your choice. Enjoy the journey!*

ESSENTIAL OILS FOR INFANTS AND THE VERY YOUNG

Great care must be taken when using essential oils around the very young. These same guidelines should also be followed with the elderly and with those who are frail or whose immune systems are severely compromised.

Children are more vulnerable than adults to environmental and topical chemicals (including essential oils), substances, and microbes. A baby's skin is just one-fifth the thickness of adult skin and does not fully mature until six years of age. Thus the barrier function of infant skin is not fully developed and more susceptible than adult skin to chemical and microbial infiltration, especially at birth and during the first three months of life. Substances easily penetrate surface tissues and quickly pass to the lower layers of the dermis. Also, while infant skin holds more water than adult skin, this quickly evaporates, so their skin is prone to dryness and is easily irritated. Essential oils can actually exacerbate this process. As well, an infant's organs of elimination are less capable of processing essential oil molecules, increasing the risk of neurotoxicity. Pregnant women are similarly susceptible, not only due to increased sensitivity, but also because essential oil molecules cross the placenta and the blood-brain barrier. For this reason my advice is *do not apply essential oils, even in dilution, to infants and toddlers under three years old, and most especially, do not use essential oils around babies*

*My two previous books, *Essential Oils for Mindfulness and Meditation* and *Essential Oils for the Whole Body,* complement the information in this book and cover the aforementioned dynamics in detail, from safe use and application of essential oils to their complementary subtle qualities, including how to use essential oils in a way that complements meditation and deep relaxation. These books also contain information about how to nurture your body, which, after all, is the vehicle of your soul, by providing information such as the basic vital nutrients you need to maintain health and well-being, breathing and relaxation exercises, how to create skin-care products using plant botanicals and many other ways you can use essential oils to enhance your well-being.

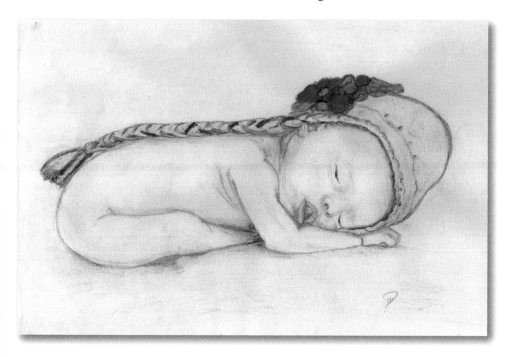

younger than three months or pregnant women. Between three and six years old, certain essential oils can be used topically on young children in very high dilution (1 drop of essential oil in about 7 ounces, or 20 ml, of carrier medium) or they can be diffused, but only provided you follow the instructions given in this section.

Organic Vegetable Oils for Infant Massage and Skin Care

Certain vegetable oils, without added essential oils, can be used as massage oils on babies and young children. These oils protect and soothe the skin and exhibit valuable healing qualities of their own. For example, sunflower oil, massaged into the skin of premature babies three times a day, has been found to enhance barrier function and thus support immunity, with a 41 percent reduction in incidences of sepsis (LeFevre et al. 2010). Note that massaging babies and infants with oil, lotion, or cream is best done on a mat on the floor rather than on an elevated surface such as a table or bed; wriggliness and slipperiness are not a good combination!

The following oils are safe to use on infants and young children.

Evening Primrose (*Oenothera biennis*) Oil

Qualities: Evening primrose oil is anti-inflammatory and balances sebum production.

Indications: Eczema and irritated skin

Marigold-Infused Olive Oil
(*Calendula officinalis* and *Olea europaea*)

Qualities: Calendula is cooling and skin-healing; it soothes skin irritation and soreness and is moisturizing.

Indications: Eczema, dry and damaged skin, diaper rash

Jojoba (*Simmondsia chinensis*) Oil

Qualities: Jojoba oil is a nonsticky, liquid plant wax that balances sebum production in the skin and improves the quality and appearance of skin, scalp, and hair.

Indications: Irritated skin and dry skin and scalp

Safflower (*Carthamus tinctorius*) Oil

Qualities: Safflower is rich in fatty acids and absorbs well into the skin.

Indications: Diaper rash

Sunflower (*Helianthus annuus*) Oil

Qualities: Sunflower is deeply moisturizing and absorbs well into the skin. It blends well with other vegetable oils.

Indications: Good for all-around skin care

Topical Application of Essential Oils for Children Aged Three Years and Over

For topical use on young children, dilute 1 drop of essential oil in 7 ounces (20 ml) of olive, evening primrose, jojoba, safflower, or sunflower oil. Select either a single essential oil or a blend of two or three of the following. *Use only one drop of this single oil or blend at a time.*

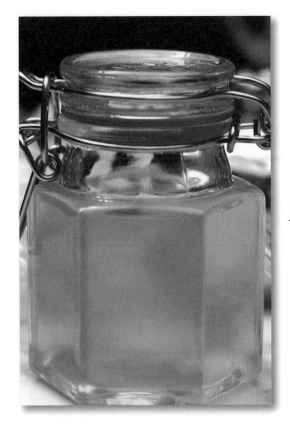

Jojoba oil

Chamomile, Roman
(*Chamaemelum nobile*)

Indications: Eczema, bruises, and dry, itchy skin; aids skin-healing, eases agitation, anger, anxiety, excitability, hyperactivity, insomnia, restlessness; calms and sedates

Application method: 1 drop of essential oil in 7 ounces (20 ml) of carrier oil for massage or skin application; 1 or 2 drops in a room diffuser

Caution: Prone to oxidation if not stored appropriately. Do not apply essential oil neat to skin. Use in moderation. Do not take or administer orally (internally).

Lavender (*Lavandula angustifolia*)

Indications: Bruises, chapped or cracked skin, eczema; also eases colds and bronchitis; aids immune system; eases agitation, anger, anxiety, insomnia, and panic attacks; balances mood, calms, and sedates

Application method: 1 drop of essential oil in 7 ounces (20 ml) of a carrier oil for massage or skin application; 3 or 4 drops in a room diffuser

Caution: Do not apply neat to children's skin; do not take or administer orally/internally.

Mandarin (*Citrus reticulata*)

Indications: Asthma, bronchitis, colds, and coughs; aids immune system; eases anxiety, hyperactivity, insomnia, panic attacks, and restlessness; uplifts mood, calms, and sedates

Application method: 3 or 4 drops of essential oil in a room diffuser

Caution: Mandarin is prone to rapid oxidation if not stored correctly; use within six months of opening the bottle; do not apply neat to child's skin; do not take or administer orally/internally.

Essential Oils Safe to Diffuse around Young Children

For children three years and older, use either a single essential oil or a blend of two or three. The essential oils indicated above can be used, as well as the following oils listed here. Remember, if diffusing around young children, always keep the diffuser away from the child's head space—eyes, nose, mouth, and airways.

Lemon (*Citrus limonum*)

Indications: Aids concentration, clears thoughts, uplifts and eases feelings of anxiety; antimicrobial

Application: 3 or 4 drops in a room diffuser

Caution: Lemon is prone to rapid oxidation if not stored correctly; use within six months of opening the bottle. Do not apply to an infant's skin. Do not take or administer orally/internally.

Neroli (*Citrus x aurantium*)

Note: This is a very expensive essential oil, but it can be purchased as a 5% blend in jojoba oil.

Indications: Eases feelings of anxiety, depression, and nervous tension;

encourages feelings of self-confidence and instills a sense of peace; tranquilizing

Application: 1 or 2 drops in a room diffuser

Caution: Neroli is often adulterated due to its high cost. The absolute is less expensive but may contain residues of solvent material used during extraction. Do not apply to the skin of a young child. Do not take or administer orally/internally.

Rose (*Rosa centifolia*)

Note: This is a very expensive essential oil, but it can be purchased as a 5% blend in jojoba oil.

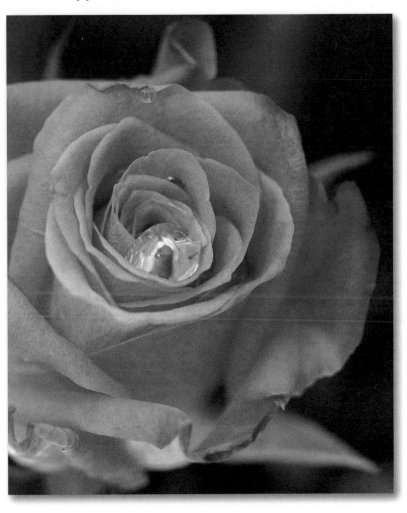

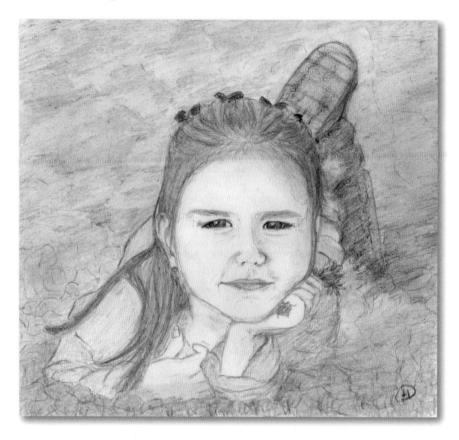

Indications: Eases feelings of agitation, anger, and anxiety; useful for insomnia, mood swings, and panic attacks; sedative yet also uplifting

Application: 1 or 2 drops in a room diffuser

Caution: Rose oil is often adulterated due to its high cost. The absolute is less expensive but may contain residues of the solvent material used during extraction. Do not apply to an infant's skin. Do not take or administer orally/internally.

Spearmint (*Mentha spicata*)

Indications: Energizing, refreshing, and uplifting

Application: 3 or 4 drops in a room diffuser

Caution: Do not apply to an infant's skin. Do not take or administer orally/internally.

Young Children:
Safety Precautions

- Do *not* use essential oils on or around babies and children under three years old.
- If used on children over three years old, essential oils must be used in extreme moderation—1 drop of essential oil in 7 ounces (20 ml) of a carrier oil such as sunflower, safflower, jojoba, marigold-infused olive, or evening primrose oil, or an unscented (organic) cream or lotion.
- Do not use herbaceous, spice, or citrus oils (with the exception of mandarin) essential oils, or oils that are strongly scented such as ylang-ylang. The skin and vital organs of babies and young children are still developing, especially the organs of elimination; essential oils are highly concentrated and can easily cause a toxic reaction in the very young.
- Do not put drops of essential oil directly onto pillows due to the risk of eye contact.
- Never apply undiluted essential oil to the skin of a young child (and definitely not a baby), and never add undiluted essential oil to bathwater.
- Never use essential oil for internal consumption by a child of any age.
- Keep essential oils out of the reach of children (good suppliers will provide childproof lids if requested), and keep them away from pets.
- When using around young children, essential oils are best diffused into the environment, away from the child's head space, to avoid irritation of the airways, to soothe restlessness, and to aid sleep.

Do not use the following essential oils around young children (because they may be toxic or irritating):

- Herbaceous oils and oils extracted from citrusy plants and fruit (with the exception of mandarin in high dilution)
- Oils derived from seeds, herbs, spices, and sensitizing florals such as ylang-ylang
- Oils that contain citral, such as lemongrass and citronella
- Oils that influence the hormonal system, including rose and clary sage

ESSENTIAL OIL SAFETY

While essential oil safety is covered extensively in my two previous books, it is necessary to repeat important points made in those books to guide appropriate application.

Use

We are reminded that although essential oils are oil-like in their behavior (that is, they do not mix with water), they are not greasy or oily like fat or vegetable oils (which are known as *fixed* oils). They are not lubricant and are, in fact, extremely drying and potentially irritating to the skin, even in small quantities. This is why essential oils are always blended in an emollient substance such as a vegetable oil, ointment, cream, or lotion before they are applied to the body. Emollients add their own unique skin-supporting qualities, and when carefully blended with essential oils, they create a very effective skin-care synergy.

Essential oil molecules more readily leave, or partition, from a water-based medium (for example, lotions, creams, and gels) to bond with lipids in the skin than they do from an oily medium or ointment. However, vegetable oils and ointments create a barrier that prevents or significantly decreases water evaporation from the skin, which increases the opportunity for essential oil molecules to penetrate, as they must be in direct contact with the skin to be absorbed.

When prescribed by a qualified herbalist or holistic doctor for internal ingestion, essential oils are administered in small, controlled amounts and are contained in a dispersant emollient and/or in a safe-to-swallow, gel-like capsule composed of hypromellose, a polymer formulated from plant cellulose. Capsules made of animal gelatin are derived from skin or bone collagen, so these are not suitable for vegans or vegetarians, although there are vegetarian capsules on the market that can be used as an alternative. I do not advocate the internal ingestion of essential oils unless they are prescribed and/or administered by a professional health-care practitioner, herbalist, pharmacist, or chemist with appropriate knowledge of the chemical constituents of essential oils and how they interact in the body and with other chemicals such as are found in medications.

Employing their antimicrobial, skin-healing, and underlying soft tissue–healing qualities, essential oils can be safely and effectively applied topically to the skin in an appropriate dilution. Always check the qualities and safety information of an essential oil before using it. When applying topically, use vegetable oil or vegetable wax* (for example, jojoba), gels (such as aloe vera gel or gels made from pectin or cellulose gum and distilled water), ointment, or compresses; this is an effective way to treat local conditions such as eczema, sprains, and insect bites and to aid repair of damaged skin tissue, improve the appearance of scars, and combat minor infections. Essential oils may be added to creams and lotions for their skin-care qualities. They can also aid the digestive system (to alleviate indigestion or symptoms of IBS) and relieve menstrual pain when applied topically as an essential oil–infused compress or essential oil–infused cream, lotion, or vegetable oil on the mid to lower back and/or abdomen.

Essential oils are quite effective, in dilution and in small quantity (one to four drops of essential oil), when inhaled using a room diffuser, which disperses an ambient room scent. As well, you can apply drops to a tissue or cotton pad or an aroma stick (a specially designed nasal inhaler) to relieve symptoms of a cold or sore throat. And essential oil therapeutic perfumes (such as those diluted in vegetable oil and dispensed using a roller bottle) can be used for their psycho-emotional benefits (uplifting, calming, energizing).

We cannot emphasize enough that essential oils are *highly concentrated volatile organic phytochemicals* with a propensity to be very drying and irritating to the skin and mucous membranes. They rapidly oxidize and degrade, especially if they are not stored correctly, which also increases their tendency to become irritating and sensitizing, toxic, and corrosive. Degradation of an essential oil occurs naturally over time but is exacerbated in the presence of heat and UV light and when exposed to oxygen. To slow these reactions and to preserve optimum quality, essential oils must be stored in a cool, dark place in

---

*The antiseptic action of phenols, the components found in clove, cinnamon, basil, and thyme, are possibly negated by fatty or oily mediums; also, remember that phenol-rich essential oils tend to be skin irritants.

noncorrodible brown or blue glass or aluminum or UV-protected bottles, with dropper-dispensing caps or tightly secured lids.

Storage and Care

Purchase essential oils only from reputable suppliers whose oils are ethically and appropriately sourced, extracted, and handled, and who provide safety data information and details about their chemical composition and source.

Purchase only essential oils stored in amber or dark blue glass bottles with dropper-top lids to ensure careful measurement and prevent spillage or accidental ingestion. Some suppliers place the essential oil–filled glass bottle in an additional canister, or sleeve, that prevents light infiltration; this guarantees the essential oil is protected from UV light.

Check the sell-by date before using and make a note of the date of purchase. Essential oils oxidize rapidly when exposed to oxygen in the atmosphere and UV light, and therefore they have a limited shelf life—two years if unopened, one year once opened (citrus oils, such as mandarin or lemon, will keep for only six months once opened). Pine oils and other oils with a high terpene content oxidize rapidly.

Discard the small amounts of essential oil left in a bottle or container unless rapidly used up from the moment of first opening the bottle. *Note:* Do not flush residue or old, unused essential oils down the sink or toilet, as their oxidized chemicals can be toxic to fish and the local aquatic microbiome.

Place the lid back on the bottle immediately after using to slow oxidation.

Never top off a bottle of essential oil with more essential oil once it has been opened for use.

Always store essential oils in a cool, dark place, away from sources of heat and direct sunlight to protect the oils from rapid oxidation, which is exacerbated by light, heat, and atmospheric oxygen. A fridge is preferable for many essential oils (although some oils, such as rose otto, will solidify when very cold, but do return to a liquid state at room temperature).

Application

Do not apply essential oils neat on the skin; always dilute in a vegetable oil or unscented lotion or cream (for example, 1 or 2 drops of essential oil to 0.17 ounce, or 5 ml, of vegetable oil). Undiluted dermal application of essential oils can lead to irritation and sensitization. Lavender and tea tree essential oils are the exception to this rule; they are often used as a first-aid remedy for insect stings, minor burns, skin abrasions, or mild skin infections. Note that repeated long-term topical application of these oils is not advisable due to the risk of sensitization.

Do not swallow or take essential oils internally (see "Accidents and Reactions," below).

To avoid sensitization, do not use the same essential oil or blend of essential oils repeatedly. Take breaks from use (every two or three weeks), and vary the essential oils you use if applying them over a long period. Also, use limited quantities—no more than six drops daily. Essential oils are highly concentrated, and very small amounts are quite effective.

Always make sure that the essential oils you select are compatible with your requirements and are otherwise not contraindicated. This is especially important if you are taking prescription medication such as painkillers like codeine or other opiate derivatives or blood-thinning medications.

Wipe up any spillages immediately; essential oils will dissolve or damage polystyrene, plastic, varnish, paint, and polished and laminated surfaces.

Accidents and Reactions

+ **Accidental ingestion:** *Do not induce vomiting.* Drink full-fat milk. Seek medical advice immediately. Keep the bottle the essential oil was stored in for identification; the label should display the Latin name, batch number, sell-by date, etc.; the bottle will have traces of the oil.

+ **Eyes:** Essential oils can be transferred from your fingers to your eyes, so always wash your hands thoroughly after using or handling. If neat essential oil enters your eyes, *immediately* flush with vegetable oil or full-fat milk, then rinse thoroughly with clean, warm water. Sometimes diluted essential oils enter the eyes during steam inhalation, bathing, or showering. If this happens, *immediately* flush eyes with clean, warm water. In either case, seek medical advice right away if irritation or stinging persists after flushing the eye(s).

+ **Skin reaction:** Apply vegetable oil to dilute the essential oil on the skin, then thoroughly wash the area with unscented soap (liquid if possible) and rinse with warm water to remove any trace of soap and the essential oil. Dry the area thoroughly and apply an unscented base cream (a vegetable oil or even butter if nothing else is available) to soothe the irritation.

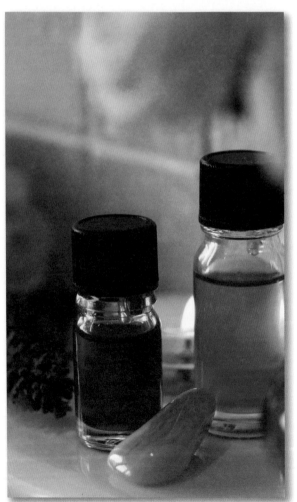

Always dilute essential oils in a carrier medium before adding them to your bath.

MEASURING ESSENTIAL OILS

Measurement percentages can seem quite complicated, especially considering that dropper-top sizes vary, and some oils are more viscose than others, which renders absolute accuracy of measurement impossible, making the quantity of essential oil released per drop variable. However, in the interest of safety, essential oil quantities do need to be carefully monitored. Therefore, as a rule of thumb, assume the averages set out in the "Safe Measurements" guide below.

Risk of sensitivity or irritation reactions increases when large amounts of essential oil are applied to very small areas of skin. In other words, applying six drops of essential oil in a carrier medium to the whole body through massage will have negligible irritant effect, yet the same quantity of essential oil applied to a small area of skin can be an irritant, particularly in sensitive areas such as the face, underarms, etc. If you experience any skin or respiratory tract irritation (itching, redness, rashes, swelling, breathing difficulty), stop using the essential oil or the blend of essential oils immediately.

Remember to use essential oils within their stipulated use-by date (found on the bottle or packaging).

Use no more than one or two drops of essential oil in a carrier medium on localized areas of the skin. Keep this in mind when making first-aid ointments or face creams or lotions. When making face creams and the like for regular use, reduce the amount of essential oils included, change the essential oil selection from time to time, and take periodic breaks from using essential oil.

Safe Measurements

+ 5 ml = 100 drops of essential oil
+ 10 ml = 200 drops of essential oil
+ Maximum amount of essential oil per twenty-four-hour period, including direct inhalation and topical use: 6 to 10 drops for a healthy adult
+ Apply for two to three weeks only, followed by one week's abstinence, and change essential oil(s) selection regularly.

+ Carrier medium: vegetable oils or unscented creams, lotions, ointments, and gels
+ 1 drop of essential oil per 5 ml of carrier medium = 1% blend
+ 2½ drops of essential oil in 5 ml of carrier medium = 2.5% blend
(round down or up, i.e., 2 or 3 drops)
+ 5 drops of essential oil in 5 ml of carrier medium = 5% blend

Appropriate Quantities

As noted previously, reduce the amount of essential oil used on young
children (over three years old), the elderly, and adults with sensitivities. Use the maximum dilution (1 drop of essential oil in 20 ml vegetable oil or unscented cream or lotion) on children over three years
old, and do not use herbaceous, spicy, or citrus oils on young children. Always make sure the genuine purity of your essential oil before
applying—100 percent pure, unadulterated essential oil purchased from
a reputable supplier who provides relevant safety information.

The following amounts are appropriate for children, for those who
are frail or elderly, and for those with sensitivities, allergies, eczema, or
asthma, as well as for facial blends.

+ 1 drop of essential oil in 5 ml of carrier medium = 1% blend
+ 2 drops of essential oil in 10 ml of carrier medium = 1% blend
+ 1 drop of essential oil in 10 ml of carrier medium = 0.5% blend
+ 2 drops of essential oil in 20 ml of carrier medium = 0.5% blend
+ 1 drop of essential oil in 20 ml of carrier medium = 0.25% blend
(for children three years or older)

The normal amount for general adult use:

+ 2½ drops of essential oil in 5 ml of carrier medium = 2.5% blend
(rounded up or down)
+ 5 drops of essential oil in 10 ml of carrier medium = 2.5% blend
+ 5 drops of essential oil in 5 ml of carrier medium = 5% blend
+ 10 drops of essential oil in 10 ml of carrier medium = 5% blend

THE SUBTLE DYNAMICS OF ESSENTIAL OILS

Besides the purely physical qualities imparted by the chemical constituents of essential oils as documented in numerous scientific studies, and being that they are living plant essences, they possess a wide range of subtle dynamics that relate to qualities such as color, the chakras, gemstones, yin and yang, and the five natural elements as delineated by traditional Chinese (Taoist) medicine, which apply to all forms of life. So when we work with essential oils it's important to realize that we're not just working with physical matter; we're tapping into the subtle energy profile of each individual plant oil. These subtle energies can be harnessed for healing, such that knowing the correspondences between an oil and its color(s) as they manifest in pure light as well as in certain gemstones, chakras, elements, and the yin/yang quality of the oil can allow us to greatly expand the healing potential of the oils we work with.

These multidynamic subtle qualities are discerned in the depths and layers of an essential oil's scent. From the moment of extraction, volatile molecules begin to evaporate and transmute. The scent profile that an essential oil starts with will alter over time as a consequence. These changes are anticipated as a natural aspect of volatility, but only within an acceptable range. Essential oils become less volatile over time, but this doesn't mean they are less reactive, as some can transmute and become toxic, sensitizing, or more irritating, such as with an herbaceous oil like basil. On the other hand, some essential oils like sandalwood, rose, and patchouli improve with age, particularly their scent.

Taking these kinds of changes into account, and the fact that essential oils are complex mixtures of many, sometimes hundreds of chemical components with different rates of volatility, some oils will have more than one subtle quality. For example, an oil may be predominantly yang with underlying yin qualities, but this dynamic may alter as the oil ages. This balance also depends on the method and time frame of extraction (i.e., whether the optimum extraction time was met), the ratio and quantity of components extracted, the age of the oil at the time of its use, how it was stored, and the rate of oxidation, among other factors.

Color

Color plays a huge role not only in the therapeutic use of essential oils, but also when it comes to working in a complementary way with gemstones and chakras. Indeed, the subtle vibrational, or energetic, principles underpinning the properties of color are expressed within the tenets of many healing modalities, including Chinese medicine, Ayurveda, and homeopathy. In Chinese medicine, for example, yellow is linked with the element earth and spleen, pancreas, and stomach energy and, through this association, the lower mind and emotional energy (see the charts on pages 168 and 174). Earth is both yin and yang (wood and fire are yang, metal and water are yin). Yellow is associated with the solar plexus chakra, which is symbolically associated with fire. The seven major chakras are located at junctures along the spine and head, while meridians thread as an interconnected network throughout the body. Both systems, however, are linked, just as all systems in the body are inseparably interconnected. The solar plexus chakra is associated with the sense and expression of personal power; personal power is seeded and grows from the base chakra and a sense of feeling grounded and safe—*earthed*. The color or hue of a person's skin reflects their state of health and illness, and thus color is used as both a diagnostic indicator and a healing tool.

Colored light is reflective and consists of three primary colors: red, blue, and green. When combined, they produce the appearance of white light. Pigment color is absorptive and produced when light waves hit objects of different densities. The three primary pigment colors are yellow, cyan, and magenta, and when combined they produce the appearance of black pigment. Both essential oils and gemstones have pigment colors but do not resonate at the same frequency as colored light; chakras resonate at the frequency of colored light.

When working with the subtle qualities of essential oils as they pertain to color, we must first understand the principle of opposites. Solar light energy (which channels into the body via the chakras) resonates at a different frequency to that of pigment color (which reflects from material objects, including crystals and gemstones). To match the resonance of colored light as closely as possible, pigment colors are paired together in opposites—for example, red with green, blue with orange, yellow with violet. Pairing opposite colors also accentuates their qualities and appearance.

In color therapy, for example, yellow is paired with violet to support and balance the solar plexus chakra. Distilled Roman chamomile essential oil resonates with the color yellow and thus can be paired with the gemstone amethyst (color: violet/purple), or a combination of amethyst and citrine (color: yellow), to enhance each other's properties. Cypress essential oil, which also resonates with the color yellow, might be selected to counterbalance a lack of self-confidence and feelings of anxiety or nervousness before an important job interview or performance, where clarity of thought and the ability to answer questions spontaneously with calm assertiveness is important. To optimize the desired qualities of this essential oil, the color yellow, as represented by citrine, may be used along with its complementary opposite gemstone, amethyst, to enhance the activity of the oil and its corresponding stone. Both gemstones could also be placed together in your hand or worn as jewelry. Or, when working with the chakras, as described further down, the citrine would be applied to the solar plexus chakra, which corresponds to the color yellow, while the amethyst, its complementary stone, would be applied to the crown chakra, which resonates with the color violet and the crown chakra. Pairing the two opposite stones with the cypress essential oil would optimize the healing properties of both the oil and the stones.

Gemstones

Gemstones—meaning crystals and semiprecious stones—are gentle in their action and safe to use alongside other therapies. Generally speaking, they are energizing, cleansing, clearing, and protective, and they can be employed to amplify the qualities of remedies such as flower essences and essential oils by providing complementary elements that support the qualities of both the minerals and the essential oils. Gemstones will not change a person's inherent, intrinsic tendencies, but they can influence and support inner potential through rebalancing (increasing and decreasing) the electromagnetic energy in the body. They are also mediums of transference for thoughts, intentions, and healing energy.

When it comes to vibration or frequency, gemstones and essential oils do not have equal or even parallel qualities; each has their own special values. However, there are certain common aspects that bring them together when correctly paired—the resonant influence of color (as in the example of pairing cypress essential oil and citrine, above) being one. When carefully matched, each can enhance the potency of the other. Of course, as with combining essential oils, there is also the risk of creating a void or antisynergistic effect by putting too many dynamics into play at once. Therefore, I recommend focusing on a small, select group of gemstones. These primary gemstones can be matched with a corresponding essential oil; the stones can be held in your hand, worn as jewelry, or placed on the corresponding chakra, in conjunction with using essential oils.

The following chart lists the small group of basic gemstones I like to work with when matching with essential oils. Your work with stones and oils may also be combined with chakra, element, and yin/yang correspondences, as described below.

QUALITIES ATTRIBUTED TO COLOR AND GEMSTONES

VIOLET (AMETHYST)

Assoicated with the third eye chakra (Ajna), spiritual awareness, and ascendance; associated with all of the elements; harmonizes yin-yang qualities; aids focus during meditation

> Physical: Supports the hypothalamus and pituitary gland and the autonomic nervous system

> Mental, emotional, spiritual: Sense and awareness of higher self and spiritual connection, unspoken understanding and knowing, erudition, intuition, conscience, justice and fairness, concentration and effective thinking, rationality and logic, inquisitive inquiry, finding fair solutions and agreement, wonder

> Associated essential oils include: Patchouli, frankincense, lavender

BLUE (LAPIS LAZULI/AQUAMARINE)

Associated with the throat chakra (Vishuddha), giving voice to feelings and emotions, effective communication, and self-expression; associated with the element ether (metal); inclines toward yin

Physical: Supports the endocrine system, throat, and mouth

Mental, emotional, spiritual: Authentic self and inner truth; self-honesty, awareness, and dignity; communication and expression of ideas, insights, and feelings; bridge between intellect, heart, and gut reaction; ability to manage conflict

Associated essential oils include: chamomile(s), lavender, yarrow

BLUE GREEN (AQUAMARINE)

Associated with the thymus (higher heart) chakra, known as the "seat of the soul," and the heart chakra (Anahata), or love and life energy; associated with the element air (wood); inclines toward yin

Physical: Supports the immune system and healthy production of T cells; also supports the heart and lungs

Mental, emotional, spiritual: Supports the higher heart/thymus energy, resilience, unconditional love, compassion, lightheartedness, forgiveness of self and others; acts as a bridge between heart and voice/expression; tranquilizing and uplifting

Associated essential oils include: Thyme (and potentially other immune-supporting essential oils)

GREEN (AVENTURINE)

Associated with the heart chakra (Anahata) and the circulatory system; associated with the liver organ and the season of spring as well as yin energy and the element wood in traditional Chinese medicine and the element air in Ayurveda. Air is vital to life, wood grows and expands, and liver energy plans and crystallizes our vision of the future.

Physical: Associated with the heart, circulatory system, and lungs

Mental, emotional, spiritual: Unconditional acceptance of self and others, tolerance and patience, enthusiasm and inspiration; equanimity, mental and emotional wisdom, maturity, and balance; equilibrium between earth self and higher self

Associated essential oils include: Cypress, frankincense, galbanum, mandarin green

PINK (ROSE QUARTZ)

Associated with the heart chakra (Anahata) and the heart organ system in Chinese medicine; associated with the element air in Ayurveda and the element fire in traditional Chinese medicine; yang moving toward yin. Air symbolizes vitality, fire, warmth, and enthusiasm.

>Physical: Associated with the heart, circulatory system, and liver

>Mental, emotional, spiritual: Self-love, a strong heart, ability to love others; helpfulness, empathy, and sensitivity; liberates from worry and overconcern; encourages emotional balance and harmony; openness and awe

>Associated essential oils include: Geranium, grapefuit, rose, spikenard

YELLOW (CITRINE)

Associated with the solar plexus chakra (Manipura) and the spleen and digestive system (particularly the stomach, gallbladder, and pancreas); associated with the element earth in both Ayurveda and traditional Chinese medicine; balances yin and yang energy.

>Physical: Digestive system

>Mental, emotional, spiritual: Self-worth, value, and belief; self-expression; courage and self-permission to face and enjoy life; desire for new experience and adventure; individuality and self-confidence

>Associated essential oils include: Caraway, cardamom, carrot seed

ORANGE (CARNELIAN)

Associated with the sacral chakra (Svadhisthana), fertility, creativity, feelings and emotions—"gut instinct"—nourishment, concentration, and focus; associated with the element earth, and warmth, in both Ayurveda and tradditional Chinese medicine; yang.

>Physical: Digestive functions, organs of the urinary system and reproductive system, and the emotional brain (limbic system)

>Mental, emotional, spiritual: Gut instinct, intuition, and emotional intelligence; courage, steadfastness, and idealism; willingness to help, supportiveness; stimulates ability to problem-solve and digest information; realism in the face of confusion; truth

>Associated essential oils include: Myrrh, sandalwood, turmeric

RED (JASPER)

Associated with the base chakra (Muladhara) and the spinal cord, earth nourishment, conception, and survival instincts (fight or flight); associated with the element fire in Ayurveda and the element earth in traditional Chinese medicine; yang.

Physical: External reproductive organs—genitals and testes; fertility; supports the circulatory system

Mental, emotional, spiritual: Earthing, grounding, roots, stability; determination, endurance, protection; honesty, uprightness, passion; transforms ideas into action; stimulates the imagination; protects

Associated essential oils include: Vetivert, rose absolute, valerian

Chakras

The chakras, which resonate at the frequency of light, are energy vortices, or portals, situated at major nerve plexuses and glandular centers of the endocrine system, which regulates hormones, metabolism, and growth and affects almost every organ, including the brain and central nervous system and every cell in the body. The seven major chakras are located from the base of the spine to the top of the head, with a number of related minor chakras spread throughout the body. Each chakra resonates at a particular frequency, which is expressed as a color (as seen in the chart above), a sound, and a particular life-force condition. As well, each chakra is associated with a particular organ, which also resonates at a similar frequency.

While each chakra resonates with the full color spectrum, one color will always dominate over the others. So, for example, red dominates the base chakra, yellow dominates the solar plexus chakra, blue dominates the throat chakra, and so forth. Ideally, each chakra resonates in harmony with the other chakras with equal strength. However, this state is in constant flux, and sometimes one chakra is weaker or more dominant than the others, which creates a physical, mental, or spiritual imbalance. The aim of chakra therapy is to rebalance and harmonize the chakras' vibration by applying light and/or pigment color via essential oils and gemstones to help strengthen or unblock the affected chakra and to bring it back into balance with the other chakras. This is where pairing with essential oils and gemstones comes into the picture, as described in the examples above.

Yin and Yang

The ancient Taoist principle of healing—i.e., coming into balance—is based on the philosophical principle that primordial energy manifests as two opposing yet complementary energetic forces. These forces, yin and yang, resonate in a perpetual state of flux, always seeking balance; this gives form and substance to the material and ethereal universe. When in perfect balance or harmony, yin and yang are symbolically represented as two equal, interlinking halves of a whole circle, each perceivable by virtue of the contrasting or complementary existence of the other. Although one may predominate over the other (as one increases, the other decreases), dominance by either is never complete or constant—there always exists an element of yang in yin, and yin in yang.

Just as all living beings express yin and yang, essential oils possess yin and yang qualities too, the balance of which depends on various factors. A plant requires soil (yang) and water (yin) to germinate. Roots (yang) reach down and spread into the earth (yin), and shoots (yin) push up through the earth toward sunlight (yang). So stems, tree trunks, buds, and fruits tend toward yin, while leaves, blossoms, and flowers tend toward yang. However, whether an essential oil is extracted from a root or a blossom does not mean it will exhibit the same tendencies; separated from the plant, the essential oil becomes an entity unto itself. Also, the chemical and energetic qualities of an essential oil alter from the moment of extraction and over time; the period of time allocated to distillation and the age and storage conditions of the essential oil, among other things, are determinant factors.

The charts in this chapter and the profiles in chapter 6 indicate an essential oil's tendency toward yin or yang or both, depending on the oil's general qualities. Using this information as a guide will assist you in determining the qualities of an essential oil at a given moment in time (as we have established, essential oils are dynamic) and how best to match that oil to a specific need.

The Elements

The five elements of traditional Chinese medicine (TCM) and ancient Taoist philosophy are wood, earth, water, fire, and metal, and in traditional Indian Ayurveda they are air, water, ether (space), fire, and earth. Each element represents a specific quality that complements and influences the movement and behavior of the others. These qualities manifest seamlessly within the mind-body-spirit and in the environment (nature, the atmosphere, the universe, and the heavens). Essential oils express one or more of these elements and balance and normalize the energetic qualities expressed by the elements. As essential oils are physiologically and energetically protective and restorative, these adaptogenic qualities promote the dispersion of energetic excess or deficiency in order to restore the natural flow between the elements.

TCM and Ayurveda

TCM and Ayurveda evolved simultaneously more than three thousand years ago; they share certain principles and philosophies, especially related to primordial energy and life force (*chi* in TCM and *prana* in Ayurveda).

The elements of wood (TCM) and air (Ayurveda) express similar qualities to each other, as do metal and ether. In the plant profiles in chapter 6, the ayurvedic elements are listed in parentheses following the comparable TCM elements.

Yet there are also subtle differences between these systems. For example, wood refers to the qualities of growth, change, and pushing through, while air refers to the qualities of motion or kinetic energy. Metal refers to the qualities of firmness, rigidity, persistence, strength, and determination, while ether refers to the qualities of space, stillness, containing, and holding.

In TCM, yin and yang represent energetic polarities (as primordial energy moves from oneness) and the manifest, contrasting motion between these two states as each increases and decreases to either dominate or give way to the other. This is observed, for example, in the rhythm of day and night, the changing seasons, the waxing and waning of the moon, and so on.

QUALITIES ATTRIBUTED TO THE FIVE ELEMENTS
OR PHASES OF MOVEMENT

New yang and new yin *denote the phase of movement created as one state gives way to the next.*

INDICATION	NEW YANG WOOD	FULL YANG FIRE	YIN/YANG EARTH	NEW YIN METAL	FULL YIN WATER
Color	green/blue	red	yellow	white	black
Season	spring	summer	change of season	autumn	winter
Climate	wind	hot	damp	dry	cold
Organs	liver, gallbladder	heart, small intestine	spleen, pancreas, stomach	lungs, large intestine	kidneys, bladder
Sensory Organs	eyes	tongue	mouth	nose	ears
Emotion	anger	happiness	love	grief/ sadness	fear
Character	creative cheerful compassionate charismatic impulsive proactive adaptable determined motivated carefree artisan extrovert	passionate enthusiastic love energetic tactical idealistic inspirational joyful ambitious strong-willed leadership extrovert	agreeable somber empathy considerate logistical guardian reliable sensitive attentive reverence innovative introvert	intuitive thoughtful reflective mindful regulator supportive focused positive high standards self-reliant artistic introvert	erudition calm wise affectionate strategist diplomatic resourceful introspective observant curious steward introvert

Fragrance Notes

Essential oils are generally categorized into three broad groups according to their fragrance profile, the behavior of their predominant chemical components, and their volatility, or rate of evaporation. These categories are called *notes* (as in the musical sense), and they identify and acknowledge the multilayered, often complex qualities and nuances expressed by the various chemicals that comprise an essential oil. Consider an orchestra harmonizing the sounds of various instruments to produce a melody; similarly, each chemical within an essential oil expresses its own unique tone and color, and each essential oil its own melody or harmony. When

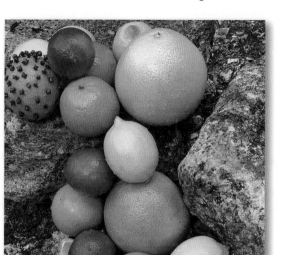

we blend essential oils, the aim is to create a particular tune, or story. In general, the fragrance notes break down as follows:

Top notes: These are quick, fast, rapid, and loud, the first scent to be experienced and the first to fade. They are the most reactive—you can detect these notes when you first open an essential oil container. Top notes tend to be stimulating, vitalizing, and uplifting. They evaporate rapidly. The corresponding color is red.

Middle notes: These are the harmonizers of the top notes and the base notes, balancing fast and slow qualities. They comprise the body of a scent and are still detectable thirty minutes after applying an essential oil. The corresponding color is blue.

Base notes: These are gentle, soft, grounding, and heavy. They are the least volatile and the most tenacious, the scent that lingers longest, sixty minutes after application. The corresponding color is green.

ESSENTIAL OIL FRAGRANCE CHARACTERISTICS

Some oils appear in more than one category; these are identified with an asterisk. They are listed first with their primary category, and then in italics for the category they move toward; this movement is determined by the characteristics of the chemical mixture of an oil—for instance, how volatile the oil is and the nature of that oil's general therapeutic properties. For example, due to its chemical composition cypress is somewhere between a middle note and a base note, going from a blue (harmonizing) to a green (grounding) influence, and so it is represented in italics in the chart. Petitgrain is a top note but may move toward a middle note, going from a red (stimulating) to a blue (harmonizing) correspondence.

The volatility rate scale (1–100), originally applied by Robert Tisserand in his book *The Art of Aromatherapy* (1977), indicates the rate of evaporation: 1–14 denotes rapid evaporation and 61–100 slow evaporation; top notes are very volatile whereas base notes are much less volatile. For example, light citrusy oils, such as orange or lemongrass, which have a high terpene content, evaporate very quickly, while cedarwood, which consists mainly of sesquiterpenes and alcohols, is more viscous and heavy and evaporates very slowly.

CHARACTERISTIC	TOP NOTE	MIDDLE NOTE	BASE NOTE
Type of Oil	lemon and other citrus fruits; leaves	herbs, flowering tops	resins, woods, roots, blossoms
Volatility Rate (Scale of 1–100)	1 to 14	15 to 60	61 to 100
Evaporation Rate	0 to 30 minutes	up to 8 hours	usually 12 to 24 hours, possibly a week, sometimes longer
Action	fastest	moderate	slowest
General Fragrance Characteristic	sharpish	round	heavy
Dry-Out Odor Quality	fresh, distinctive, cluster of odors, obvious, light, potentially intense due to rapid evaporation	lingering traces of top notes, heart of the bouquet, character, softer edges	lingering traces of middle notes, faint, faded, subtle, nondescript, heavy, tenacious residue
Therapeutic Effects	uplifting, stimulating, revitalizing, aids memory and function of the brain and head	balancing, harmonizing, rejuvenating	relaxing, earthing, sedating, calming
Skin Penetration	½ to 1 hour	2 to 3 hours	4 to 6 hours or more
May Support/ Ease (General Indications)	extreme lethargy, melancholy, lack of interest, apathy, acute depression	bodily functions, metabolism, digestion, menstruation, circulation (blood pressure)	nervous, erratic, or flighty behavior; hyperactivity; chronic and/or longstanding conditions, the elderly, anxiety

CHARACTERISTIC	TOP NOTE	MIDDLE NOTE	BASE NOTE
Essential Oils	basil*	basil*	benzoin
	bergamot	black pepper	cedarwood
	cajeput	caraway*	cinnamon leaf/bark*
	caraway*	cardamom*	clove bud
	cardamom*	carrot seed*	frankincense*
	carrot seed*	chamomile(s)	jasmine*
	citronella*	chaste tree	jasmine absolute
	clary sage*	cinnamon leaf/bark*	myrrh
	coriander*	citronella*	neroli*
	eucalyptus	clary sage*	patchouli*
	fennel*	coriander*	rose otto*
	galbanum	cypress	sandalwood*
	ginger*	fennel*	spikenard
	grapefruit	frankincense*	turmeric*
	lavender*	geranium	valerian
	lemon	ginger*	vetivert
	lemongrass	helichrysum/	ylang-ylang*
	mandarin	immortelle	
	may chang*	hyssop	
	melissa*	jasmine*	
	myrtle*	juniper	
	niaouli*	lavender*	
	nutmeg*	marjoram	
	orange (bitter/sweet)	may chang*	
	palmarosa*	melissa*	
	peppermint*	myrtle*	
	petitgrain*	neroli*	
	rosewood*	niaouli*	
	tea tree*	nutmeg*	
	thyme, white/red*	oregano	
		palmarosa*	
		patchouli*	
		peppermint*	
		petitgrain*	
		pine	
		rosemary	
		rose otto*	
		rosewood*	
		sandalwood*	
		spikenard*	
		tea tree*	
		thyme, white/red*	
		turmeric*	
		yarrow	
		ylang-ylang*	

◆ ◆ ◆

Along with all the information provided in this chapter, your own nose will guide you when assessing an oil's subtle qualities. If in any doubt about a particular essential oil, for whatever reason, then do not use it; you can always find an alternative among those listed in this book. A carefully selected single essential oil can be just as effective as a blend, and sometimes more so. Remember also that essential oils are complementary gifts (just as they are within the plant) that work well as team players and as part of a holistic well-being strategy.

Essential oils work best when they are carefully honed and matched to a specific need, taking into account the whole person. Essential oils are very effective in their own right, yet their properties can be gently enhanced or amplified when they are complementarily combined with the subtle qualities of gemstones, colors, and chakras and/or when observing and aligning their elemental properties—especially when dealing with psycho-emotional-spiritual issues or events. Sometimes, a gentle approach is what is required, such as, for example, when someone is frail, is recovering from illness, is very young or elderly, or has underlying chronic conditions or an autommimune disease. In such circumstances, essential oils are best applied in reduced amounts or in high dilution, or avoided altogether; the subtle qualities of gemstones and colors may be used as an alternative, or to support the subtle properties of an essential oil.

The ancient Chinese observed that excessive, imbalanced emotional states, when prolonged and unchecked, can systematically erode health. For example, excessive grief injures the lungs, excessive fear injures the kidneys, excessive anger injures the liver, excessive joy injures the heart, and excessive worry injures the spleen. Here is another instance where essential oils may offer support.

As an example, someone experiencing loss or bereavement (perhaps of a job, a person, a relationship, or even an opportunity) may benefit from oils such as frankincense and cypress, which support the lungs and regulate breathing, and rose and spikenard, which support the heart; the lungs and heart are physiologically and energetically connected. The color red (jasper; base chakra) or pink (rose quartz; heart chakra) can be applied to add warmth and a sense of being earthed, grounded, and nurtured while the person travels through their grief. Green (aventurine; heart chakra) heals and regenerates the heart. Frankincense and cypress are associated with the heart and solar plexus chakras. Yellow dominates the solar plexus chakra and is related to the element earth in traditional Chinese medicine, and therefore it is also grounding. Rose and spikenard are also associated with the heart and solar plexus; spikenard is also associated with the sacral chakra, which instills courage and fortifies the nerves. Cypress eases uncontrollable crying, and frankincense eases sadness and despair, as does rose, while spikenard is grounding and eases insomnia; all four essential oils ease grief. What a team!

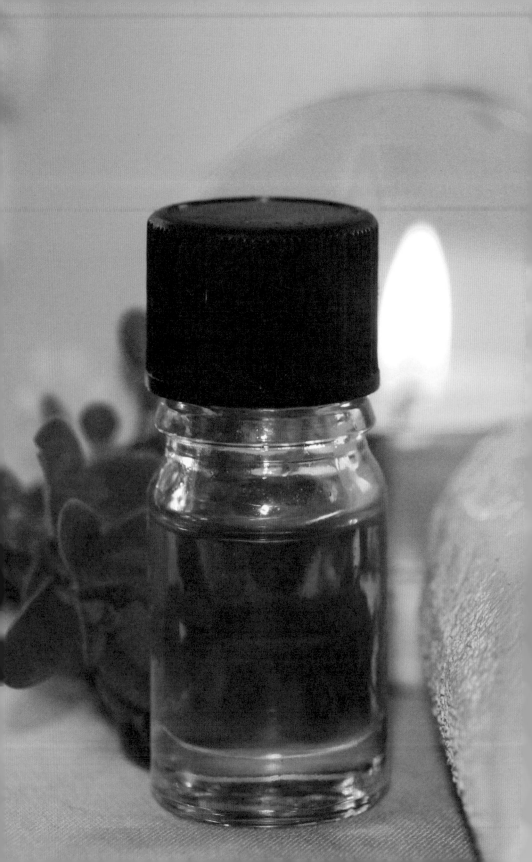

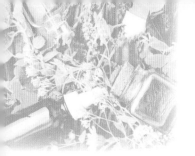

6

Essential Oil Profiles

The Antiviral, Restorative,
and Life-Enhancing Properties
of 58 Plants

Many factors can affect an essential oil's composition and characteristic chemical profile and therapeutic actions. The location of growth, the plant species, and the length of distillation time will influence the resultant oil's chemical composition, qualities, and properties. The range and quantity of chemical constituents comprising an essential oil can vary tremendously; the minutest, barely detectable constituent can procure significant synergistic influence on other constituents. Some essential oils are composed of two hundred constituents—far too many to include here. The following fifty-eight essential oil profiles, therefore, include examples of the main chemical components. Each example relates to the relevant plant species—for instance, *Ocimum basilicum* ct. linalool for basil and *Carum carvi* for caraway. Sometimes, where there might be significant differences between types of oil, two examples are given—for instance, both bitter and sweet fennel for *Foeniculum vulgare* and Nepalese and Indian spikenard for *Nardostachys grandiflora*. The main chemical constituents are set in **bold** for ease of identification.

Citrus aurantium var. *amara,* the bitter orange tree, produces three distinct essential oils, which, while complementary, express their own therapeutic and odor personalities and profiles. For example, petitgrain, from the leaves and twigs, is woody, mossy, citrusy, and sweet; neroli, from the blossoms, is sweet and floral with citrusy undertones; and bitter orange, from the fruit, is fresh, citrusy, and orange-like. These essential oils are therefore presented here individually.

The 58 Essential Oils

1. Basil	30. Lemongrass
2. Benzoin	31. Mandarin
3. Bergamot	32. Marjoram, Sweet
4. Cajeput	33. May Chang
5. Caraway	34. Melissa/Lemon Balm
6. Cardamom	35. Myrrh
7. Carrot Seed	36. Myrtle
8. Cedarwood Atlas (Atlantic)	37. Neroli/Orange Blossom
9. Chamomile, German (Blue)	38. Niaouli
10. Chamomile, Roman	39. Nutmeg
11. Chaste Tree	40. Orange, Bitter
12. Cinnamon Leaf/Bark	41. Palmarosa
13. Citronella	42. Patchouli
14. Clove Bud	43. Pepper, Black
15. Coriander	44. Peppermint
16. Cypress	45. Petitgrain/Orange Leaf
17. Eucalyptus	46. Pine Needle, Scotch
18. Fennel	47. Rosemary
19. Frankincense/Olibanum	48. Rose Otto
20. Galbanum	49. Sage, Clary
21. Geranium	50. Sandalwood
22. Ginger	51. Spikenard
23. Grapefruit	52. Tea Tree
24. Helichrysum/Immortelle	53. Thyme
25. Hyssop	54. Turmeric
26. Jasmine	55. Valerian
27. Juniper Berry	56. Vetivert
28. Lavender	57. Yarrow
29. Lemon	58. Ylang-Ylang

German chamomile (*Matricaria recutita*) and Roman chamomile (*Chamaemelum nobile*), while sharing similar qualities, derive from two different species that produce oils that differ in chemical composition. Distilled German chamomile, for example, is deep green-blue in appearance with herbaceous medicinal-like odor tones, while Roman chamomile is transparent to yellow or blue in appearance with sweet, fruity apple-like odor tones. These oils are also presented here individually.

The following profiles include essential oils extracted from plant species that are ecologically vulnerable or at risk due to commercial over-harvesting, among other reasons—for instance, spikenard, frankincense, galbanum, cedarwood Atlas, sandalwood, and Scotch pine. These oils can be purchased with buyer's discretion from sustainable sources or they can be substituted with other essential oils with similar profiles (see chapters 2 and 4).

BASIL, FRENCH AND SWEET
(Ocimum basilicum)

Geographical location: Native to India, where it has grown and been cultivated for over five thousand years as a culinary herb, and to tropical Asia and Africa, basil is now widely cultivated throughout Europe, the Mediterranean, the Pacific Islands, and North and South America. There are over 150 varieties currently found around the world, grown mainly for their distinctive culinary flavor and essential oil. The word *basil* derives from the Greek *basileus,* meaning "king." It is also known as St. Joseph's wort, Thai basil, and sweet basil. The European, French, or true sweet basil is produced in France, Italy, Egypt, Bulgaria, Hungary, and the United States; the oil is produced in Greece, Indonesia, Israel, and Morocco.

Plant description: A strongly aromatic and tender annual herb with an erect square stem growing up to 24 inches (60 centimeters), it has very dark green leaves that are grayish green underneath and whorls of small, two-lipped greenish or light pinkish or white flowers. The leaves and flowering tops are gathered as the plant comes into flower. There are numerous cultivars and chemotypes, of which only a few are used for aromatherapy—for example, holy basil (*Ocimum sanctum*), sweet basil (*Ocimum basilicum*), and pungent basil (*Ocimum gratissimum*).

Botanical family: Lamiaceae (Labiatae)

Extraction method: Steam distillation of the flowering tops and leaves

Appearance of essential oil: Clear to pale yellow or yellow to pale green liquid

Odor of essential oil: Type: anisic; strength: medium; characteristics: fresh, sweet, herbaceous, aniseed-like, tarragon-like, slightly green with warm balsamic-woody undertone and lingering faint, sweet to nondistinctive dry-out notes

Compatible essential oils for blending: Bergamot, black pepper, citronella, clary sage, geranium, grapefruit, hyssop, lavender, lime, orange, peppermint, petitgrain, sandalwood, violet leaf (absolute)

Safety data: Basil is relatively nontoxic and nonirritant but has the potential for sensitization in some people, as oxidation of linalool may render the oil as a skin irritant. Use fresh and store appropriately, in a cool, dark spot with a tightly secured lid, and discard small amounts remaining in the bottle. Avoid using on sensitive skin. Avoid during pregnancy. Do not consume orally.

Perfume note: Top to middle

Principal chemical constituents: CAS No: 8015-73-4

Ocimum basilicum ct. linalool (least irritant): beta-pinene (trace amount to 1%), beta-myrcene (trace amount to 1.5%), limonene (trace amount to 0.5%), 1,8-cineole (2 to 10%), trans-beta-ocimene (trace amount to 2%), camphor (trace amount to 2%), **linalool (45 to 62%),** bornyl acetate (trace amount to 2%), trans-alpha-bergamotene (1–5%), beta-elemene (1 to 3.5%), alpha-guaiene (trace amount to 0.5%), beta-caryophyllene (trace amount to 0.3%), terpeninol-4-ol (trace amount to 1%), estragole (trace amount to 2%), alpha-humulene (trace amount to 1%), alpha-terpiniol (trace amount to 1.5%), germacrene D (trace amount to 0.6%), beta-selinene (trace amount to 0.2%), alpha-bulnesene (trace amount to 2%), geraniol (trace amount to 0.3%), epi-cubenol (trace amount to 0.4%), **eugenol (2 to 15%)**

Subtle Connections

Colors: Green (*opposite: red*), pink (*opposite: pale aqua green*), yellow (*opposite: violet*)

Chakras: Solar plexus, heart, crown (said to balance all chakras)

Gemstones: Citrine (*opposite: amethyst*), aventurine (*opposite: jasper*), rose quartz (*opposite: aquamarine*), sugalite (*opposite: carnelian*)

Energy: Yang

Element: Fire

Actions and Uses

General actions: Antidepressant, anti-infectious, antimicrobial, antiseptic, antispasmodic, antiviral, cephalic, emmenagogue, expectorant, nervine, tonic

Skin: Acne, dry skin, eczema, infections, insect bites (insect repellent), shingles, tonic

Respiratory: Asthma, bronchitis, coughs, sinusitis

Muscles: Aches and pains, arthritis

Immune system: Infections, viral infections

Endocrine system: Premenstrual tension (may increase menstrual bleeding)

Potential psycho-emotional and spiritual support: Aids clarity of thought; eases depression and low mood, feelings of anxiety and agitation; encourages intuition; relieves insomnia and mental and emotional fatigue (encourages emotional strength); relieves premenstrual tension; strengthens memory; uplifts mood and emotion

BENZOIN
(Styrax benzoin, Ricinus communis)

Geographical location: Native to Sumatra, Borneo, Thailand (Siam), and Java, where it grows in tropical rain forests, benzoin is also cultivated in Laos, Vietnam, Cambodia, and China. The main regions of production are Sumatra, Java, and Malaysia (and their benzoin is referred to as Sumatra benzoin and Siam benzoin).

Plant description: A fast-growing, shrubby, deciduous tree from 15 to 100 feet (4.5 to 30 meters) high, it has pointed, oval, pale green, citrus-like leaves that are whitish underneath and clusters of silky-white bell-shaped flowers that produce hard-shelled fruits that contain one or two round seeds. The tree's bark is covered in a silky, whitish down. Incisions are made in the bark when the tree is around six or seven years old, from which exudes a thick, resinous, white to yellow juice, or balsam, that hardens with exposure to air; this is chipped from the tree and collected. Resin produced during the first three years of tapping is the purest; after this, for a period of about seven or eight years, an inferior yellowish-red to brown resin is produced. The trees are then cut down and any remaining resin is scraped from the logs; this resin is very dark and hard and also includes scrapings of wood. Resin tears from different trees of various ages are often mixed together. Benzoin is widely used as an incense and fixative in perfumes.

Botanical family: Styracaceae

Extraction method: Solvent extraction

Siam benzoin: Pebble or tear-shaped orangish-brown pieces, with a sweet-balsamic, vanilla-like scent (a more refined odor than that of the Sumatra type)

Sumatra benzoin: Grayish-brown, brittle lumps with reddish streaks, with a styrax-like odor.

Benzoin resinoid is produced from either the crude Siam or Sumatra types, or a mix of the two. Solvents used during extraction include benzene and alcohol. Commercial benzoin is usually sold dissolved in ethyl glycol or a similar solvent.

Appearance of essential oil: A sticky, solid mass that is made pourable by diluting it in alcohol, ethyl glycol, or another solvent. The absolute produced is a brown or orangish-brown viscous mass or liquid.

Odor of essential oil: Type: balsamic; strength: medium; characteristic: intensely rich, sweet-balsamic, vanilla-like, camphoraceous, medicinal

Compatible essential oils for blending: Coriander and other spice oils, cypress, frankincense, jasmine, juniper, lemon, orange, rose, sandalwood

Safety data: Nontoxic, nonirritant, but possibly sensitizing (for example, benzoic and cinnamic acid are strong sensitizers); mainly used in perfumes; not recommended for use on skin. Do not consume orally.

Perfume note: Base

Principal chemical constituents: CAS No: 9000-05-9 *(Sumatra benzoin)*

benzyl benzoate (60%), benzyl alcohol (45%), trans-(Z)-cinnamyl (2%), cinnamic acid (2%), ethyl cinnamate (1%), benzoic acid (0.1%)

CAS No: 9000-72-0 *(Siam benzoin)*

benzyl benzoate (40%), benzyl alcohol (39%), benzoic acid (19%), ethyl cinnamate (1%)

Subtle Connections

Colors: Red *(opposite: green)*, orange *(opposite: blue)*

Chakras: Base, sacral

Gemstones: Jasper *(opposite: aventurine)*, carnelian *(opposite: lapis lazuli/aquamarine)*

Energy: Yin

Element: Earth

Actions and Uses

General actions: Resinoid and absolute: anti-inflammatory, antioxidant, antiseptic, sedative

Skin: Although indicated in many books, benzoin absolute is *not* recommended here for skin care due to its solvent content and the risk of sensitization.

Respiratory: Bronchitis, respiratory infections (at low dose)

Environmental: Incense and perfume

Potential psycho-emotional and spiritual support: Relieves nervous tension; sedative, warming

BERGAMOT
(Citrus bergamia)

Geographical location: Native to tropical Asia, bergamot is extensively cultivated in Calabria, in southern Italy, for its essential oil (accounting for approximately 80 percent of growth), and also, to a lesser extent, in southern France and the Ivory Coast, Turkey, Spain, Argentina, Brazil, and Russia. Italy is the main essential oil–producing country. Oils produced from fruits grown in southern Italy are considered superior to oils extracted from fruits grown on the Ivory Coast.

Plant description: A small evergreen tree growing to about 15 to 30 feet (4.5 to 10 meters) tall, with oval, pointed leaves and fragrant white flowers that bear small, round, sour fruits that have an aromatic peel that ripens from green to yellow (like miniature oranges). Historically, bergamot is probably a hybrid created from bitter orange (*Citrus limetta*) and sour orange (*Citrus aurantium*). Bergamot orange is mainly grown to produce essential oil for the food (for example, Earl Grey tea and Turkish delight tea), pharmaceutical, and cosmetics industries; bergamot essential oil also features as an ingredient in eau de cologne. The fruit is not grown commercially for its juice production but is grown in Mauritius as a local food source, and in southern Turkey and France for marmalade production. A terpeneless or rectified oil produced from bergamot, known as FCF (furocoumarin-free), is, due to the reduction of phototoxic components, considered safer to use, especially when used topically, but is not to be confused with the herb bergamot or bee balm (*Monarda didyma*).

Botanical family: Rutaceae

Extraction method: Cold expression of the fruit rind. The rectified or terpeneless oil is produced by vacuum distillation or solvent extraction.

Appearance of essential oil: Golden yellow or yellow to green liquid that turns to a brownish-olive color as the oil ages

Odor of essential oil: Type: citrus; strength: medium; characteristics: citrus, fresh, lemony orange, sweet-fruity, green, slightly spicy–balsamic undertones

Compatible essential oils for blending: Chamomile (German and Roman), coriander, cypress, frankincense, geranium, jasmine, juniper, lavender, lemon, lemongrass, violet absolute

Safety data: Nontoxic and generally nonsensitizing. Use the furocoumarin-free (FCF) type for topical application; also use fresh and within six months of opening the bottle; store in a cool, dark spot with a tightly secured lid. Do not expose skin to sunlight or sunbed rays for at least twelve hours after skin application. Non-FCF bergamot oils may be photocarcinogenic. Avoid using old or oxidized oils. Do not consume orally.

Perfume note: Top

Principal chemical constituents: CAS No: 8007-75-8

alpha-pinene (1 to 3%), alpha-thujene (trace amount to 0.5%), beta-pinene (1 to 10%), sabinene (1 to 10%), beta-myrcene (0.5 to 2%), **limonene (30 to 50%),** beta-phellandrene (trace amount to 0.2%), **gamma-terpinene (5 to 12%),** trans-beta-ocimene (trace amount to 0.3%), para-cymene (trace amount to 0.2%), **linalool (3 to 15%), linalyl acetate (22 to 36%),** trans-alpha-bergamotene (trace amount to 0.3%), bergapten (0.5 to 0.35%), neryl acetate (0.1 to 1.5%), beta-bisabolene (0.3 to 0.6%), geranial (0.3 to 0.5%), geranyl acetate (0.3 to 0.5%)

Bergamot FCF: alpha-pinene (0.5 to 1.5%), alpha-thujene (trace amount to 0.5%), beta-pinene (5 to 10%), sabinene (0.5 to 2%), beta-myrcene (0.5 to 2%), **beta-limonene (30 to 50%), gamma-terpinene (6 to 10%),** para-cymene (trace amount to 0.5%), terpinolene (trace amount to 0.5%), **linalool (3 to 15%), linalyl acetate (22 to 36%),** trans-alpha-bergamotene (trace amount to 0.2%), beta-caryophyllene (trace amount to 0.3%), neryl acetate (trace amount to 0.3%), geranial (0.3 to 0.5%), geranyl acetate (trace amount to 0.3%)

Subtle Connections

Color: Yellow (*opposite: violet*), green (*opposite: red*), pink (*opposite: pale aqua-green*)

Chakras: Solar plexus, heart

Gemstones: Citrine (*opposite: amethyst*), aventurine (*opposite: jasper*), rose quartz (*opposite: aquamarine*)

Energy: Yang, yin

Elements: Fire, earth

Actions and Uses

General actions: Analgesic, antidepressant, antifungal (moderate), anti-infectious, antimicrobial, antiseptic, antispasmodic, antitoxic, antiviral, deodorant, diuretic, febrifuge (reduces fever), rubefacient (reduces redness of skin), stimulant, tonic

Skin: Acne, boils, chickenpox, cold sores, eczema, insect repellent, insect bites, nerve and muscular pain, oily skin, psoriasis, scar tissue, shingles, spots, wounds

Respiratory: Colds, flu, halitosis, mouth infections, sore throat

Potential psycho-emotional and spiritual support: Allays frustration, balances mood and emotions, eases feelings of anger and frustration, eases feelings of anxiety and depression, eases feelings of apathy, relieves insomnia, refreshing, sedative, addresses stress and stress-related conditions, uplifting

CAJEPUT
(Melaleuca cajuputi)

Geographical location: Native to Australia, cajeput also grows in China, Malaysia, Indonesia, the Philippines, Vietnam, Java, Southeast Asia, and North America. A species was introduced to Florida as an ornamental tree and to control swamp erosion; it is now considered invasive. The main essential oil–producing countries are Indonesia and the Philippines.

Plant description: An aromatic evergreen tree that grows to about 98 to 130 feet (30 to 40 meters) high, cajeput has pale green, oval leaves with pointed tips and white, cream, or greenish-yellow flowers carried on many-flowered spikes. The spongy, flexible bark easily flakes from the trunk (and is used by Australian Aborigines for shields, canoes, roofing material, and timber). Other common names include paper bark tree, punk tree, and white bottle-brush tree. The name *cajeput* derives from the Indonesian *kayu putih,* or "white wood." Other family species include *M. linariifolia, M. viridiflora,* and *M. quinquenervia* species. Cajeput is related to *Melaleuca alternifolia,* which produces tea tree essential oil.

Botanical family: Myrtaceae

Extraction method: Steam distillation of fresh leaves and twigs

Appearance of essential oil: Colorless to pale yellow or green-tinted liquid

Odor of essential oil: Type: herbal; strength: medium; characteristics: mild, sweet-fruity, fresh, rosemary, camphoraceous, menthol, metallic, with an herbaceous green, woody odor, then very faint herbaceous dry-out notes

Compatible essential oils for blending: Bergamot, cedarwood, cypress, juniper berry, lavender, lemon, marjoram, petitgrain, pine, rose, rosemary, thyme

Safety data: Nontoxic and nonsensitizing; may be irritant to skin and mucous membranes; avoid use during pregnancy or while breastfeeding; may be adulterated with additional eucalyptus oil and *M. quinquenervia* and *M. symphyocarpa* oils and occasionally fixed oils or kerosene (Tisserand and Young 2014, 224); assure authenticity and purity with your essential oil supplier. Do not consume orally.

Perfume note: Top

Principal chemical constituents: CAS No: 8008-98-8

1,8-cineole (41 to 71%), alpha-terpineol (6 to 9%), para-cymene (0.5 to 7%), terpinolene (0 to 6%), gamma-terpinene (1 to 5%), linalool (0.3 to 5%), dextro-limonene (3 to 5%), alpha-pinene (1 to 5%), beta-myrcene (0.1 to 3%)

Subtle Connections

Colors: Green (*opposite: red*), pink (*opposite: pale aqua-green*), yellow (*opposite: violet*)

Chakras: Heart, solar plexus

Gemstones: Aventurine (*opposite: jasper*), rose quartz (*opposite: aquamarine*), citrine (*opposite: amethyst*)

Energy: Yin

Elements: Metal (ether), water

Actions and Uses

General actions: Analgesic, antiarthritic, antimicrobial, antiseptic, antispasmodic, bactericidal, expectorant

Skin: Acne, chapped and cracked skin, oily skin, pimples, psoriasis, insect bites

Respiratory: Asthma, bronchitis, catarrhal infections, colds/flu, coughs, hay fever, laryngitis, sinusitis, sore throat, upper respiratory tract infections and pain

Joints and muscles: Arthritis, joint and muscle pain

Circulatory: Supports venous and arterial tissues and varicose veins

Fungal Infections: Addresses *Trichophyton* species (ringworm, athlete's foot, etc.)

Potential psycho-emotional and spiritual support: Aids concentration, bracing, clears and stimulates the mind and thoughts, eases apathy and low mood, helps one find courage in finding new pathways and managing change, strengthens the spirit

CARAWAY
(Carum carvi)

Geographical location: Caraway is native to Europe, where it grows wild, as well as North Africa and western Asia, and it is naturalized in North America. It is now widely cultivated in Germany, the Netherlands, Scandinavia, and Russia. Finland supplies 28 percent of the world's caraway production. It prefers warm, sunny climates and well-drained soils and grows in sites up to 6,600 feet (2,000 meters) above sea level. The seeds are harvested ripe in late summer. The plant is also known as meridian fennel and Persian cumin. The main essential oil–producing countries are Egypt, Hungary, India, Iran, Morocco, the Netherlands, Poland, and Russia.

Plant description: An aromatic annual herb growing up to 2 feet (60 centimeters), caraway has a ridged stem, feathery leaves that have threadlike divisions, and umbels of small white or pink flowers that appear in midsummer, which produce exploding seed capsules. Each capsule contains two small, narrow seeds that are curved, with five distinct ridges. It is similar in appearance to other members of the Apiaceae botanical family, such as aniseed, fennel, and cumin.

Botanical family: Apiaceae (Umbelliferae)

Extraction method: Steam distillation of the dried, ripe seeds or fruits, which are crushed before distillation

Appearance of essential oil: Colorless to pale or yellowish-brown liquid (darkens with age)

Odor of essential oil: Type: herbal; strength: medium; odor characteristics: fresh, herbal, spicy, minty, balsamic, rye bread, carvones, seedy, carroty

Compatible essential oils for blending: Jasmine; cinnamon, cassia, and other spices; very overpowering, use in small doses

Safety data: Nontoxic, nonsensitizing (although sensitizing to skin if oxidized or old), nonirritant; store in a cool, dark spot with a tightly secured lid; avoid use on sensitive or damaged skin; avoid during pregnancy. Do not consume orally.

Perfume note: Top to middle

Principal chemical constituents: CAS No: 8000-42-8
beta-myrcene (0.2 to 1%), **dextro-limonene (35 to 50%),** beta-phellandrene (trace amount to 1%), *cis-* and *trans-*dihydrocarvone (0.3 to 2%), **dextro-carvone (45 to 60%)**, *cis-* and *trans* carveol (0.2 to 1%)

Subtle Connections

Colors: Yellow (*opposite: violet*), orange (*opposite: blue*)

Chakras: Solar plexus, sacral

Gemstones: Citrine (*opposite: amethyst*), carnelian (*opposite: lapis lazuli/ aquamarine*)

Energy: Yang, yin

Elements: Fire, earth

Actions and Uses

General actions: Antimicrobial, antiseptic, astringent, carminative, emmenagogue, expectorant, stimulant, tonic

Skin: Acne, boils, bruises, itchy scalp, wounds

Respiratory: Bronchitis, coughs, laryngitis

Potential psycho-emotional and spiritual support: Relieves dizziness, eases irritability and intolerance, eases mental strain and stress, eases fatigue, replenishes lost energy, stimulating, tonic to nerves, relieves vertigo, warming to emotions

CARDAMOM
(Elettaria cardamomum)

Geographical location: Cardamom is native to tropical Asia, especially southern India, Sri Lanka, Indonesia, Nepal, Pakistan, Bangladesh, and Bhutan, where it grows abundantly in forests at 2,500 to 5,000 feet (800 to 1,500 meters) above sea level. Cardamom is cultivated extensively in India, Sri Lanka, Laos, Guatemala, and El Salvador. It was historically imported and used in ancient Egypt to make perfumes. The main essential oil–producing countries are now Sri Lanka and Guatemala.

Plant description: A perennial, reedlike herb that grows up to 13 feet (4 meters) high, cardamom has long, silky, blade-shaped leaves. Its long sheathing stems bear small yellowish flowers with purple tips that produce pods of oblong, dark red to brown seeds. Cardamom seedpods are harvested by hand in autumn, just before they start to open; they are then dried in the sun. The seedpods are triangular in cross-section, spindle-shaped, and small, with a thin, papery outer shell; each pod contains up to twenty aromatic seeds. Cardamom plants are propagated from seed in autumn or by root division in spring and summer, in rich, moist, and well-drained soil, in shady locations. Cardamom is one of the oldest spices in the world and currently one of the most expensive, after vanilla and saffron. Cardamom has the same properties as ginger, which is in the same family, but it is less irritating. There are numerous related species that are used locally as spices and medicine, such as, for example, round or Siam cardamom (*Amomum cardamomum*), found in India and China. An essential oil is also produced from wild cardamom (*Elettaria cardamomum* var. *major*).

Botanical family: Zingiberaceae

Extraction method: Steam distillation from the dried, ripe fruit/seeds

Appearance of essential oil: Colorless to pale yellow liquid that becomes thicker and deeper yellow as it matures or ages

Odor of essential oil: Type: spicy; strength: medium; characteristics: warm, camphoraceous, medicinal, eucalyptus, sweet and spicy, warming, with a woody-balsamic undertone

Compatible essential oils for blending: Caraway, cedarwood, cinnamon, clove, cypress, frankincense, ginger, neroli, rose, ylang-ylang

Safety data: Nontoxic, nonirritant, nonsensitizing, although possibly sensitizing when applied to hypersensitive skin. 1,8-cineole presents a low risk of irritation or sensitization (Tisserand and Young 2014, 232). It is sometimes adulterated by the addition of 1,8-cineole, alpha-terpinol acetate, or linalyl acetate (Burfield 2003).

Perfume note: Middle to top

Principal chemical constituents: CAS No: 8000-66-6
alpha-pinene (1 to 2%), beta-pinene (trace amount to 0.4%), sabinene (2 to 4%), beta-myrcene (trace amount to 3%), limonene (3 to 7%), **1,8-cineole (23 to 45%),** gamma-terpinene (trace amount to 0.5%), para-cymene (trace amount to 1%), trans-thujenol (trace amount to 5%), linalool (2 to 7%), linalyl acetate (0.5 to 9%), terpinen-4-ol (1 to 4%), alpha-terpineol (0.3 to 7%), **terpenyl acetate (32 to 42%),** geraniol (0.3 to 2%), nerolidol (0.5 to 2%)

Subtle Connections

Color: Yellow (*opposite: violet*)

Chakra: Solar plexus

Gemstone: Citrine (*opposite: amethyst*)

Energy: Yin, yang

Elements: Earth, wood (air)

Actions and Uses

General actions: Antiseptic, antispasmodic, cephalic, digestive, nerve tonic, stimulant

Respiratory: Bronchitis, coughs

Muscles/joints: Arthritis

Potential psycho-emotional and spiritual support: Relieves mental fatigue, nervous tension, and exhaustion; uplifting, refreshing and invigorating, restorative (especially during recovery from illness)

CARROT SEED
(*Daucus carota*)

Geographical location: *Daucus carota* is native to Europe, southwest Asia, North Africa (Egypt, Morocco, Algeria, Tunisia), and tropical Africa (Eritrea, Ethiopia) and is naturalized in North America and Australia. The main essential oil–producing countries are France and Hungary.

Plant description: *Daucus carota* is a herbaceous annual (cultivated) and a biannual (wild). It has a small, inedible, tough, whitish root (cultivated species have edible, fleshy, orange taproots) with a stiff, hairy stem. It grows up to 3 feet (1 meter) high. The leaves are tripinnate, finely divided, and lacy, and the flowers are small and dull white, appearing in a cluster of flat, dense umbels, which are sometimes pink in bud and reddish at the center of the umbel. The seeds/fruits are flat and green. Note that the wild plant looks very similar to the deadly, poisonous hemlock! It is also known as wild carrot or Queen Anne's lace. Domestic (edible) carrots are produced from cultivars of the subspecies *Duacus carota* subsp. *sativus.*

Botanical family: Umbelliferae (Apiaceae)

Extraction method: Steam distillation of the dried fruit/seeds

Appearance of essential oil: Pale yellow to clear or straw-yellow to amber liquid

Odor of essential oil: Type: herbal; strength: high; characteristic: dry, carrotlike, sweet, fresh, cumin, spicy, green, woody, earthy, fungal-like, slightly herbaceous to slightly peppery at dry-out

Compatible essential oils for blending: Cedarwood, geranium, lavender, mandarin and other citrus oils, patchouli, rose, sandalwood, spice oils

Safety data: Nontoxic, nonsensitizing, nonirritating; avoid during pregnancy and breastfeeding. Do not consume orally.

Perfume note: Middle to top

Principal chemical constituents: CAS No: 8015-88-1

alpha-pinene (**0.5 to 12%**), sabinene (trace amount to 4%), beta-pinene (trace amount to 2%), myrcene (trace amount to 2%), limonene (trace amount to 2%), daucene (0.5 to 6%), beta-caryophyllene (0 to

6%), beta-1-cubenene (trace amount to 2%), (E)-alpha-bergamotene (0.5 to 3%), (E)-beta-farnesene (0.1 to 3%), gamma-muurolene (trace amount to 1%), (E)-alpha-farnesene (trace amount to 1%), **beta-bisabolene (1 to 65%),** cedrene oxide (trace amount to 1%), **carotol (19 to 74%)**

Subtle Connections
Colors: Orange (*opposite: blue*), yellow (*opposite: violet*)
Chakras: Sacral, solar plexus
Gemstones: Carnelian (*opposite: lapis lazuli/aquamarine*), citrine (*opposite: amethyst*)
Energy: Yin, yang
Element: Earth

Actions and Uses
General actions: Analgesic, antiarthritic, anti-infectious, anti-inflammatory, antioxidant (skin), antiviral, bactericidal, smooth muscle relaxant, tonic

Skin: Abscesses, acne, chapped and cracked skin, dermatitis, dry skin, eczema, mature skin, psoriasis; detoxifying; revitalizes and improves the appearance of skin and scar tissue

Respiratory: Aids chronic pulmonary conditions, bronchitis, and coughs; strengthens mucous membranes

Joints and muscles: Accumulation of toxins, arthritis

Digestive system (topical application): Colic, IBS, indigestion (inhalation or as an external applicaton in a compress or ointment or cream)

Immune system: Myalgic encephalomyelitis (ME), chronic fatigue syndrome, allergies

Potential psycho-emotional and spiritual support: Calms feeling of stress, confusion, and indecision; eases anxiety, apathy, and inability to move on; eases mental and emotional exhaustion; provides mental clarity; nervous system sedative; relaxant; revitalizing

CEDARWOOD ATLAS
(Cedrus atlantica)

Geographical location: This species of cedarwood is native to the Atlas mountains of Morocco (the Middle and High Atlas) and Algeria, where forests are comprised either purely of cedarwood or of a mixture of cedarwood, Algerian fir, oak, and *Acer* species. These forests are currently in decline due to overharvesting and environmental challenges (wildfires, pests, disease, drought), and thus cedars growing in this region are now classified as vulnerable, and in some areas endangered. Fortunately, extensive reforestation programs have been set up to protect and regenerate these ancient forests. Cedarwood Atlas is also referred to as Atlas cedar and Moroccan cedarwood. A related species, Port Orford cedar (*Chamaecyparis lawsoniana*), is distributed along the coast of California and Oregon and is also classified as a near-threatened species. Cedars classified as being of least concern include Himalayan cedar (*Cedrus deodora*), western red cedar (*Thuja plicata*), eastern white cedar (*Thuja occidentalis*), Texas cedar (*Juniperus ashei*), and Virginia cedar (*Juniperus virginiana*). (Texas and Virginia cedars belong to a different botanical family, Cupressaceae.) The main cedarwood essential oil–producing countries are China and the United States.

Plant description: *Cedrus atlantica* is a pyramid-shaped, cone-bearing evergreen tree with dark green, needlelike leaves that grow up to 115 to 131 feet (35 to 40 meters) high. The wood, which contains a high percentage of essential oil, is hard and durable and is used extensively as building material and to make furniture and tools. *Cedrus atlantica* is believed to have originated from Lebanon cedars (*Cedrus libani*), which grow wild in Lebanon and on the island of Cyprus. It is a close botanical relation to the Himalayan deodar cedarwood (*Cedrus deodora*), which produces a very similar essential oil.

Botanical family: Pinaceae

Extraction method: Steam distillation from the wood, stumps, and sawdust. A resinoid and absolute are also produced in small quantities.

Appearance of essential oil: Yellowish-amber to deep amber–tinted, viscous liquid

Odor of essential oil: Type: woody; strength: medium; characteristics: dry, woody, spicy, warm, herbaceous, with camphoraceous top notes and sweet, tenacious wood-balsamic undertones, with a mild wood dry-out scent

Compatible essential oils for blending: Bergamot, clary sage, cypress, frankincense, grapefruit, jasmine, juniper, neroli, rose, rosemary, vetivert, ylang-ylang

Safety data: Nonsensitizing, nontoxic, nonirritant (although may be irritant when used in high concentration). Avoid using during pregnancy.

Perfume note: Base

Principal chemical constituents: CAS No: 8023-85-6

A complex essential oil with numerous components, most of which are present in small quantities: **alpha-himachalene (10 to 17%), gamma-himachalene (6 to 11%), beta-himachalene (30 to 50%),** beta-cadinene (0.5 to 3%), alpha-cedrene (0.5 to 2%), alpha-curcumene (0 to 2%), trans-alpha-bisabolene (trace amount to 0.6%), beta-himachalene oxide (0 to 2%), deodarone (1 to 7%), isocedranol (1 to 3.5%), cubenol (0.5 to 3%), himachalol (0.5 to 4%), atlantone isomer (trace amount to .2%), alpha-atlantone (1 to 4%), beta-atlantone (0.1 to 2%), allo-himacholol (trace amount to 1%), (E)-alpha-atlantone (1 to 4%), deodarone (1 to 7%), isocedranol (1 to 3.5%), gamma-cadinene (1 to 2%), cedranone (0.5 to 2%), beta-calacorene (0.03 to 2%), beta-vetiverenen (0 to 1.5%), cadalene (0 to 1.5%)

Subtle Connections

Colors: Orange (*opposite: blue*), yellow (*opposite: violet*)

Chakras: Sacral, solar plexus

Gemstones: Carnelian (*opposite: lapis lazuli/aquamarine*), citrine (*opposite: amethyst*)

Energy: Yang, yin

Elements: Earth, water

Actions and Uses

General actions: Antiseptic, aphrodisiac, astringent, diuretic, expectorant, fungicidal, mucolytic, sedative, stimulant (circulatory), tonic

Skin: Acne, dandruff, dermatitis, eczema, fungal infections, greasy skin, skin eruptions, ulcers

Respiratory: Bronchitis, catarrh, coughs, respiratory infections

Joints and muscles: Arthritis

Immune system: Immune stimulant

Potential psycho-emotional and spiritual support: Aids meditation, calming, eases feelings of agitation, anger, anxiety, sense of disconnectedness, nervous tension, stress and stress-related conditions; instills feelings of peace and sense of connection; sedative

CHAMOMILE, GERMAN (BLUE)
(Matricaria recutita)

Geographical location: German chamomile is native to Europe and temperate Asia and was introduced to temperate North America and Australia. It grows near roads, around landfills, and in cultivated fields as a weed and is also cultivated, particularly in Hungary and eastern Europe. It is also known as Hungarian chamomile, wild chamomile, false chamomile, and scented mayweed. The main essential oil–producing countries are Germany, Morocco, the United Kingdom, and the United States.

Plant description: A strongly aromatic annual herb growing up to 24 inches (60 centimeters) tall, German chamomile has a smooth, erect, branching stem; delicate, feathery leaves; and simple, daisylike white flowers with a central yellow floret disk presented on a single stem. The German variety is similar in appearance to Roman chamomile, but the flower heads are smaller and have fewer petals. Under cultivation, the seeds are sown in spring or autumn, and the flower heads are picked in full bloom in summer—an expensive, time-consuming operation as the staggered blooming of German chamomile flowers means that the harvest has to be repeated over three to four weeks. There are numerous species of German chamomile, each producing an essential oil of varying composition; for example, Egyptian, German, Dutch, Brazilian, Bulgarian, and Finnish. The name is derived from the Greek *chamamelon,* which means "apple on the ground"—an accurate description, as when crushed or stood on the plant exudes an apple-like scent.

Botanical family: Asteraceae (Compositae)

Extraction method: Steam distillation of the flowering heads. Matricin, a sesquiterpene found in the plant, decomposes during this process to form the blue-colored compound chamazulene. An absolute is also produced in small quantities; it is deeper blue in color, with greater tenacity and fixative properties.

Appearance of essential oil: Deep greenish blue, turning to a deep inky blue and moderately viscous liquid

Odor of essential oil: Type: herbal; strength: high; characteristics: herbaceous, sweet, medicinal, phenolic, fruity, green, warm, intense, haylike, with warm, tobacco like dry-out notes

Compatible essential oils for blending: Bergamot, geranium, lavender, lemon, patchouli, petitgrain, rose

Safety data: Nontoxic, nonirritant, and nonsensitizing, although it may cause sensitization in some individuals; prone to oxidation if not stored in a cool, dark spot with a tightly secured lid. Poor-quality versions are sometimes adulterated with bisabolol and azulenes, which creates natural and synthetic mixtures. Use in moderation. A possible CYP2C9, CYP1A2, and CYP34A enzyme interaction or drug substrate inhibition can occur, although those interactions are seen mostly through oral ingestion (Tisserand and Young 2014, 58).

Perfume note: Middle

Principal chemical constituents: CAS No: 8002-66-2

A complex essential oil with numerous components, most of which are present in small quantities. There are various chemotypes of German chamomile, each identified by its predominant chemical—alpha-bisabolol, the farnesene, or chamuzulene. The following constituents relate to the farnesene chemotype: alpha-pinene (trace amount to 0.5%), beta-ocimene (0.2 to 2%), cis-beta-ocimene (trace amount to 0.3%), trans-beta-ocimene (trace amount to 2%), beta-caryophyllene (0 to 3%), **(E)-trans-beta-farnesene (40 to 58%), chamazulene (0 to 4%), germacrene (4 to 15%),** alpha-bisabolol (0.05 to 10%), delta-cadinene (0.1 to 6%), alpha-bisabolol oxide (2 to 5%)

Subtle Connections

Colors: Green (*opposite: red*), pink (*opposite: pale aqua-green*), blue (*opposite: orange*)

Chakras: Heart, throat

Gemstones: Aventurine (*opposite: jasper*), rose quartz (*opposite: aquamarine*), lapis lazuli/aquamarine (*opposite: carnelian*)

Energy: Yin

Elements: Water, metal (ether)

Actions and Uses

General actions: Analgesic, antiallergic, antiarthritic, anti-infectious, anti-inflammatory, antispasmodic, bactericidal, moderate fungicidal, skin-healing

Skin: Abscesses, acne rosacea, burns, chapped and cracked skin, dry skin/oily skin (balancing), infection, inflammation, psoriasis, puffiness; skin-healing (very effective when applied in low dose)

Respiratory: Asthma, catarrh, colds and flu, hay fever, mouth ulcers, teething, tonsillitis

Joints and muscles: Arthritis, inflamed joints, muscular aches and pain, neuralgia, rheumatism, sprains

Immune system: Immune stimulant

Digestive system (topical application): Colic, indigestion, nausea (effective with inhalation, compress, or ointment or cream)

Other: Headache, painful periods/PMS

Potential psycho-emotional and spiritual support: Calms stress, mental sedative (calms an active mind), nervous system sedative; eases depression and low mood, agitation, anger, anxiety, headaches caused by tension, hypersensitivity, impatience, insomnia, irritability and intolerance, mental exhaustion, migraine, mood swings

CHAMOMILE, ROMAN
(Chamaemelum nobile)

Geographical location: Native to southern and western Europe and naturalized in North America, Roman chamomile is also cultivated in England, Belgium, Hungary, Italy, France, North America, and

Argentina. The flowers are harvested as they begin to open in summer (June and July). Chamomile is a soothing herbal tea. Other common names include English chamomile, garden chamomile, ground apple, low chamomile, and whig plant. The main essential oil–producing countries are Germany, Morocco, the United Kingdom, and the United States.

Plant description: Roman chamomile is an aromatic perennial flowering plant growing from 10 to 20 inches (25 to 50 centimeters) high, with feathery, finely dissected bipinnate leaves and solitary, terminal, white, daisylike flower heads with a prominent central yellow disk. The flowers of Roman chamomile are larger than those of German chamomile.

Botanical family: Asteraceae (Compositae)

Extraction method: Steam distillation of the flowering heads

Appearance of essential oil: Pale blue to straw-yellow or transparent to bluish-green liquid

Odor of essential oil: Type: herbal; strength: high; characteristics: sweet, fruity (like ripe apple), herbaceous, green, spicy, woody, and cognac-like, with warm, tealike dry-out notes

Compatible essential oils for blending: Bergamot, clary sage, cypress, geranium, jasmine, lavender, lemon, neroli, petitgrain, rose

Safety data: Nontoxic, nonirritant, nonsensitizing; prone to oxidation if not stored appropriately (in a cool, dark spot with tightly secured lid). Poor-quality versions are sometimes adulterated with angelate and bisabolols (Tisserand and Young 2014, 245; Burfield 2003) or synthetic isobutyl angelate and bisabolols (Burfield 2003), so assure authenticity and purity with your essential oil supplier.

Perfume note: Middle to top

Principal chemical constituents: CAS No. 8015-92-7

A complex essential oil with numerous components, most of which are present in small quantities: **isobutyl angelate (0 to 38%), butyl angelate (0 to 35%), 3-methylpentyl angelate (0 to 23%), isobutyl isobutyrate (0 to 23%), isoamyl angelate (8 to 18%),** methyl angelate (0 to 14%), 2-methyl butyl angelate (3 to 7%), camphene (0 to 6%), borneol (0.5%), pinocarvone (2 to 7%), alpha-pinene (1 to 5%), alpha-terpinene (0 to 6%), chamazulene (0 to 5%), (E)-pinocarveol

(0 to 5%), alpha-thunene (0 to 4.5%), hexyl butyrate (0 to 4%),
terpinolene (0 to 4%), anthemol (0 to 3.5%), gamma-terpinene (0
to 3.5%), isoamyl isobutyrate (2.5 to 5%), delta-3-carene (0 to 3%),
isoamyl 2-methylbutyrate (0 to 3%), 2-methylbutyl 2-methylbutyrate
(0 to 3%), isoamyl butyrate (0 to 3%), beta-myrcene (0 to 2.5%), rho-
cymene (0 to 2%), beta-pinene (0 to 2%), isomyl methacrylate (0 to
2%), beta-phellandrene (0 to 2%), propyl angelate (0 to 1.5%)

Subtle Connections

Colors: Yellow (*opposite: violet*), green (*opposite: red*), pink (*opposite: pale aqua-green*), blue (*opposite: orange*)

Chakras: Solar plexus, heart, throat

Gemstones: Citrine (*opposite: amethyst*), aventurine (*opposite: jasper*), rose quartz (*opposite: aquamarine*), lapis lazuli/aquamarine (*opposite: carnelian*)

Energy: Yin, yang

Elements: Water, wood (air)

Actions and Uses

General actions: Analgesic, antiarthritic, anti-infectious, antineuralgic, antiseptic, antispasmodic, bactericidal, nerve sedative, skin-healing

Skin: Abscesses, acne, bruises, burns, chapped and cracked skin, dry skin/oily skin (balancing), eczema, dermatitis, itchy skin, psoriasis, puffiness, sensitive skin; toner, skin-healing

Respiratory: Asthma (especially nervous), mouth ulcers, teething

Joints and muscles: Antispasmodic; helps with neuralgia, arthritis, inflamed joints, muscular pain, sprains

Digestive system: Relieves IBS, colic, indigestion (topical/external application via compress, ointment, or cream; internal application via herbal tea, inhalation)

Immune system: Supports immune function

Endocrine system: Eases painful periods

Potential psycho-emotional and spiritual support: Eases agitation, anger, anxiety, depression and low mood; emotional sedative; calms fear, hyperactivity, hypersensitivity, insomnia, irritability, intolerance, impatience; mental sedative (calms an active mind); nervous-system sedative; eases nervous tension, panic attacks, stress, premenstrual tension, restlessness, solar plexus tension

CHASTE TREE
(Vitex agnus-castus)

Geographical location: Also known as vitex, chaste berry, Abraham's balm, lilac chaste tree, and monk's pepper, chaste tree is native to the Mediterranean region (especially Crete), as well as western Asia; it is cultivated and naturalized in warm-temperate and subtropical areas around the world. Crete is the main essential oil–producing country, and the oil is also produced in Turkey, Italy, Cyprus, Croatia, and China.

Plant description: A fragrant, deciduous shrub or tree growing from 3 to 16 feet (1 to 5 meters) high, chaste tree, or vitex, has palmate leaves composed of five or six entire leaflets and small, sweet-scented, white to pinkish-lilac to deep blue flowers arranged racemose in long, terminal spikes that produce small, fleshy, reddish-black fruit or berries. The ripe berries are collected in autumn.

Botanical family: Lamiaceae (formerly Verbenaceae)

Extraction method: Steam distillation or hydrodistillation of the fruits or leaves. Essential oil produced from the leaves has a milder affect compared to that from the berries.

Appearance of essential oil: Colorless to pale yellow, clear, mobile liquid

Odor of essential oil: Type: herbal; strength: medium; characteristics: cannabis-like and eucalyptusy top notes, with floral, warm, fresh, peppery, sweet, spicy body notes and lemonlike, woody undertones and dry-out notes

Compatible essential oils for blending: Geranium, lavender, mandarin, rose

Safety data: Nontoxic, nonirritating, nonsensitizing. The herb has been used with success for hundreds of years, but the essential oil is relatively new. It exhibits dopaminergic activity, lowers serum estrogen, and increases progesterone levels. Avoid during pregnancy and while breastfeeding, and also during menstruation (it may increase bleeding). May cause unpleasant side effects in some women. Also avoid in prepubescent children. There is a theoretical risk of interaction between chaste tree leaf oil and drugs metabolized by CYP2D6, an enzyme expressed in the liver and central nervous system (Tisserand and Young 2014, 247).

Perfume note: Middle

Principal chemical constituents: CAS No: 91722-47-3

Leaf oil: **1,8-cineole (10 to 36%), sabinene (5 to 17.5%),** alpha-pinene (1 to 15%), alpha-terpineol (1 to 10%), gamma-elemene (0 to 10%), beta-selinene (0 to 10%), beta-caryophyllene (2 to 10%), beta-farnesene (0 to 9%), citronellyl acetate (0.5 to 8%), citronellic acid (0 to 7%), dextro-limonene (0 to 5%), terpenen-4-ol (1 to 4%), beta-myrcene (0 to 4%), alpha-bisabolol (0 to 3%), (E)-beta-farnesene (0 to 3%), (E)-nerolidol (0 to 3%), beta pinene (0 to 3%), (Z)-beta-ocymene (0 to 2.5%), spathulenol (0 to 2%), (E)-dihydroterpineol (0 to 2%), gamma-terpenene (0.5 to2%), alpha-gurjunene (0.1 to 2%), guaiol (0 to 1.5%), manool (0 to 1.5%), alpha-guiaiene (0 to 1.5%), dodecane (0 to 1%), thymol (0 to 1%)

Subtle Connections

Colors: Orange (*opposite: blue*), yellow (*opposite: violet*)
Chakras: Sacral, solar plexus
Gemstones: Carnelian (*opposite: lapis lazuli*), citrine (*opposite: amethyst*)
Energy: Yin
Element: Metal (ether)

Actions and Uses

General actions: Antianxiety, antidepressant, emmenagogue, progesterone-like
Reproductive system: Menstrual and menopausal problems
Potential psycho-emotional and spiritual support: Eases anxiety and depression; calms erratic moods; eases premenstrual tension

CINNAMON LEAF/BARK
(Cinnamomum verum, C. zeylanicum)

Geographical location: This small evergreen tree is native to Sri Lanka (Ceylon) and India, where cinnamon grows in tropical forests at altitudes of up to 1,500 feet (500 meters), with numerous species cultivated throughout the tropical regions of the world, especially in the Philippines, West Indies, and Madagascar; each region grows its own particular species. The main *C. verum* and *C. zeylanicum* essential oil–producing countries are India (bark) and Sri Lanka (Ceylon cinnamon leaf and bark).

Plant description: A tropical evergreen tree that grows up to 49 feet (15 meters) high, cinnamon has a thick, scabrous bark; strong branches; young, speckled, greenish-orange shoots; leathery, shiny leaves; and small white flowers that produce oval, bluish-white berries. The leaves smell spicy when bruised. The tree is propagated from cuttings, and every second to third year the young trees are cut back to just above ground level during the rainy season. The bark is harvested from the many stump shoots; these are then left to ferment for twenty-four hours before being processed. The outer bark is scraped away to reveal the inner bark. Cassia (*Cinnamomum cassia*), known as Chinese cinnamon or false cinnamon, is native to China, where it is grown and cultivated, mainly as a spice (bark). Cassia essential oil contains up to 95% cinnamaldehyde and is not recommended for general aromatherapy use. *C. verum* and *C. zeylanicum* contain up to 2% cinnamaldehyde and a high quantity of eugenol (up to 88%); cinnamaldehyde is a strong dermal irritant, whereas eugenol is a relatively mild dermal irritant (Tisserand and Young 2014, 561). See safety data on the following page.

Botanical family: Lauraceae

Extraction method: Steam distillation of the leaves and twigs. Both the leaf and bark oils are used for their fragrant and antimicrobial properties (for example, in nasal sprays, cough medicine, and dental preparations). However, cinnamon bark essential oil is extremely irritating to the skin and mucous membranes and is not recommended for general aromatherapeutic use.

Appearance of essential oil: Yellow to yellowish-brown or brownish, clear, oily liquid

Odor of essential oil: Type: spicy; strength: medium; characteristics: woody, spicy, clove, cinnamon, with a warm but slightly harsh tone, and warm-spicy, clove-like dry-out notes.

Compatible essential oils for blending: Benzoin, clove, coriander, frankincense, ginger, grapefruit, lavender, mandarin, nutmeg, orange, petitgrain, ylang-ylang. Add oils high in monoterpenes, such as grapefruit and orange, to a blend to soften the scent and quell the irritant effect of eugenol and cinnamaldehyde.

Safety data (leaf oil): Relatively nontoxic, but a possible dermal irritant due to eugenol and cinnamaldehyde content (eugenol is irritant to mucous membranes); a sensitizer. Avoid using during pregnancy and while breastfeeding, and do not use on sensitive or damaged skin.

Safety data (bark oil): A dermal toxin, irritant, and sensitizer, and also irritant to the mucous membranes; may inhibit blood clotting; may interact with pethidine, a synthetic opioid pain medication found in antidepressent medications (SSRIs), and with anticoagulant medications. Use in moderation; may be adulterated by the addition of clove fractions such as eugenol or cinnamic aldehydes (Burfield 2003; Tisserand and Young 2014, 249).

Perfume note: Base to middle

Principal chemical constituents: CAS No: 8015-91-6

> *Leaf oil:* **eugenol (68 to 88%),** eugenyl acetate (1 to 8%), linalool (1.5 to 5%), (E)-cinnamyl acetate (0.5 to 4.5%), benzyl benzoate (trace amount to 4%), beta-caryophyllene (1.5 to 4%), (E)-cinnamaldehyde (0.5 to 2%), safrole (0 to 1.5%), cinnamyl alcohol (0 to 6%)

Subtle Connections

Colors: Orange (*opposite: blue*), yellow (*opposite: violet*)

Chakras: Sacral, solar plexus

Gemstones: Carnelian (*opposite: lapis lazuli/aquamarine*), citrine (*opposite: amethyst*)

Energy: Yang

Elements: Fire, earth

Actions and Uses

General actions: Analgesic, antibacterial, anti-infectious, anti-inflammatory, antimicrobial, antiseptic, antispasmodic, antiviral, aphrodisiac, astringent, carminative and digestive (topical application), emmenagogue, hemostatic, stimulant (cardiac, circulatory, respiratory)

Skin: Lice, tooth and gum infections/hygiene, wasp stings, insect bites

Respiratory system: Bronchitis, coughs, respiratory tract infections, sore throats

Immune system: Flu, infectious diseases, viral infections

Environmental diffusion: Antimicrobial

Potential psycho-emotional and spiritual support: Arouses senses and creativity; eases sense of isolation and emotional coldness, fear, and depression; relieves feelings of mental and emotional weakness, tension, and nervous exhaustion; stimulant; strengthening; addresses stress-related conditions

CITRONELLA
(Cymbopogon winterianus, C. nardus)

Geographical location: Native to Sri Lanka and Indonesia and now extensively cultivated throughout the tropics, including Africa and Central America, citronella is a grasslike plant whose leaves and stems produce an essential oil. The main essential oil–producing countries are China, Java, India, Indonesia, and Vietnam.

Plant description: Also known as citronella grass, fever grass, and silky head, this tall, erect, aromatic perennial grass probably developed from the wild-growing managrass found in Sri Lanka. The plant grows in bushes to about 6.6 feet (1 to 2 meters) high and has green to yellowish-green leaves and magenta-colored base stems with dense or loose clusters of reddish flowers. The leaves are narrow, long, and shiny; the dried leaves curl down at the base of the bush. There are a number of other related species of scented grass.

Botanical family: Poaceae (Gramineae)

Extraction method: Steam distillation of fresh or partially dried leaves. Java citronella (*C. winterianus*) yields twice as much essential oil as the Sri Lanka type (*C. nardus*).

Appearance of essential oil: Colorless to pale yellow (*C. winterianus*) to dark yellowish-brown (*C. nardus*) liquid

Odor of essential oil: Type: citrus; strength: medium; characteristics: fresh, sweet, geraniol, lemony, green, grassy-woody

Compatible essential oils for blending: Bergamot, cedarwood, geranium, grapefruit, lemon, lime, orange, pine

Safety data: Nontoxic; may cause sensitization or irritation (use in moderation); sometimes adulterated with lemongrass or *Eucalyptus citriodora* (lemon-scented gum). Do not use on sensitive or damaged skin.

Perfume note: Top to middle

Principal chemical constituents: CAS No: 8000-29-1

C. winterianus: dextro-limonene (3 to 4%), **citronellal (35 to 45%),** geranyl acetate (2 to 4%), laevo-citronellol (10 to 15%), **geraniol (22 to 24%),** elemol (2 to 4%)

C. nardus: **dextro-limonene (2 to 12%), citronellal (4 to 48%), geraniol (15 to 30%), laevo-citronellol (3 to 22%),** (E)-methyl isoeugenol (0 to 11%), camphene (7 to 10%), citronellyl acetate (0 to 7.5%), borneol (4 to 7%), elemol (1 to 5%), alpha-pinene (2 to 5%), geranyl formate (0 to 4.5%), beta-cubebene (0 to 4%), geranyl acetate (2 to 7%), beta-caryophyllene (0 to 4%), alpha-bergamotene (0 to 2.5%), (Z)-beta-ocimene (0 to 2.5%), isopulegol (0 to 2.5%), guatene (0 to 2%), (E)-beta-ocimene (0 to 2%), trans-methyleugenol (0 to 11%), delta-cadinene (0 to 2%), linalool (0.5 to 2%), tricylene (0 to 1.5%), geranyl butyrate (0 to 2%), alpha-cadinene (0 to 1.5%), (Z)-methyl isoeugenol (0 to 1.5%)

Subtle Connections

Colors: Orange (*opposite: blue*), yellow (*opposite: violet*)

Chakras: Sacral, solar plexus

Gemstones: Carnelian (*opposite: lapis lazuli/aquamarine*), citrine (*opposite: amethyst*)

Energy: Yin, yang

Elements: Earth, fire

Actions and Uses

General actions: Analgesic, anti-infectious, anti-inflammatory, antifungal, antimicrobial, antiseptic, antispasmodic, antiviral, bactericidal, deodorant, diuretic, emmenagogue, febrifuge (fever-reducing), insecticide, tonic

Skin: Excessive perspiration, oily skin and hair

Immune system: Colds, flu, minor infections

Potential psycho-emotional and spiritual support: Clearing and uplifting; eases feelings of depression, fatigue, headaches, migraine, and neuralgia

CLOVE BUD
(Syzygium aromaticum, Eugenia caryophyllus)

Geographical location: Native to the Moluccas Islands, Indonesia, and the southern Philippines, the clove tree is now extensively grown in India, Pakistan, Sri Lanka, Zanzibar, Tanzania, Brazil, and Madagascar. The main essential oil–producing countries are Brazil, Indonesia, Madagascar, Sri Lanka, and Tanzania.

Plant description: A slender evergreen tree that grows up to 39 feet (12 meters) high, clove has a smooth, gray trunk and strongly aromatic, smooth, bright green, shiny leaves that are arranged in pairs on short stalks. At the start of the rainy season, long, tiny, highly aromatic buds appear with a yellow to rosy-pink corolla at the tip that turns fiery red over time (the buds are not allowed to mature and blossom). The buds are picked twice a year and dried in the sun, during which time they turn deep reddish brown. The tree is grown from seed in spring or from semiripe cuttings in the summer.

Botanical family: Myrtaceae

Extraction method: Steam distillation of dried flower buds, leaves, or stalks and stems

Appearance of essential oil: *Bud:* colorless to pale yellow liquid (favored in perfumery); *leaf:* dark brown liquid; *stalk and stems:* pale yellow to light brown liquid

Odor of essential oil: Type: spice; strength: medium; characteristics: *bud:* fresh, fruity top note, sweet, spicy, balsamic, woody, minty, phenolic, with warm, spicy, woody dry-out notes; *leaf:* spicy, aromatic, woody, balsamic, minty, peppery, phenolic, and powdery, with clove-like dry-out notes; *stalks and stems:* spicy, aromatic, woody, minty, fatty, phenolic, and powdery, with clove-like dry-out notes

Compatible essential oils for blending: Bergamot, clary sage, grapefruit, lavender, mandarin, orange, rose

Safety data: All clove oils can cause skin and mucous-membrane irritation and sensitization (moderate risk). Do not use on hypersensitive, diseased, or damaged skin. Oil may cause dermatitis, inhibit blood clotting, or interact with pethidine, a synthetic opioid pain medication, and anticoagulant medications (Tisserand and Young 2014, 256). Clove bud is considered the least irritant/sensitizing. Use in moderation.

Perfume note: Base

Principal chemical constituents: CAS No: 8000-34-8

Bud oil: **eugenol (75 to 97%),** beta-caryophyllene (0.5 to 12.5%), eugenyl acetate (0.5 to 15%), alpha-caryophyllene (0 to 1.5%), alpha-humulene (0 to 0.7%), delta-cadinene (0 to 0.25%), calamenene (0 to 0.11%), caryophyllene oxide (0 to 0.35%), chavicol (0 to 0.15%), methyleugenol (0 to 0.05%)

Subtle Connections

Colors: Orange (*opposite: blue*), yellow (*opposite: violet*)

Chakras: Sacral, solar plexus

Gemstones: Carnelian (*opposite: lapis lazuli/aquamarine*), citrine (*opposite: amethyst*)

Energy: Yang

Elements: Fire, earth

Actions and Uses

General actions: Analgesic, antiarthritic, antibiotic, antifungal, anti-irritant, antineuralgic, antimicrobial, antioxidant, antiseptic, antispasmodic, antiviral, carminative, stimulant

Skin: Acne, athlete's foot and fungal infections, bruises, insect repellent, toothache and nerve pain, wounds, burns, ulcers (used in low dose only)

Respiratory: Asthma, bronchitis, mouth ulcers, respiratory tract infections

Muscles/joints: Arthritis

Immune system: Herpes, shingles, viral infections

Environmental diffusion: Antimicrobial

Potential psycho-emotional and spiritual support: Aids memory and recall; aphrodisiac (impotence, frigidity); eases depression, mental and emotional fatigue, headaches, lethargy, and tension; general stimulant; stimulates mental functions; uplifting

CORIANDER
(Coriandrum sativum)

Geographical location: Native to the Mediterranean, regions of the Middle East, and western Asia and Africa, this herb, the leaf of which is commonly known as cilantro, is naturalized in North America and cultivated throughout the world. The main essential oil–producing countries are India, Russia, Morocco, Canada, Bulgaria, Romania, and Ukraine; smaller producers include Iran, Turkey, Israel, Egypt, South Africa, the United Kingdom, Poland, the Netherlands, China, Canada, the United States, Argentina, and Mexico.

Plant description: A strongly aromatic annual herb growing to about 20 inches (50 centimeters) in height, the coriander plant has bright-green, delicate leaves that are variable in shape and broadly lobed at the base of the plant. The upper leaves of the plant are finely cut and feathery and appear higher on the flowering stem, and it produces umbels of small white or very pink flowers, followed by a mass of rounded green (turning brown) seeds in beige seed coats. The seeds are gathered when ripe in late summer.

Botanical family: Apiaceae (Umbelliferae)

Extraction method: Steam distillation of crushed, ripe seeds. Cilantro essential oil, produced from fresh and dried leaves, contains a high proportion of decyl adehyde (decanal).

Appearance of essential oil: *Seed:* colorless to straw-colored or pale yellow liquid; *leaf:* colorless to pale yellow clear liquid

Odor of essential oil: *Seed type:* spice; strength: medium; characteristics: fresh, sweet, floral, herbal, rosewoody, woody-spicy, blueberry, green, terpenic. *Leaf type:* green; strength, medium; characteristics: green, fatty, aldehydic, citruslike, with brown (woody-nutty) herbal nuances

Compatible essential oils for blending: *Seed:* Bergamot, cinnamon, citronella, clary sage, cypress, frankincense, grapefruit, ginger, jasmine, lemongrass, neroli, petitgrain, pine, sandalwood, lemon-scented tea tree. *Leaf:* Basil, bergamot, black pepper, clary sage, coriander, geranium, lemon, marjoram, tea tree, ylang ylang

Safety data: Nontoxic, nonirritant, possible sensitization on sensitive or damaged skin; cross-sensitivity reported with fennel and anise; may be adulterated with natural or synthetic linalool. Cilantro is an irritant when applied to skin (Tisserand and Young 2014, 260).

Perfume note: Top to middle

Principal chemical constituents: CAS No: 8008-52-4

Seed: **linalool (55 to 88%), alpha-pinene (3 to 11%),** gamma-terpinene (0 to 10%), beta-pinene (1 to 9%), para-cymene (0 to 9%), beta-myrcene (0.5 to 1.5%), terpinolene (trace amount to 1%), camphor (0 to 8%), geraniol (0 to 6%), camphene (trace amount to 4.5%), dextro-limonene (2 to 5%), geranyl acetate (0 to 3.5%), terpinen-4-ol (trace amount to 3%), alpha-terpineol (0.5 to 2.5%)

Leaf: **linalool (0 to 30%), decanal (3 to 20%), (E)-2-decanal (1 to 46%), (E)-2-decen-1-ol (0 to 24%), 1-decanol (2 to 36%),** (*E*)-2-undecenal (0 to 6%), (*E*)-2-dodecen-1-ol (0 to 18%), (*E*)-2-tetradecenal (0 to 13%), (*E*)-2-pentadecenal (0 to 5%)

Subtle Connections

Colors: Orange (*opposite: blue*), yellow (*opposite: violet*), green (*opposite: red*), pink (*opposite: pale aqua-green*)

Chakras: Sacral, solar plexus, heart

Gemstones: Carnelian (*opposite: lapis lazuli/aquamarine*), citrine (*opposite: amethyst*), aventurine (*opposite: jasper*), rose quartz (*opposite: aquamarine*)

Energy: Yang, yin

Elements: Fire, earth

Actions and Uses

General actions: Analgesic, antiarthritis, antimicrobial, antioxidant, antispasmodic, aphrodisiac, bactericidal, carminative, digestive, fungicidal, stimulant (cardiac, circulatory, nervous system)

Joints and muscles: Arthritis, neuralgia, muscle aches and pains
Immune system: Colds, flu, infections, viruses (measles)
Digestive system: Eases digestive discomfort (topical application)
Potential psycho-emotional and spiritual support: Aids and restores memory and recall; eases debility, nervous exhaustion, insomnia, migraine, shock; a mental stimulant (gentle)

CYPRESS
(Cupressus sempervirens)

Geographical location: This coniferous tree or shrub is native to northern Persia, Syria, Turkey, Cypress, and the Greek islands and was introduced by the Romans to Europe, where it became naturalized in eastern Mediterranean regions (it is also known as Mediterranean cypress), northeast Libya, southern Albania, Greece, Crete, Italy, northern Europe, Lebanon, Israel, Malta, and Jordan, as well as Great Britain. Other cypress family members are found in the United States and Canada, including western red cedar (*Thuja plicata*) and Monterey cypress (*Hesperocyparis macrocarpa*). Western red cedar has a high thujone content (60 to 85%), and Monterey cypress has a high carvacrol content (68 to 90%); neither of these constituents is found in *Cupressus sempervirens*. Cypress is famous for its longevity—some trees are a thousand years old! Other common names include Italian cypress, Tuscan cypress, graveyard cypress, and pencil pine.

Plant description: This statuesque, cone-shaped tree is a medium-sized coniferous evergreen growing up to 115 feet (35 meters) tall. It possesses dense, dark green foliage sprays with tiny, dark green, needlelike leaves. The small flowers produce oblong or ovoid seed cones (both male and female) that are initially green but turn brown when mature, up to two years after pollination. Many cypress species produce essential oil; however, *C. sempervirens* essential oil is considered to be of superior quality. The main essential oil–producing countries are France and Spain.

Botanical family: Cupressaceae
Extraction method: Steam distillation of twigs and needles, and sometimes cones

Appearance of essential oil: Colorless to pale yellow to green-tinted liquid

Odor of essential oil: Type: terpenic; strength: medium; characteristics: fresh, pine, woody, earthy, dry, spicy, cedar-like, and gently camphoraceous, with sweet, balsamic dry-out notes.

Compatible essential oils for blending: Benzoin, bergamot, cardamom, cedarwood, chamomile (Moroc and Roman), clary sage, frankincense, juniper, lavender, lemon, mandarin, marjoram, orange, pine, sandalwood, spikenard, lemon-scented tea tree

Safety data: The oil is nontoxic, nonirritant, and nonsensitizing, although it can be sensitizing when oxidized, so be sure to include antioxidant ingredients such as avocado oil, vitamin E oil, or cold-pressed carrot seed oil and carrot seed essential oil to a cypress blend that you intend to store. Sometimes cypress oil is adulterated with cheap, nature-identical synthetics such as alpha-pinene, delta-3-carene, and beta-myrcene (Burfield 2003); assure authenticity and purity with your essential oil supplier.

Perfume note: Middle

Principal chemical constituents: CAS No: 8013-86-3

alpha-pinene (20 to 53%), delta-3-carene (15 to 22%), cedrol (1 to 7%), alpha-terpinyl acetate (0 to 6.5%), alpha-terpinolene (2 to 6.5%), dextro-limonene (2 to 6%), beta-pinene (0.5 to 3%), sabinene (0.5 to 3%), germacrene (0 to 2%), beta-myrcene (2 to 4%), delta-cadinene (0.5 to 3%), terpineol acetate (2 to 5%), terpinen-4-yl-acetate (1 to 3%), alpha-terpineol (0.5 to 2%), rho-cymene (0 to 1.5%), gamma-terpinene (0.2 to 2%), terpinen-4-ol (1 to 3.5%), borneol (trace amount to 1%)

Subtle Connections

Colors: Yellow (*opposite: violet*), green (*opposite: red*), pink (*opposite: pale aqua-green*)

Chakras: Solar plexus, heart

Gemstones: Citrine (*opposite: amethyst*), aventurine (*opposite: jasper*), rose quartz (*opposite: aquamarine*)

Energy: Yin

Elements: Water, metal (ether)

Actions and Uses

General actions: Antiarthritic, anti-infectious, anti-inflammatory, antiseptic, antispasmodic, antitussive (cough-relieving), astringent, bactericidal, deodorant, mucolytic

Skin: Dry and oily skin (balancing), mature skin, perspiration (excessive), puffiness

Respiratory system: Asthma, bronchitis, colds, flu, dry throat, hoarseness, laryngitis, pulmonary infections, sinusitis, sore throat, spasmodic cough, upper respiratory-tract infections and pain, whooping cough

Joints and muscles: Aching muscles, arthritis, muscle cramps, muscular aches and pains

Circulatory system: Addresses blood-pressure problems (helps the body with regulation, but do not use if taking medication) and poor circulation

Immune system: Immune stimulant

Other: Eases painful periods/PMS (but note that cypress may encourage bleeding)

Potential psycho-emotional and spiritual support: Relieves confusion and indecision, dwelling on unpleasant events; eases anger, anxiety, fear, grief, bereavement, impatience, uncontrolled crying; shifts inability to move on, feeling stuck, irritability and intolerance, lack of concentration; eases nervous tension, premenstrual tension; regulates autonomic nervous system; sedative; eases stress and stress-related conditions

EUCALYPTUS
(Eucalyptus globulus)

Geographical location: Native to Australia, Tasmania, and surrounding islands, as well as New Guinea and Indonesia, this tree is also known as blue gum. Just fifteen species grow outside of Australia. It is propagated widely in tropical and temperate areas, including North, South, and Central America (particularly California), as well as Europe, Africa, the Mediterranean, the Middle East, China, and the Indian subcontinent. Planting eucalyptus can cause ecological problems because these trees absorb huge quantities of water and prevent the growth of native plants; in some instances, however, this can be beneficial, as they dry up marshy areas in the process. Due to their high 1,8-cineole content, which easily becomes gaseous and highly flammable when hot, eucalyptus trees can cause devastating wildfires. The main essential oil–producing countries are Australia, Austria, Brazil, China, India, Paraguay, Portugal, South Africa, and Spain.

Plant description: *Eucalyptus* is a diverse genus of flowering trees and shrubs. *E. globulus* is a tall evergreen tree growing up to 295 feet (90 meters) in height. The young trees have bluish-green, oval leaves, and the mature trees develop long, narrow, yellowish leaves, creamy-white flowers, and a smooth, pale gray bark that is often covered with a white powder. The leaves are harvested for essential oil. Of the 700 different species of eucalyptus, at least 500 produce a type of essential oil. They are classified into three groups or categories: medicinal oils, industrial oils, and perfumery oils. Because there are so many species, the oils are easy to muddle, mix up, or adulterate.

Botanical family: Myrtaceae

Extraction method: Distillation of freshly or partially dried leaves and young twigs

Appearance of essential oil: Colorless to pale yellow (turning darker yellow with age) mobile liquid

Odor of essential oil: Type: herbal; strength: high; characteristics: herbal, eucalyptus, camphoraceous, medicinal, with a woody undertone

Compatible essential oils for blending: Cedarwood, geranium, grapefruit, lavender, lemon, marjoram, peppermint, pine, rosemary, thyme

Safety data: Applied topically, this oil is nontoxic, nonirritant, and nonsensitizing. However, it can cause central nervous system and breathing problems in young children (due to 1,8-cineole). *Safety note:* When taken internally, eucalyptus is highly toxic; ingesting as little as 4–5 ml has been reported as being fatal. This oil must be kept out of the reach of children (Tisserand and Young 2014, 273).

Perfume note: Top

Principal chemical constituents: CAS No: 8000-48-4

1,8-cineole (60 to 85%), alpha-pinene (3 to 17%), beta-pinene (0 to 1%), dextro-limonene (1.5 to 9%), globulol (trace amount to 6%), (E)-pinocarveol (2 to 5%), pinocarvone (0.1 to 1%), beta-caryophyllene (0 to 1%), para-cymene (0.1 to 3.5%), aromadendrene (0.1 to 4.5%), pinocarvone (trace amount to 1%), geranial (0 to 1%)

Subtle Connections

Colors: Yellow (*opposite: violet*), green (*opposite: red*), pink (*opposite: pale aqua-green*)

Chakras: Solar plexus, heart

Gemstones: Citrine (*opposite: amethyst*), aventurine (*opposite: jasper*), rose quartz (*opposite: aquamarine*)

Energy: Yin, yang

Elements: Metal (ether), earth

Actions and Uses

General actions: Analgesic, anti-infectious, antimicrobial, antineuralgic, antiseptic, antispasmodic, antiviral, cicatrizant, decongestant, deodorant, stimulant

Skin: Blisters, burns, cuts, herpes, insect bites, insect repellent, lice, skin infections, shingles (with geranium and peppermint), wounds

Respiratory system: Asthma, bronchitis, catarrh, coughs, sinusitis, throat infections

Immune system: Immune stimulant; flu, viral infections, microbial infections

Potential psycho-emotional and spiritual support: Aids concentration; bracing; clears head; eases fatigue and debility; assists in moving on from past trauma; soothes neuralgia, headaches

FENNEL
(Foeniculum vulgare)

Geographical location: This flowering plant species in the carrot family is native to the Mediterranean region, where it is found growing along roadsides and in pastures in many regions, extending from coastal and inland to mountain areas. It has been naturalized in the United States, southern Canada, Bulgaria, Germany, Greece, France, Italy, and much of Asia and Australia. The main essential oil–producing countries are Hungary, France, Spain, and the United States.

Plant description: An aromatic biennial or perennial herb, fennel grows from 5 to 6 feet (1.5 to 2.5 meters) high. It is an erect plant with hollow stems and feathery, finely dissected leaves with threadlike ultimate segments (filiform), which are similar in appearance to those of dill, although thinner. The flowers are produced in terminal compound umbels (2 to 6 inches, or 5 to 15 cm wide), with each umbel consisting of twenty to fifty tiny, golden-yellow flowers on short pedicels. There are two main varieties of fennel: bitter or common fennel, which is slightly taller with less divided leaves (occurs in a cultivated or wild form), and sweet fennel, also known as Roman, garden, or French fennel, a variety that is always cultivated. There are many cultivated varieties; *F. vulgare* is closely related to Florence fennel (*F. axoricum*). The flowers produce dry, grooved seeds, 4 to 10 mm long and half as wide. The seeds are gathered in the autumn.

Botanical family: Apiaceae (Umbelliferae)

Extraction method: Distillation of crushed seeds (or in the case of bitter fennel, the seeds or the whole herb)

Appearance of essential oil: Colorless to pale yellow liquid (both sweet and bitter fennel)

Odor of essential oil: Type: anise; strength: medium; *characteristics, sweet fennel:* very sweet, earthy, anise-like, green, peppery, herbal, spicy, with warm, aniseed-like dry-out notes; *characteristics, bitter fennel:* sharp, warm, camphoraceous

Compatible essential oils for blending: Geranium, lavender, rose, sandalwood

Safety data: Nonirritant, nonsensitizing, and relatively nontoxic, although prone to rapid oxidation, particularly if not stored correctly, rendering the oil potentially sensitizing; may be adulterated with monoterpene hydrocarbons such as limonene and synthetic anethole, which contain more toxic (Z)-isomers. Bitter fennel is sometimes passed off as sweet fennel (Burfield 2003). Fennel is potentially carcinogenic due to its estragole content and may inhibit blood clotting. There is a possible drug interaction in the presence of hormone modulation. Do not use during pregnancy or breastfeeding, or in presence of estrogen-dependent cancers or endometriosis. Use very moderately. Do not use bitter fennel on the skin, although bitter fennel is considered medicinally superior to sweet fennel, according to Tisserand and Young (2014, 277).

Perfume note: Top to middle

Principal chemical constituents: CAS No: 8006-84-6

Sweet fennel: **trans-anthole (55 to 74%),** limonene (0.5 to 21%), fenchone (2 to 8%), estragole (1 to 5%), alpha-pinene (0.1 to 8.5%), alpha-phellandrene (0.1 to 2.0%), cis-anethole (trace amount to 7%)

Bitter fennel: alpha-phellandrene (0.3 to 13%), alpha-pinene (trace to 19%), **anethole (47 to 85%),** estragole (2 to 9%), **fenchone (3 to 24%),** dextro-limonene (0.5 to 10%)

Subtle Connections

Color: Yellow (*opposite: violet*)
Chakra: Solar plexus
Gemstone: Citrine (*opposite: amethyst*)
Energy: Yin
Elements: Metal (ether), earth

Actions and Uses

General actions: Analgesic (mild), antiarthritic, antifungal, anti-infectious, anti-inflammatory, antimicrobial, antiseptic, antispasmodic, antiviral, bactericidal, carminative, detoxifying, diuretic, emmenagogue, expectorant, immune-boosting, laxative, splenic, stimulant (circulatory), stomachic, tonic

Skin: Bruises; dull or oily, mature complexions

Joints and muscles: Arthritis, edema, pain (slightly analgesic)

Respiratory system: Asthma, bronchitis

Digestive system: Constipation, flatulence, nausea (topical application only; use compress, cream, lotions, gel, vegetable oil); steam inhalation

Potential psycho-emotional and spiritual support: Gives courage and instills a sense of protection; eases nervous tension and stress; tonic to nerves

FRANKINCENSE / OLIBANUM
(Boswellia carteri, B. sacra, B. neglecta)

Geographical location: The aromatic, resinous trees in the *Boswellia* genus are native to the Red Sea region (Egypt, Sudan, Eritrea, Saudi Arabia, and Yemen), Somalia, Oman, parts of India, and Pakistan. It grows in desert-woodland areas, on rocky limestone slopes and gullies, particularly along the southern coastal mountains of the Arabian Peninsula, Somalia, Ethiopia, Southeast Asia, India, Sri Lanka, and China. The species vary from region to region. The main essential oil–producing countries are China, India, Kenya, Saudi Arabia, and Somalia.

Plant description: This small tree has a papery, peeling bark and tangled branches with abundant leaves at the end. The oleo gum resin is extracted from the living tree by tapping the tree trunk via incisions made in the bark; yellow-tinted, golden, or amber-brown exudes are left to dry, then removed. Distillation of the dried exudes takes place in Europe, Somalia, Yemen, and India. Dried exudes have been used as ceremonial incense in churches and temples (smoldered or smoked) and in indigenous rituals for thousands of years. The trees are endangered in some areas due to overharvesting of the oleo gum resin, thereby reducing the reproductive capacity of the trees, so ensure that your essential-oil supplier obtains their essential oil from a sustainable source.

Botanical family: Burseraceae

Extraction method: Steam distillation of the dried oleo gum resin

Appearance of essential oil: Colorless to pale amber, yellow, or greenish clear liquid

Odor of essential oil: Type: terpenic; strength: medium; characteristics: fresh, terpenic, lemony, green, resinous, with persistent, balsamic-herbaceous dry-out notes

Compatible essential oils for blending: Basil, bergamot, black pepper, geranium, grapefruit, lavender, mandarin, neroli, orange, petitgrain, pine, sandalwood, spikenard, vetivert

Safety data: Nontoxic, nonirritant, nonsensitizing (although it can be sensitizing when oxidized, so be sure to include antioxidant ingredients such as avocado oil, vitamin E oil, or cold-pressed carrot seed oil and carrot seed essential oil when blending). Some frankincense essential oils are derived from a mixture of resins or oils from various species (Tisserand and Young 2014, 288).

Perfume note: Base to middle

Principal chemical constituents: CAS No: 8016-36-2

B. neglecta: **alpha-thujene (14 to 20%), alpha-pinene (16 to 54%),** sabinene (1 to 3%), beta-pinene (0.5 to 1%), delta-3-carene (0.1 to 4%), **rho-cymene (5 to 10%),** limonene (1 to 3%), **terpinene-4-ol (5 to 13%),** alpha-terpineol (0.5 to 2%), alpha-copene (trace to 1%)

B. carti/sacra (a very complex oil with over 170 consitituents): **alpha-pinene (10 to 55%),** camphene (0 to 2%), sabinene (0 to 6%), beta-pinene (0 to 10%), delta-3-carene (0 to 5%), **beta-myrcene (0 to 21%), alpha-phellandrene (0 to 42%),** sabinene (0 to 6%), **limonene (6 to 22%),** rho-cymene (0 to 8%), terpinen-4-ol (0.4 to 7%), verbenone (trace to 6.5%), beta-caryophyllene (0 to 8%), linalool (0 to 6%) alpha-thujene (0 to 5%), delta-cadinene (0 to 2.5%), thujole (0 to 1.5%), 1,8-cineole (0 to 1%)

Subtle Connections

Colors: Yellow (*opposite: violet*), green (*opposite: red*), pink (*opposite: pale aqua-green*)

Chakras: Solar plexus, heart, crown

Gemstones: Citrine (*opposite: amethyst*), aventurine (*opposite: jasper*), rose quartz (*opposite: aquamarine*), sugalite (*opposite: carnelian*)

Energy: Yin, yang

Elements: Metal (ether), fire, earth

Actions and Uses

General actions: Antifungal, anti-inflammatory, antimicrobial (mild), antiseptic, antiviral, astringent, bactericidal, cicatrizant, expectorant, toner

Skin: Burns, dermatitis, eczema, mature skin, dry skin (balancing), oily skin, scars (toning), wound care

Respiratory system: Asthma, catarrh, colds, coughs, flu, laryngitis, bronchitis, sore throat, upper respiratory-tract infections; eases shortness of breath, calms breathing, encourages deep breathing

Circulatory system: Helps the body regulate blood pressure

Immune system: Chronic fatigue syndrome, myalgic encephalomyelitis; general immune stimulant

Other: PMS, menopausal problems

Potential psycho-emotional and spiritual support: Eases confusion, indecision, inability to move on, dwelling on unpleasant events; eases anger, anxiety, depression, low mood, fear, grief, bereavement; eases end-of-life agitation; helps in letting go of unwanted thoughts and memories; calms hyperactivity, impatience, insomnia, irritability, and intolerance; balances mood swings; relieves nervous tension, panic attacks (calms and relaxes breathing), premenstrual tension, feelings of resentment and disappointment, sadness, and despair; sedative; eases stress and stress-related conditions; supports meditation and finding inner tranquility

GALBANUM
(Ferula gummosa)

Geographical location of growth: Indigenous to Persia (Iran) and to other countries in the Middle East and western Asia, this plant grows abundantly on mountain slopes and the desert in northern Iran and is also cultivated in Afghanistan, Madagascar, Lebanon, and Turkey. Iran is the main producer of the essential oil.

Plant description: This is a large perennial herb with a smooth, hollow stem; shiny, finely toothed or serrated compound ovate leaflets; and umbels of small white flowers. The whole plant contains a milky-white juice produced in resinous ducts, which exudes from the base of the stem when cut down. Incisions made in the harvested roots makes the most of this juice, which hardens into a translucent white or sometimes light brown, yellowish, or greenish-yellow resinous tears or lumps that are waxy in texture—soft when warm, brittle when cold. Distillation is undertaken in Europe and America.

Botanical family: Apiaceae (Umbelliferae)

Extraction method: Steam distillation of the oleo gum resin

Appearance of essential oil: Clear to yellowish-brown or olive-tinted liquid

Odor of essential oil: Type: green; strength: high; characteristics: fresh, green, earthy, rooty, woody, balsamic, metallic, with balsamic agrestic to dry-earthy and spicy dry-out notes

Compatible essential oils for blending: Sweet, rich, floral oils such as jasmine, rose, and ylang-ylang; also frankincense, geranium, lavender, and pine

Safety data: Nontoxic, nonirritant (when diluted, but potentially very irritating when undiluted), nonsensitizing (although can be sensitizing when oxidized, so be sure to include antioxidant ingredients such as avocado oil, vitamin E oil, or cold-pressed carrot seed oil and carrot seed essential oil to a galbanum blend that you intend to store)

Perfume note: Top

Principal chemical constituents: CAS No: 8023-91-4
beta-pinene (40 to 60%), delta-3-carene (3 to 10%), alpha-pinene (5 to 12%), sabinene (0 to 7%), beta-myrcene (0 to 5%), dextro-limonene (2 to 5%), gamma-elemene (0 to 3%), 1,3,5,-undercatriene (1 to 3%), (Z)-beta-ocimene (0 to 2%), guaiol (0 to 2%)

Subtle Connections

Colors: Yellow (*opposite: violet*), green (*opposite: red*), pink (*opposite: pale aqua-green*)

Gemstones: Citrine (*opposite: amethyst*), aventurine (*opposite: jasper*), rose quartz (*opposite: aquamarine*)

Chakras: Solar plexus, heart

Energy: Yang, yin

Elements: Earth, metal (ether)

Actions and Uses

General actions: Analgesic, antiarthritic, anti-infectious, anti-inflammatory, antimicrobial, antispasmodic, astringent, decongestant, expectorant, restorative, skin-healing

Skin: Abscesses, acne, boils, mature skin, pimples, psoriasis, scars; tones the skin

Respiratory system: Asthma, bronchial spasms, catarrh, chronic coughs, colds, flu, mucus congestion

Joints and muscles: Arthritis; improves circulation, eases muscular pain

Other: Painful periods, menopausal symptoms

Potential psycho-emotional and spiritual support: Balancing, both sedative and stimulant; calming; eases anxiety, depression, low mood, erratic moods; calms nervous tension, premenstrual tension, and menopausal symptoms; restorative to the nerves; eases stress and stress-related conditions; tonic, uplifting

GERANIUM
(Pelargonium graveolens, P. x asperum)

Geographical location: This popular flowering plant is native to South Africa and widely cultivated in Russia, Egypt, the Democratic Republic of the Congo, Morocco, Madagascar, Japan, Central America, Europe (Spain, Italy, and France), and China. The main essential oil–producing countries are Egypt and China, and to a lesser extent, South Africa and Morocco.

Plant description: There are more than 250 named species (mostly cultivated for ornamental purposes), but only *P. graveolens* and *P. x asperum* are used for essential oil extraction. Rose geranium (*P. graveolens* var. *roseum*) was originally derived from the Bourbon geranium cultivar (*P. graveolens* var. *bourbon*), grown in Réunion, France; the essential oil from this species is now only produced in very small quantities, so it is rare. *Pelargonium* x *asperum* is a cross between *P. capitatum* and *P. radens.* These are hairy perennial shrubs that grow up to 3 feet (1 meter) high, with pointed leaves that are serrated at the edges and small pink flowers. The whole plant is aromatic. It is also known as rose geranium and rose-scented geranium. The cultivated plants are harvested twice a year for essential oil extraction, in the spring and late autumn.

Botanical family: Geraniaceae

Extraction method: Steam distillation of the leaves and stalks

Appearance of essential oil: Pale yellow to golden yellowish-green liquid. (By comparison, Bourbon geranium is a greenish-olive liquid.)

Odor of essential oil: Type: floral; strength: medium; characteristics: rich, floral, roselike, sweet, and minty, with a hint of lemon and greens, finishing with green and roselike dry-out notes

Compatible essential oils for blending: Bergamot, carrot seed, clove, frankincense, galbanum, grapefruit, jasmine, lavender, lemongrass, mandarin, neroli, patchouli, petitgrain, Roman chamomile, rose, sandalwood, tea tree

Safety data: Nontoxic, nonirritant, nonsensitizing (except in rare cases, and then more particularly with the highly perfumed Bourbon type [*P. graveolens* var. *bourbon*], which is rarely found in the aromatherapy market; use in moderation as a caution). Indian geranium oil, which may contain diphenyl oxide, a synthesized chemical mixture with a geranium-like odor, is used as an ingredient in perfumery and is sometimes added to Chinese geranium oil to increase profits (Burfield 2003). Assure authenticity and purity with your essential oil supplier.

Perfume note: Middle

Principal chemical constituents: CAS No: 8000-46-2

Pelargonium graveolens, Egyptian rose geranium: cis-trans-rose oxide (0.5 to 2.5%), oxide-trans-rose (0 to 1%), menthone (0 to 2%), isomenthone (trace to 6%), linalool (4 to 9%), **citronellyl formate (6 to 9%),** guaia-6,9-diene (0.1 to 2%), geranyl formate (1 to 4%), alpha-terpeniol (0.5 to 1%), **citronellol (20 to 36%), geraniol (12 to 18%),** geranyl butyrate (1 to 2%), geranyl tiglate (1 to 2%), 10-epi-gamma-eudesmol (3 to 6%), 2-phenylethyl tiglate (1 to 2%)

Pelargonium graveolens var. *bourbon*: cis-rose oxide (0.5 to 1.5%), trans-rose oxide (0.1 to 0.6%), menthone (trace to 2%), **isomenthone (5 to 10%),** beta-bourbonene (0 to 1%), **linalool (4 to 10%),** alpha-guaiene (0 to 1%), beta-caryophyllene (0 to 1.5%), **6,9-guiaiadiene (5 to 9%), citronellyl formate (6 to 11%),** alpha-terpineol (0.3 to 1%), geranyl formate (3 to 7%), **citronellol (18 to 26%), geraniol (10 to 20%),** geranyl butyrate (1 to 2%), geranyl tiglate (1 to 2%), 2-phenylethyl tiglate (0.4 to 1%)

Subtle Connections

Colors: Yellow (*opposite: violet*), green (*opposite: red*), pink (*opposite: pale aqua-green*)

Chakras: Solar plexus, heart

Gemstones: Citrine (*opposite: amethyst*), aventurine (*opposite: jasper*), rose quartz (*opposite: aquamarine*)

Energy: Yin

Elements: Water, metal (ether)

Actions and Uses

General actions: Analgesic, antiarthritic, antifungal, anti-infectious, anti-inflammatory, antimicrobial, antiparasitic, antispasmodic, antiviral, astringent, bactericidal, decongestant, deodorant, expectorant, restorative, skin-healing

Skin: Abscesses, acne, bruises, burns, chapped and cracked skin, dermatitis, dry and oily skin (balances sebum), eczema, herpes simplex, mature skin, shingles

Respiratory system: Asthma, colds and flu, congestion, infections, sore throat, tonsillitis

Joints and muscles: Cellulitis, edema

Immune system: Chronic fatigue syndrome, myalgic encephalomyelitis, viral infections (including shingles); immune stimulant

Fungal infections: *Candida* species (ringworm, fungal nail infection, athlete's foot)

Other: Painful periods, PMS, menopausal problems

Potential psycho-emotional and spiritual support: Both sedative and stimulant; eases anger, anxiety, depression, low mood; endocrine stimulant (hormonelike); eases feelings of fear; relieves headache, insomnia (low dose); eases nervous tension and fatigue; balances nerves and solar plexus; relieves premenstrual tension and menopausal symptoms; sedative; helps stress and stress-related conditions; uplifting

GINGER
(Zingiber officinale)

Geographical location: Native to southeastern Asia (and used in India and China as a food and medicinal spice since ancient times), ginger is cultivated in other southern areas of Asia, in West Africa, and in the Caribbean and is now grown in many tropical and mild areas around the world. The oil is mostly distilled in Britain (imported from Nigeria), the Netherlands, China, and India. India is the largest producer of ginger. Other essential oil–producing countries include Indonesia, Java, Madagascar, and the West Indies.

Plant description: Ginger is a reedlike perennial that grows to about 3 to 4 feet (1 meter) in height, with erect, annual leaves and white and pink flower buds that bloom to become pinkish purple or yellowish green, with thick, tuberous, spreading, very pungent rhizome roots. The rhizomes are gathered when the sprouting stalk withers. Ginger flourishes in fertile soil and needs plenty of rain. The rhizome is unearthed when the plant is ten months old. The roots are divided to propagate the plant.

Botanical family: Zingiberaceae

Extraction method: Steam distillation of the unpeeled, dried, and ground roots

Appearance of essential oil: Pale yellow to light orange or greenish liquid

Odor of essential oil: Type: spicy; strength: medium; characteristics: fresh, slightly green, spicy-woody, terpenic, warm, citrusy, and mellow, with coriander-like tones and warm, balsamic, floral-woody dry-out notes

Compatible essential oils for blending: Cedarwood, cinnamon, clove, coriander, frankincense, grapefruit, lemon, lime, mandarin, neroli, orange, patchouli, petitgrain, rose, rosemary, sandalwood, vetivert

Safety data: Nontoxic, nonirritant, nonsensitizing. Has a very low level of phototoxicity but is not regarded as significant; mildly antioxidant (Tisserand and Young 2014, 295).

Perfume note: Middle to top

Principal chemical constituents: CAS No: 8007-08-7

Madagascar: alpha-pinene (1 to 4%), camphene (4 to 8%), beta-myrcene (0 to 1%), limonene (0 to 1.5%), beta-phellandrene (0.1 to 5%),

1,8-cineole (1 to 3.5%), **alpha-zingiberene (25 to 40%)**, beta-bisabolene (2 to 6%), geranial (2 to 4%), Z,E-alpha-farnesene (0 to 6%), **beta-sesquiphellandrene (7 to 13%)**, curcumene (3 to 5%), geraniol (trace to 1%)

Subtle Connections

Colors: Orange (*opposite: blue*), yellow (*opposite: violet*), green (*opposite: red*), pink (*opposite: pale aqua-green*)

Chakras: Solar plexus, heart

Gemstones: Carnelian (*opposite: lapis lazuli*), citrine (*opposite: amethyst*), aventurine (*opposite: jasper*), rose quartz (*opposite: aquamarine*)

Energy: Yang, yin

Elements: Fire, wood (air), earth

Actions and Uses

General actions: Analgesic, antiarthritic, antioxidant, antiseptic, antispasmodic, antitussive, aperitif, aphrodisiac, bactericidal, carminative, cephalic, decongestant, expectorant, febrifuge (reduces fever), stimulant (circulatory), stomachic (nausea) (topical use: skin; internal use: inhalation only)

Respiratory system: Chronic bronchitis, congestion, cough, sinusitis, sore throat, tonsillitis

Joints and muscles: Arthritis, injury, muscle fatigue and aches, pain, sprains

Potential psycho-emotional and spiritual support: Eases debility, emotional pain, nervous exhaustion, tiredness; stimulating yet grounding; aids memory and recall; warms cold emotions; offers emotional and psychic protection

GRAPEFRUIT
(Citrus x paradisi)

Geographical location: The grapefruit tree is native to tropical Southeast Asia and the West Indies and was introduced to Jamaica in the seventeenth century. It is now cultivated in the United States (Arizona, California, Florida, Texas), Mexico, Brazil, Thailand,

South Africa, Israel, Turkey, Argentina, India, and Sudan. China and the United States are major growers. The essential oil is mostly produced in the United States, Argentina, Brazil, and Israel.

Plant description: A cultivated evergreen tree that usually grows to around 16 to 20 feet (5 to 6 meters) tall but can reach up to 40 to 43 feet (13 to 15 meters), the grapefruit tree has spreading branches and thorny twigs; glossy, dark green, long, thin leaves; and large, white, four-petaled, sweet-smelling flowers that yield large fruits with yellowish-orange skins. The fruits can vary in color depending on cultivars (fruit pulps, for example, can be white, pink, or red, red being the sweetest). *Citrus* x *paradisi* is a cross between sweet orange (*Citrus sinensis*) and pomelo/shaddock (*Citrus maxima* or *Citrus grandis*).

Botanical family: Rutaceae

Extraction method: Expression of fresh fruit peel. The rinds are often steam-distilled after expression to extract any remaining oil; the oil yield from secondary extraction is of poorer quality.

Appearance of essential oil: Yellow to reddish or greenish mobile liquid

Odor of essential oil: Type: citrus; strength: medium; characteristics: fresh, sweet, dry, citrus, with faint, nondistinct dry-out notes

Compatible essential oils for blending: Bergamot, cardamom and other spice oils, cedarwood, cypress, frankincense, geranium, lemon and lemon-scented oils, neroli, lemon-scented tea tree, vetivert

Safety data: Nontoxic, nonirritant, nonsensitizing. Grapefruit has a short shelf life as it oxidizes rapidly. When oxidized, this oil becomes irritating and sensitizing. Ensure that you store this oil correctly in an amber-colored glass bottle, preferably in a cool, dark place, and discard residue amounts remaining in the bottle. It may be adulterated with orange terpenes (Burfield 2003) or with purified limonene (Tisserand and Young 2014, 297).

Perfume note: Top

Principal chemical constituents: CAS No: 8016-20-4

  dextro-limonene (85 to 96%), beta-myrcene (1.3 to 2%), alpha-pinene (0.2 to 1%), sabinene (0.1 to 1%), nookatone (0.1 to 0.15%), bergapten (trace amount to 1%), linalool (trace amount to 0.5%), neral (trace amount to 0.05%), geranial (trace amount to 0.1%), beta-caryophyllene (trace amount to 0.5%)

Subtle Connections

Colors: Yellow (*opposite: violet*), green (*opposite: red*), pink (*opposite: pale aqua-green*)

Chakras: Solar plexus, heart

Gemstones: Citrine (*opposite: amethyst*), aventurine (*opposite: jasper*), rose quartz (*opposite: aquamarine*)

Energy: Yang

Element: Wood (air)

Actions and Uses

General actions: Antiseptic, antitoxic, astringent, bactericidal, depurative, diuretic, stimulant, tonic

Skin: Acne, oily skin; tones and tightens skin

Respiratory system: Airborne disinfectant (in high dose); colds, flu

Muscles: Eases muscle fatigue and stiffness

Antifungal: Athlete's foot, candida

Immune support: Bacterial and fungal infections

Potential psycho-emotional spiritual support: Eases feelings of depression and low mood; relieves headache; improves sense of self-confidence; eases nervous exhaustion, emotional fatigue, stress; supports withdrawal from addiction (especially when combined with vetivert and/or frankincense); uplifting

HELICHRYSUM / IMMORTELLE
(Helichrysum angustifolium, H. italicum)

Geographical location: A species of the sunflower family, helichrysum is native to the eastern Mediterranean regions, including Crete and parts of Asia, as well as North Africa. It grows and is cultivated in both the north and the south of Africa, Madagascar, Australasia, Spain, France, and the United States; it is mainly cultivated in Italy, the former Yugoslavia (Bosnia, Serbia, Croatia, Montenegro,

Macedonia), and Slovenia. The main essential oil–producing countries are France (including Corsica) and Slovenia.

Plant description: A strongly aromatic herb, helichrysum grows up to 24 to 35 inches (60 to 90 centimeters) high and has a much-branched stem that is woody at the base; each plant produces sixty to seventy stems, and each stem produces on average twenty flowers. The leaves are oblong to lanceolate and flat. The brightly colored, daisylike flowers become dry as the plant matures yet retain their color, which can be any color other than blue. There are a number of varieties, which are sometimes distilled together, and therefore the essential-oil composition can vary considerably from region to region. There are several other *Helichrysum* species: *H. arenarium* is used in floristry; *H. stoechas* (found in France, Corsica, and Yugoslavia) is used to produce an absolute, though the chemical composition varies according to the location of growth; and *H. orientale* is grown for its essential oil. Other oil-producing species include *H. gymnocephalum* and *H. bracteaflorum* (both varieties from Madagascar).

Botanical family: Asteraceae (Compositae)

Extraction method: Steam distillation of fresh flowers and flowering tops. The absolute and concrete are produced by solvent extraction.

Appearance of essential oil: Pale yellow to red oily liquid

Appearance of absolute: Yellow to brown viscous liquid

Odor of essential oil: Type: herbal; strength: medium; characteristics: sweet, fruity, honey-like, warm, herbal, woody, floral, coumarinic, with delicate, tealike undertones and dry-out notes

Odor of absolute: Rich, floral, tealike

Compatible essential oils for blending: Cedarwood, chamomile, citrus oils, clary sage, clove, frankincense, geranium, juniper, lavender, Peru balsam, rose

Safety data: Nontoxic, nonsensitizing, nonirritant

Perfume note: Middle

Principal chemical constituents: CAS No. 8023-95-8 (the absolute CAS no. is 90045-56-0)

Helichrysum italicum essential oil: **alpha-pinene (21 to 30%)**, limonene (2 to 4%), alpha-copaene (0.1 to 2%), isoitalicene (1 to 2%), linalool (to 2%), italicene (0.1 to 4%), alpha-cis-bergamotene

(0.1 to 2%), alpha-trans-bergamotene (1 to 2%), beta-caryophylene (1 to 6%), gamma-selinene (0.1 to 3%), **gamma-curcumene (10 to 13%),** neryl acetate (5 to 7%), beta-selinene (1 to 7%), alpha-selinene (1 to 5%), alpha-curcumene (1 to 3%), italidions (5 to 12%), 10-epi-gamma-eudesmol (0.1 to 0.4%)

Subtle Connections

Colors: Yellow (*opposite: violet*), orange (*opposite: blue*), red (*opposite: green*)

Chakras: Solar plexus, sacral, base

Gemstones: Citrine (*opposite: amethyst*), carnelian (*opposite: lapis lazuli/ aquamarine*), jasper (*opposite: aventurine*)

Energy: Yin

Element: Earth

Actions and Uses

General actions: Antiallergic, antifungal, anti-inflammatory, antimicrobial, antiparasitic, antiseptic, antitussive (relieves coughs), antiviral, astringent, cicatrizant, diuretic, expectorant, fungicidal, insecticidal, nervine, vulnerary (wound-healing)

Skin: Abscesses, acne, allergic conditions, boils, broken capillaries, bruises, burns, cuts, dermatitis, eczema, inflammation, scar tissue and stretch marks, spots, wounds; stimulates new cell growth

Respiratory system: Asthma, bronchitis, chronic coughs, colds, flu, sinusitis

Muscles and joints: Arthritis, muscular aches and pains, sprains; supports tissue regeneration

Immune support: Allergies, bacterial and viral infections (herpes)

Potential psycho-emotional and spiritual support: Eases feelings of depression, mental and emotional debility, burnout, exhaustion; relieves headaches (especially those caused by liver congestion); eases nervous exhaustion; good for meditation; relieves shock, stress, and stress-related conditions; aids one's ability to let go of the past and move on

HYSSOP
(Hyssopus officinalis)

Geographical location: This shrub is native to southern Europe, eastern (temperate) Asia, and the Middle East; it also grows in the Mediterranean countries, especially Turkey and the Balkans, and is naturalized in the United States. Hyssop is cultivated mainly in Hungary, France, and Morocco. The main essential oil–producing countries are France, Hungary, and Morocco.

Plant description: This small, semievergreen perennial shrub or subshrub grows from 1 to 2 feet (30 to 60 centimeters) tall. The stem is woody at the base, from which a number of straight, slim, woody, quadrangular branches or stems grow, with dark green, lance-shaped leaves about 0.8 to 1.2 inches (2 to 3 centimeters) long, arranged in pairs along the stem. The plant produces bunches or clusters of leafy, whorl-like spikes of little double-tipped flowers during summer that are violet to blue, pink, red, or, more rarely, white and fragrant. The flowering tops are harvested in the summer.

Botanical family: Lamiaceae (Labiatae)

Extraction method: Steam distillation of leaves and flowering tops (must be distilled immediately after harvest)

Appearance of essential oil: Pale yellow or yellowish-green to almost colorless liquid

Odor of essential oil: Type: herbal; strength: medium; characteristics: herbal, like sage and clary sage, camphoraceous, green, piney, terpenic, woody, with warm, spicy-herbaceous body notes and fading undertones and dry-out notes

Compatible essential oils for blending: Bay leaf, citrus oils, clary sage, geranium, lavender, myrtle, rosemary, sage

Safety data: Nonirritant, nonsensitizing, nontoxic (linalool chemotype). Avoid using during pregnancy and while breastfeeding, and do not use on children. Do not take internally (Tisserand and Young 2014, 308).

Perfume note: Middle

Principal chemical constituents: CAS No: 8006-83-5

Hyssopus officinalis ct. linalool: **linalool (48 to 53%), 1,8-cineole**

(12 to 15%), dextro-limonene (5 to 6%), gamma-pinene (2 to 4%), caryophyllene oxide (1 to 4%), alpha-pinene (2 to 3%), camphene (1 to 3%), beta-myrcene (1 to 2%), isopinocamphone (1 to 2%), beta-bourbonene (1 to 2%), sabinene (1 to 2%), pinocamphone (0.5 to 1.5%)

Hyssopus officinalis ct. cineol: alpha-pinene (1 to 3%), **beta-pinene (12 to 15%),** sabinene (1 to 4.5%), myrcene (1 to 3%), limonene (1 to 3%), **1,8-cineole (40 to 48%),** beta-ocimene (3 to 5%), para-cymene (0.1 to 1%), mytenyl methyl ether (0.1 to 1%), bourbonene (1 to 2.5%), isopinocamphone (0.1 to 2%), pinocarvone (3 to 7%), delta-terpineol (0.1 to 1%), alpha-terpineol (0.1 to 2%), linalool (0.1 to 1%), germacrene D (0.1 to 2%)

Subtle Connections

Color: Yellow (*opposite: violet*), green (*opposite: red*), pink (*opposite: pale aqua-green*)

Chakras: Solar plexus, heart

Gemstones: Citrine (*opposite: amethyst*), aventurine (*opposite: jasper*), rose quartz (*opposite: aquamarine*)

Energy: Yin

Element: Metal (ether)

Actions and Uses

General actions: Antiseptic, antispasmodic, antiviral, astringent, bactericidal, cephalic, cicatrizant, emmenagogue, expectorant, febrifuge, hypertensive, nervine, sedative, sudorific (causes sweating), tonic (circulatory system), vulnerary (heals wounds and sores)

Skin: Bruises, cuts, dermatitis, eczema, fungal infections, inflammation, wounds

Respiratory system: Asthma, bronchitis, catarrh, chest infections, cough, sinusitis, sore throat, tightness of chest, tonsillitis

Joints and muscles: Arthritis, gout pain

Potential psycho-emotional and spiritual support: Aids concentration and focus; eases anxiety, depression, low mood, grief, mental and emotional fatigue; instills a sense of spirituality; relieves nervous tension, stress, and stress-related conditions

JASMINE
(Jasminum grandiflorum, J. sambac)

Geographical location: Jasmine is a viney shrub native to tropical and subtropical regions of Africa, Asia, and Europe (particularly northern India, Pakistan, and the northwest Himalayas), Australasia, and Oceania. Jasmine is also cultivated and naturalized in Mediterranean Europe (for example, Spanish jasmine, *Jasminum grandiflorum,* originated in Iran and southern Asia) and in the United States. The concrete is mostly produced in Italy, France, Morocco, Egypt, China, Japan, Algeria, and Turkey, and the absolute mainly in France.

Plant description: Jasmines (there are over three hundred species) are either deciduous (leaves falling in autumn) or evergreen. They may be erect, spreading, or climbing shrubs or vines, growing up to 20 feet (6 meters) high, with delicate, bright to dark green trifoliate or pinnate leaves and star-shaped, tubular, white or yellow, sometimes reddish flowers, borne in cymose clusters, sweetly scented and very fragrant. The flowers produce berries that turn black when ripe. Most species are cultivated as fragrant ornamental plants. The fragrant flowers of *Jasminum officinale* (native to Iran) are used to produce the attar (fragrance) favored in perfumery, and the dried flowers of Arabian jasmine (*Jasminum sambac*) are used to make jasmine tea.

Botanical family: Oleaceae

Extraction method: Solvent extraction. Distilled jasmine is very rare due to the plant's very low oil yield and extremely high cost.

Appearance of essential oil: Dark orangish-brown or pale yellow to rich orangish-yellow viscous liquid (absolute)

Odor of essential oil: Type: floral; strength: medium; characteristics: intensely rich yet delicate, ethereal, sweet, warm, balsamic, fruity, and green, with tenacious, floral, tealike undertones and dry-out notes

Compatible essential oils for blending: Bitter orange, clary sage, galbanum, grapefruit, lavender, lime, mandarin, sandalwood, rose. Jasmine rounds out any rough or sharp notes and aromatically blends with most other oils.

Safety data: Nontoxic, moderate risk of skin sensitization, generally nonirritant (however, may cause irritation in those with a history of allergy or proneness to sensitization as a reaction to fragrance materials, which is also the case for most absolutes; Tisserand and Young 2014, 312)

Perfume note: Base to middle

Principal chemical constituents: CAS No. 8022-96-6

Absolute (solvent extraction) (*J. grandiflorum*): cis-3-hexenol (0 to 2%), trans-2-hexenol (0 to 1%), cis-3-hexyl acetate (0 to 2%), benzyl alcohol (0.5 to 2%), **linalool (3 to 12%), benzyl acetate (15 to 25%),** indole (0.5 to 4%), eugenol (0.5 to 3.5%), cis-jasmone (1 to 3%), jasmolactone (0.1 to 1.5%), cis-3-hexenyl benzoate (0.1 to 1%), methyl jasomate (0.1 to 2%), **benzyl benzoate (8 to 20%),** neo phytadiene (0 to 4%), 2-hexadecen-1-ol,3,7,11,15-tetramethyl (0 to 2%), methyl palmitate (0.1 to 1.5%), isophytol (4 to 8%), geranyl linalool (1 to 8%), **phytol (3 to 13%),** methyl linolenate (0 to 1%), **trans-phytol (6 to 13%),** 2-hexadecen-1-ol,3,7,11,15-tetramethyl-1 acetate (1 to 4%)

Subtle Connections

Colors: Orange (*opposite: blue*), yellow (*opposite: violet*)

Chakras: Sacral, solar plexus

Gemstones: Carnelian (*opposite: lapis lazuli/aquamarine*), citrine (*opposite: amethyst*)

Energy: Yin, yang

Elements: Water, fire

Actions and Uses

General actions: Antidepressant, aphrodisiac, sedative

Potential psycho-emotional and spiritual support: Eases feelings of anxiety, depression, low mood, fear, and nervous tension; euphoric; improves sense of self-confidence; uplifts mood and emotions

JUNIPER BERRY
(Juniperus communis)

Geographical location: Juniper is native to and widely distributed throughout the northern hemisphere—the Arctic regions,

Scandinavia, Siberia, Canada, northern Europe, northern Asia, Tibet and the Himalayas, and North and Central America. Juniper adapts morphologically to its surrounding climate conditions, for example, adopting a slender shape in flatlands or becoming a creeping plant in mountainous territory. The main essential oil–producing countries are Austria, Canada, the Czech Republic, Slovakia, France, Germany, Bosnia, and Croatia.

Plant description: A coniferous evergreen shrub that differs in shape and size depending on its environment, juniper ranges from a tall tree 20 to 50 feet (6 to 15 meters) high to columnar or low-spreading shrubs with long, trailing branches. It has slender twigs with whorls of bluish-green, needlelike or scalelike leaves, with small yellow (male) and blue (female) flowers on separate plants, with spherical, berrylike fruit produced on female trees, which are green in the first year and bluish black in the second and third year, although some berries are reddish brown or orange. The male trees have cones similar to those produced by other Cupressaceae trees. The berries are gathered in autumn when they are ripe. There are various other species of juniper, such as *J. oxycedrus,* which produces cade oil, *J. virginiana,* which produces the so-called Virginia cedarwood oil, and *J. sabina,* which produces savin oil.

Botanical family: Cupressaceae

Extraction method: Steam distillation of the berries (an oil is also extracted from the needles and wood). The berries are sometimes fermented before being distilled, usually as a by-product of gin or Slovakian brandy manufacturing; the oil produced in this way is of inferior quality.

Appearance of essential oil: Water-like to pale yellow or greenish mobile liquid

Odor of essential oil: Type: terpenic; strength: medium; characteristics: fresh, balsamic, terpenic, warm and woody, carrot-seedy and peppery, with sweet, warm, balsamic dry-out notes

Compatible essential oils for blending: Benzoin, bergamot, cedarwood, clary sage, cypress, galbanum, geranium, grapefruit, lavender, lemon, lime, mandarin, myrrh, orange, pine, rosemary, sandalwood, vetivert

Safety data: Nontoxic, nonsensitizing, nonirritant (although can become sensitizing and irritant if the oil is oxidized or old). Use this oil in moderation.

Perfume note: Middle

Principal chemical constituents: CAS No: 1812-91-7

alpha-pinene (25 to 45%), beta-myrcene (3 to 22%), sabinene (4 to 20%), germacrene D (1 to 6.5%), dextro-limonene (2 to 8%), beta-pinene (1 to 12%), gamma cadinene (1 to 3.5%), alpha-terpinene (0.1 to 1%), gamma-terpinene (0.1 to 3%), para-cymene (0.1 to 1.5%), terpinolene (0.1 to 1%), alpha-cubulene (0.1 to 1%), alpha-humulene (1 to 4%), terpinen-4-ol (1 to 6%), germacrene B (1 to 3%), beta-caryophyllene (1.5 to 5%), alpha-caryophyllene (0.1 to 2%), beta-elemene (0.5 to 2%)

Subtle Connections

Colors: Yellow (*opposite: violet*), green (*opposite: red*), pink (*opposite: pale aqua-green*)

Chakras: Solar plexus, heart

Gemstones: Citrine (*opposite: amethyst*), aventurine (*opposite: jasper*), rose quartz (*opposite: aquamarine*)

Energy: Yin

Element: Water

Actions and Uses

General actions: Antiseptic, antispasmodic, antitoxic, aphrodisiac, astringent, cicatrizant, diuretic, emmenagogue, nervine, rubefacient (causes skin redness), sedative, tonic, vulnerary (wound-healing)

Skin: Acne, dermatitis, eczema, hair loss, hemorrhoids, inflammation, oily complexion, water retention, ulcers, wounds; skin toner

Respiratory system: Airborne disinfectant; colds, flu

Joints and muscles: Arthritis, gout pain

Potential psycho-emotional and spiritual support: Quells confusion and indecision; dispels negative energy; eases feelings of anxiety, fear, nervous tension, fatigue, hypersensitivity; aids memory; good for insomnia; strengthening; addresses stress-related headaches and other stress-related conditions; uplifting

LAVENDER—ENGLISH AND SPIKE
(Lavandula angustifolia, L. latifolia)

Geographical location: Lavender species are native to countries bordering the Mediterranean, particularly France and the Pyrenees Mountains in northern Spain. They have been cultivated in the United Kingdom, Norway, Italy, Greece, Turkey, Bulgaria, the former Yugoslavian countries (Croatia, Bosnia, and so on), Russia, Australia, Tasmania, and the United States. The main essential oil–producing countries are Australia, Bulgaria, China, France, Portugal, Russia, Spain, and the United Kingdom.

Plant description: *L. angustifolia* is a small, woody, evergreen shrub that grows up to 3.3 feet (1 meter), with narrow, grayish-green leaves and small, tubular, pale to deep purple flowers on dense, blunt spikes. The stems are four-square. The whole plant is highly aromatic and is harvested just before the end of flowering and distilled while fresh (although it is also dried for use as an herb or a fragrant additive to potpourri). Cultivated lavender does not produce seeds and is propagated by cuttings or by dividing the roots. The botanical name *Lavendula angustifolia* is used interchangeably with *L. officinalis* (its historical name); common names include English lavender (although it is not native to England), common lavender, true lavender, narrow-leafed lavender, lavender vera, and fine lavender. Spike lavender (*L. latifolia*) is similar in appearance to *L. angustifolia,* but with pale, grayish-blue flowers at the top of single-stemmed, leafless spikes and broad, grayish-green leaves. It grows up to 32 inches (80 cm), at lower altitudes, and it has a higher plant yield than *L. angustifolia.*

Botanical family: Lamiaceae (Labiatae)

Extraction method: Steam distillation of the fresh flowering tops

Appearance of essential oil: Colorless to pale yellow or yellowish-green liquid

Odor of essential oil: *L. angustifolia* type: floral; strength: medium; characteristics: fresh, floral, fruity to herbaceous, spicy, camphoraceous, aldehydic, and balsamic-woody undertones to nondescript dry-out notes. English lavender is characterized by softer,

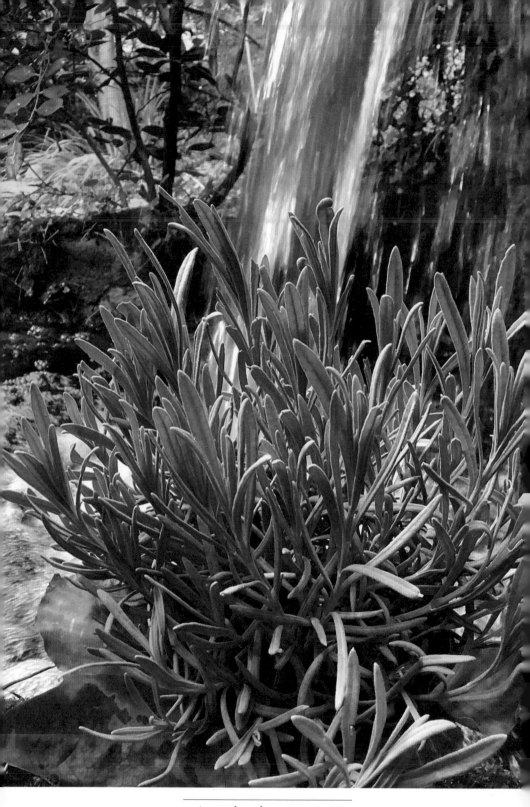

Lavender plant in autumn

mellower, slightly rounder notes compared to French lavenders and other lavender oils.

L. latifolia: fresh and strongly camphoraceous, with herbaceous-woody dry-out notes (sometimes described as a cross between sage and lavender)

Compatible essential oils for blending: Bergamot, cajeput, carrot seed, chamomile (Roman and German), clary sage, cypress, frankincense, galbanum, geranium, grapefruit, mandarin, orange, lemon, lime, patchouli, peppermint, spikenard, tea tree, vetivert, ylang-ylang; in fact, blends well with most other essential oils

Safety data: Nontoxic, nonirritant, nonsensitizing (although there is moderate risk of sensitization if overused). English lavender may be adulterated with cheaper lavandin (*Lavandula* x *intermedia*), spike lavender, rectified ho oil (*Cinnamomum* spp.) and acetylated ho or acetylated lavandin oils, Spanish sage oil, synthetic linalool, and linalyl (Tisserand and Young 2014, 327; Burfield 2003). Assure authenticity and purity with your essential-oil supplier.

Perfume note: Middle to top

Principal chemical constituents: Lavender is a complex oil with over 150 chemical constituents. The chemical constituents listed below provide an overview.

CAS No: 8016-78-2 (spike lavender, *L. latifolia*): alpha-pinene (0.5 to 2%), camphene (0 to 1%), beta-pinene (0.5 to 3%), sabinene (0.5 to 1%), beta-myrcene (0.5 to 1%), alpha-terpinene (0.5 to 1%), limonene (0.5 to 3%), **1,8-cineole (16 to 40%),** cis-beta-ocimene (0 to 1%), terpinolene (0 to 0.5%), trans-thujanol (0 to 0.5%), camphor (8 to 16%), **linalool (34 to 50%),** linalyl acetate (0.5 to 2%), bornyl acetate (0 to 0.5%), beta-caryophyllene (0.5 to 2%), terpinene-4-ol (0 to 0.5%), trans-sabinyl acetate (0 to 0.1%), E-beta-farnesene (0 to 0.5%), zonearene (0 to 0.2%), terpineol (0 to 0.5%), neral (0 to 1%), borneol (0 to 1%), alpha-terpiniol (1 to 2%), germacrene D (0 to 1%), geranyl acetate (0 to 0.2%), alpha-bisabolenen (1 to 5%), geraniol (0 to 0.1%), para-cymene-8-ol (0 to 0.1%), caryophyllene oxide (0 to 0.5%), T-cadinol (0 to 0.2%), coumarin (0 to 0.1%)

CAS No: 8000-28-0 (French high-altitude *L. angustifolia*): limonene

(0.5 to 26%), 1,8-cineole (0 to 1.5%), cis-beta-ocimene (4 to 10%), trans-beta-ocimene (1.5 to 6%), 3-octonone (0.01 to 3%), camphor (0.01 to 0.5%), **linalool (25 to 45%), linalyl acetate (25 to 45%)**, beta-caryophyllene (1 to 6%), terpinen-4-ol (1.5 to 6%), lavandulyl acetate (2 to 6%), E-beta-farnesene (2 to 3%), lavandulol (0.3 to 2%), alpha-terpineol (0.01 to 1%), geranyl acetate (0 to 0.5%)

Subtle Connections

Colors: Yellow (*opposite: violet*), green (*opposite: red*), pink (*opposite: pale aqua-green*), blue (*opposite: orange*)

Chakras: Solar plexus, heart, throat, brow

Gemstones: Citrine (*opposite: amethyst*), aventurine (*opposite: jasper*), rose quartz (*opposite: aquamarine*), lapis lazuli/aquamarine (*opposite: carnelian*)

Energy: Yin, yang

Elements: Metal (ether), wood (air)

Actions and Uses

General actions: Analgesic, antiarthritic, antidepressant, antifungal, anti-infectious, anti-inflammatory, antimicrobial, antiseptic, antispasmodic, antitoxic, antiviral, bactericidal, cicatrizant, cleansing, deodorant, hypotensive, skin-healing, toner

Skin: Abscesses (spike lavender), acne, bruises, burns, chapped and cracked skin, dermatitis, dry skin, eczema, insect bites, itchy skin, mature skin, oily skin, pimples, psoriasis, ringworm, scars, shingles

Respiratory system: *L. angustifolia* (English)*:* asthma, bronchitis, catarrh, colds, flu, gingivitis, halitosis, hay fever, laryngitis, panic attacks (relaxes and eases breathing), pulmonary infections and viruses, sore throat, teething (calming), upper respiratory infections *L. latifolia* (spike): anti-inflammatory, mucolytic; asthma, bronchitis, hay fever, laryngitis, sinusitis, tonsillitis

Joints and muscles: Arthritis (spike lavender), muscle aches and pains, sciatica, sprains

Circulatory system: Helps the body regulate blood pressure

Immune system: Chronic fatigue syndrome, myalgic encephalomyelitis; immune stimulant (spike lavender), immune support (English lavender)

Fungal infections: *C. malassezia* species (spike lavender)

Other: Allergies, headache, migraine, painful periods, PMS, menopausal problems

Potential psycho-emotional and spiritual support: Central nervous system sedative (sedative at low dose, stimulant at high dose); eases agitation, anger, anxiety, depression and low mood, grief and bereavement, feelings of hopelessness, insomnia, irritability, intolerance and impatience, mood swings, nervous tension, panic attacks, premenstrual tension, shock, solar plexus tension, stress and stress-related conditions

LEMON
(Citrus limonum)

Geographical location: Believed to have originated in northeast India, northern Burma, or China, lemon was cultivated in Italy during the second century AD, then throughout the Mediterranean and Arab world, and later in North and South America. Today it is grown in China, India, Mexico, Argentina, Brazil, the United States (California, Arizona, Florida), Turkey, Spain, Iran, and Italy. The main essential oil–producing countries are Argentina, Australia, Brazil, Greece, Italy, Peru, Spain, and the United States.

Plant description: A small evergreen tree or spreading bush, lemon grows 10 to 20 feet (3 to 6 meters) high, with young leaves that have a reddish tint, then mature to green. In some species the branches are angular. The evergreen leaves are oval and serrated, with some species producing sharp thorns at the axil of the leaves, and very fragrant flowers forming small clusters that bear thick-skinned, oval fruits that turn from green to yellow upon ripening. The flowers are reddish-tinted in bud, with petals that are white above and reddish purple underneath. Lemon trees usually bloom throughout the year, and the fruits are picked six to ten times a year. There are around forty-seven or so varieties developed in cultivation. Lemon is believed to be a hybrid between bitter orange and citron and is closely related to lime, cedrat (or citron), and bergamot.

Botanical family: Rutaceae

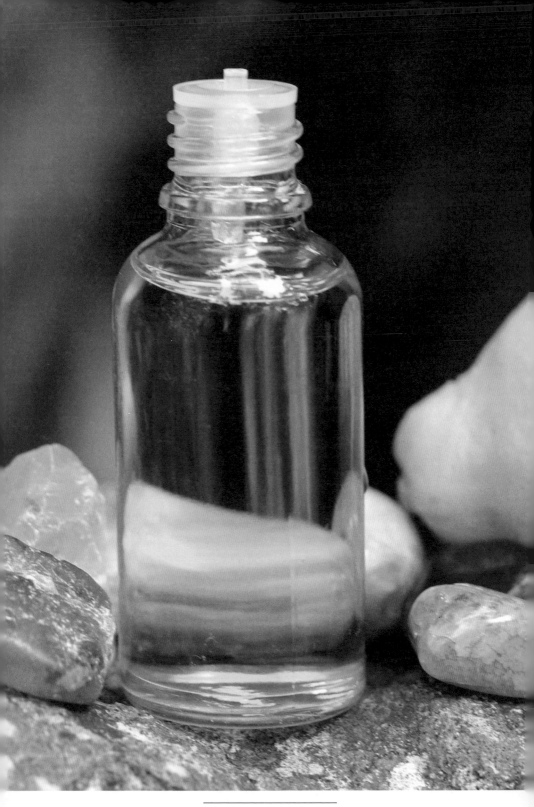

Lemon essential oil

Extraction method: Cold expression of the outer peel of the fresh fruit

Appearance of essential oil: Pale straw yellow to dark yellow to midgreen liquid (turning brown with age)

Odor of essential oil: Type: citrus; strength: medium; characteristics: light, fresh, citrus scent reminiscent of lemon peel

Compatible essential oils for blending: Benzoin, chamomile, eucalyptus, fennel, frankincense, geranium, ginger, juniper, lavender, neroli, petigrain, rose, sandalwood, lemon-scented tea tree, ylang-ylang, other citrus oils

Safety data: Nontoxic. Old or oxidized oil can cause skin sensitization. There is a low risk of phototoxicity if the skin is exposed to sunlight after application. The oil may be adulterated with natural or synthetic limonene, citral, and numerous other cheap products such as orange terpenes, lemon terpenes, or other by-products (Burfield 2003).

Perfume note: Top

Principal chemical constituents: CAS No: 8008-56-8
alpha-pinene (1.5 to 5%), alpha-thuyene (0.2 to 0.5%), **beta-pinene (6 to 17%),** sabinene (0.5 to 3%), **dextro-limonene (55 to 78%),** gamma-terpinene (3 to 13%), para-cymene (0.05 to 2.5%), alpha-terpineol (0.1 to 8%), neral (0.1 to 2%), neryl acetate (0.05 to 1.5%), beta-bisabolene (0.4 to 1%), geranial (0.5 to 5%), geranyl acetate (0.1 to 1%), terpinen-4-ol (trace amount to 2%)

Subtle Connections

Colors: Yellow (*opposite: violet*), green (*opposite: red*), pink (*opposite: pale aqua-green*)

Chakras: Solar plexus, heart

Gemstones: Citrine (*opposite: amethyst*), aventurine (*opposite: jasper*), rose quartz (*opposite: aquamarine*)

Energy: Yin

Element: Earth

Actions and Uses

General actions: Antiarthritic, antifungal, anti-inflammatory, antimicrobial, antiseptic, antispasmodic, antitoxic, antiviral, astringent, bactericidal, cicatrizant, depurative (detoxifying), febrifuge (combats fever), hypotensive, insecticidal, rubefacient (causes skin redness), tonic

Skin: Acne, boils, brittle nails, chilblains, corns, cuts, oily and greasy skin (balances sebum), spots, varicose veins, warts

Respiratory system: Asthma, bronchitis, catarrh, colds, flu, throat infections

Muscles and joints: Arthritis, cellulitis, muscle tension

Antifungal: *Microsporum* species (ringworm and superficial fungal infections)

Antimicrobial: Viral and bacterial infections

Immune system: General immune support—contagious infections, fever; immune stimulant

Potential psycho-emotional and spiritual support: Aids concentration and clears thoughts; eases feelings of apathy; mental stimulant; eases stress and stress-related conditions; uplifts and eases feelings of anxiety

LEMONGRASS
(Cymbopogon citratus, C. flexuosus)

Geographical location: This plant is native to the tropics and subtropics of Asia (particularly southern India and Sri Lanka), Africa, Australia, and Pacific tropical islands and was introduced to warm regions in the Americas (North, Central, South). It is cultivated as a medicinal herb and culinary ingredient, as well as for its essential oil. *Cymbopogon citratus,* West Indian lemongrass, is cultivated in Sri Lanka, northeast and southern India, and southeast Asia. *Cymbopogon flexuosus,* East Indian lemongrass, is cultivated on the Indian continent and in Indochina. It is similar to and sometimes confused with citronella (*Cymbopogon nardis, Cymbopogon winterianus*). All species of lemongrass are cultivated in the United States, provided they are planted in warm areas of the the country. The main essential oil–producing countries include Brazil, China, Guatemala, Haiti, India, Nepal, Russia, and Sri Lanka.

Plant description: Lemongrass is an aromatic, sweet, lemon-scented perennial that grows in dense clumps up to 5 to 6 feet (1.5 to 1.8 meters) high, with several stiff stems and slender, narrow, bladelike, bluish-green to red leaves that droop toward the tips. Plants that grow in the tropics produce large, compound flowers on spikes, but lemongrass rarely flowers in northern latitudes. The plant produces a network of roots and rootlets that rapidly exhaust the soil. Some plants grow for several years. There are up to fifty-two species of lemongrass; East and West Indian species are the most common. It is also known as barbed wire grass, silky heads, Cochin grass, and Malabar grass. Lemongrass belongs to the same botanical family as citronella and palmarosa, which are similarly citrusy and lemon-like.

Botanical family: Poaceae (Gramineae)

Extraction method: Steam distillation of the fresh or partially dried, finely chopped leaves or grass

Appearance of essential oil: Clear to pale yellow, amber, or reddish brown, or straw yellow to reddish yellow

Odor of essential oil: Type: citrus; strength: medium; characteristics: fresh, sweet, lemony, grassy, rosy, tomato leaf, with earthy undertones, with lemony, herbal, green tea–like body notes and herbaceous, oily, dry-out notes

Compatible essential oils for blending: Basil, bergamot, cedarwood, floral oils, geranium, lemon, lime, neroli, niaouli, orange, pine, sandalwood, tea tree

Safety data: Nontoxic; can cause skin irritation and sensitization. Avoid using on hypersensitive, diseased, or damaged skin. Do not use on children under two years old. Use in moderation. Possible interaction with diabetic medication. Do not take internally (Tisserand and Young 2014, 118, 334).

Perfume note: Top

Principal chemical constituents: CAS No: 8007-82-1

Sri Lanka: limonene (0.5 to 3.5%), 6-methyl-5-hepten-2-one (0.1 to 3%), beta-caryophyllene (0 to 3%), neral (25 to 35%), **geranial (35 to 47%),** geranyl acetate (0.5 to 6%), geraniol (1.5 to 8%)

West Indian: limonene oxide (0 to 7%), 6-methylhept-5-en-2-one (0.1 to 3%), **geraniol (35 to 56%), neral (25 to 36%),** beta-myrcene (5 to 20%), geraniol (0 to 7%), 1,8-cineole (0 to 3%), geranyl acetate (0.1 to 2%), linaool (0.1 to 2%)

Subtle Connections

Colors: Yellow (*opposite: violet*), orange (*opposite: blue*), red (*opposite: green*)

Chakras: Solar plexus, sacral, base

Gemstones: Citrine (*opposite: amethyst*), carnelian (*opposite: lapis lazuli/ aquamarine*), jasper (*opposite: aventurine*)

Energy: Yang

Elements: Fire, wood (air)

Actions and Uses

General actions: Analgesic, antidepressant, antifungal, anti-inflammatory, antimicrobial, antioxidant, antiparasitic, antiseptic, antiviral, astringent, bactericidal, decongestant, deodorant, expectorant, febrifuge (reduces fever), fungicidal, insecticidal, nervine, sedative, tonic

Skin: Acne, excessive perspiration, oily skin and hair; aids hydration

Muscles and joints: Arthritis, muscular aches and pains, sprains; improves muscle tone

Antifungal: Athlete's foot, most species of fungal infections

Potential psycho-emotional and spiritual support: Eases feelings of apathy and mental and emotional fatigue, irritability, and intolerance; helps with lack of concentration and nervous exhaustion; sedative; eases stress, stress-related headaches, and other stress-related conditions; awakens

MANDARIN
(Citrus reticulata)

Geographical location: Native to southeastern Asia and the Philippines, especially southern China, Japan, and the East Indies, mandarin was introduced to Europe and then America in the 1800s (where it was renamed tangerine). It is now cultivated and produced mainly in Italy, Spain, Algeria, Cypress, Greece, the Middle East, Brazil, and the United States (Alabama, Florida, Mississippi, Texas, Georgia, California, Arizona). There are many cultivars within this species. The names *tangerine, satsuma,* and *mandarin* are sometimes used interchangeably, even though each represents a different chemotype.

Plant description: A small, evergreen, usually thorny tree, mandarin grows up to 24 feet (6 to 7.5 meters) high. Mandarin trees are usually smaller than sweet orange trees, depending on the variety. The leaves are broad or slender, lanceolate, and glossy, with minute, rounded teeth, and the very fragrant flowers are single or clustered. The fleshy fruits are deep green or bright orange or reddish orange and have a loose peel. The tangerine is larger than the mandarin and rounder, with a yellowish skin, more like the original Chinese mandarin type. It is also known as mandarin orange.

Botanical family: Rutaceae

Extraction method: Cold expression of the outer peel

Appearance of essential oil: Midgreen to dark olive liquid

Odor of essential oil: Type: citrus; strength: medium; characteristics: citrus, floral, terpenic, aldehydic, intensely fruity, sweet, fresh, deep, softly citrusy with obvious mandarin peel odor fading to a faintly fruity, tangeriney, soft and round, herbaceous-fruity scent, until barely detectable

Compatible essential oils for blending: Black pepper, carrot seed, cinnamon, clove, cypress, frankincense, geranium, ginger, neroli, patchouli, petitgrain, tea tree, other citrus oils

Safety data: Nontoxic, nonirritating, generally nonsensitizing. It can become sensitizing when oxidized, so be sure to include antioxidant ingredients, such as avocado oil, vitamin E oil, or cold-pressed carrot seed oil and carrot seed essential oil to a mandarin blend that you intend to store.

Perfume note: Top

Principal chemical constituents: CAS No: 8008-31-9

alpha-pinene (1.5 to 3%), beta-pinene (1 to 2.2%), beta-myrcene (1.2 to 2%), **dextro-limonene (65 to 75%), gamma-terpinene (15 to 23%),** para-cymene (0.1 to 1.5%), octanal (trace amount to 0.2%), decanal (trace amount to 0.2%), linalool (0.05 to 0.2%), beta-caryophyllene (trace amount to 2%), alpha-terpineol (trace amount to 0.3%), alpha-sinensal (0.2 to 0.5%)

Subtle Connections

Colors: Green (*opposite: red*), pink (*opposite: pale aqua-green*)

Chakra: Heart

Gemstones: Aventurine (*opposite: jasper*), rose quartz (*opposite: aquamarine*)

Energy: Yang, yin

Elements: Fire, earth

Actions and Uses

General actions: Antiseptic, antispasmodic, bactericidal, cleansing, hydrating, tonic

Skin: Skin-healing, toning; acne, congested and oily skin, scars, spots, stretch marks

Respiratory system: Asthma, bronchitis, colds, flu, coughs

Joints and muscles: Arthritis, fluid retention

Circulatory system: Helps the body regulate blood pressure

Immune system: Allergies, chronic fatigue syndrome, myalgic encephalomyelitis; immune stimulant

Other: PMS, menopausal problems

Potential psycho-emotional and spiritual support: Awakens, brings out the inner child; eases anxiety, depression, low mood, hyperactivity (while orange can encourage hyperactivity, mandarin is calming); relieves insomnia, nervous tension, panic attacks (combine with frankincense), premenstrual tension, restlessness, stress and stress-related conditions; uplifting; sedative

MARJORAM, SWEET
(Origanum majorana, Majorana hortensis)

Geographical location: This culinary and medicinal herb is native to Asia and North Africa and naturalized in Europe and the United States, where it grows wild and is also cultivated. In some areas marjoram and oregano are referred to synonymously. The main essential oil–producing countries are Egypt, Hungary, and Spain.

Marjorams and Oregano

While often confused with oregano, marjoram does not contain phenols (carvacrol). Wild marjoram (*Origanum majorana* ct. carvacrol) has a high carvacrol content (70 to 85%) and is synonymous with oregano, which also has a high carvacrol content (60 to 85%) and may be irritant to skin. Also, Spanish marjoram (*Thymus mastaichina*), confusingly, has little in common with true marjoram and has a high 1,8-cineole content, large amounts of which can cause central nervous system and breathing problems (Tisserand and Young 2014, 346); this oil is sometimes confused with thyme. Sweet marjoram, or true marjoram, on the other hand, contains no carvacrol and contains a large amount of the alcohol terpinen-4-ol (16 to 32%); sweet marjoram is prefable for topical aromatherapeutic application. Wild marjoram, Spanish marjoram, and oregano are not recommended for topical application; these oils, however, are strongly antibacterial and antiviral and as such may be valuable additions to antimicrobial blends for use in environmental diffusers or as disinfectants (do not use around babies and young children).

Plant description: A bushy, herbaceous plant that grows up to 20 to 24 inches (50 to 60 centimeters) high, marjoram has square, frequently branching stems that are covered in small, fine hairs and tiny, hair-covered, ovate, grayish-green leaves arranged oppositely in pairs. Clusters of small purplish to pale red to white flowers grow from spikes at the top of the plant, blooming from mid- to late summer (July to September). Marjoram is an annual but grows as a perennial in some warmer locations, and it is much favored by bees and butterflies.

Botanical family: Lamiaceae (Labiatae)

Extraction method: Steam distillation of the flowering leaves and tops

Appearance of essential oil: Clear to pale yellow or amber liquid (darkens to brown with age)

Odor of essential oil: Type: spicy; strength: medium; characteristics: spicy, fresh, green, herbal, minty, camphoraceous, then warm and woody, with camphoraceous-spicy dry-out notes

Compatible essential oils for blending: Cedarwood, chamomile, cypress, eucalyptus, lavender, neroli, rosemary, sandalwood, tea tree, vetivert

Safety data: Nontoxic, nonsensitizing, nonirritant. Avoid using during menstruation and pregnancy (may irritate uterus) as a precaution. Avoid or apply with caution with low blood pressure. Use moderately when there is a history of depression (very sedative).

Perfume note: Middle

Principal chemical constituents: CAS No: 8015-01-8

Marjoram (sweet): alpha-thuyene (0.1 to 2%), **sabinene (5 to 14%),** beta-myrcene (0 to 2%), alpha-terpinene (5 to 10%), limonene (0.1 to 2.5%), beta-phellandrene (0.1 to 2.5%), **gamma-terpinene (7 to 16%),** para-cymene (1 to 2%), terpinolene (2 to 4%), trans-thuyanol (0.1 to 3%), linalool (0.01 to 2%), cis-thuyanol (10 to 12%), linalyl acetate (2 to 5%), **terpinen-4-ol (16 to 32%),** alpha-terpineol (3 to 8.5%), geranyl acetate (0.05 to 0.2%)

Subtle Connections

Colors: Yellow (*opposite: violet*), orange (*opposite: blue*)

Chakras: Solar plexus, sacral

Gemstones: Citrine (*opposite: amethyst*), carnelian (*opposite: lapis lazuli/ aquamarine*)

Energy: Yin, yang

Elements: Earth, wood (air)

Actions and Uses

General actions: Analgesic, anaphrodisiac (inhibits sexual desire), antioxidant, antiseptic, antispasmodic, antiviral, bactericidal, cephalic, emmenagogue, expectorant, fungicidal, hypotensive, nervine, sedative, tonic, vulnerary

Skin: Chilblains, bruises; wound healing

Respiratory system: Asthma, bronchitis, colds, coughs, infections, sinusitis

Joints and muscles: Arthritis; muscle aches, pains, and stiffness; sprains, strains

Circulatory system: Lowers blood pressure

Immune system: Immune stimulant

Fungal infections: Candida, athlete's foot

Potential psycho-emotional and spiritual support: Eases mild depression and anxiety, grief and heartache, irritability and agitation, nervous tension, stress and stress-related conditions, trauma, headache, hypertension, insomnia, migraine; stimulates parasympathetic nervous system; calms hyperactivity; reassuring and steadying; soothes an overactive mind

MAY CHANG
(Litsea cubeba)

Geographical location: An evergreen tree or shrub, may chang is native to southeastern Asia, especially China, Indonesia, and the Taiwan Region. China is the main producer and consumer. The plant is also cultivated in the Taiwan Region and Japan.

Plant description: A small evergreen tropical tree or shrub growing 16 to 39 feet (5 to 12 meters) high, with fragrant, lemongrass-scented leaves and small creamy-white flowers that produce pepper-like, lemon-scented fruits—hence the name *Litsea cubeba,* or "mountain pepper"; it is also called pheasant pepper tree.

Botanical family: Lauraceae

Extraction method: Steam distillation. Commercially, the essential oil is mainly produced to extract its derivatives (citral, ionone, methyl ionone, vitamins A, E, and K). An essential oil is distilled from the leaves and is produced in Java (one of the Indonesian islands), mainly for local consumption (Tisserand and Young 2014, 350).

Appearance of essential oil: Pale yellow to pale brown liquid

Odor of essential oil: Type: citrus; strength: medium; characteristics: intense, lemony, green, grassy, lemongrass like, aldehydic, with sweet, fresh undertones and sharp, lemony dry-out notes.

Compatible essential oils for blending: Bergamot, cedarwood, geranium, grapefruit, lemon, orange, pine, sandalwood, rose, most floral oils

Safety data: Nontoxic; potential skin irritant and sensitizer. Do not use on damaged, diseased, or hypersensitive skin. Use in moderation at low dose to avoid skin sensitization. Do not use on children under two years old. May be adulterated with synthetic citral (Tisserand and Young 2014, 349).

Perfume note: Top to middle

Principal chemical constituents: CAS No: 68855- 99-2
alpha-pinene (0.5 to 1.5%), beta-pinene (0.5 to 1.5%), myrcene (0.1 to 1.5%), dehydro-1,8-cineole (0.1 to 2%), dextro-limonene (8 to 23%), eucalyptol (0 to 0.6%), rose furan (0 to 0.03%), linalool (1 to 2%), citronellal (0.1 to 0.8%), iso-neral (0.1 to 1.4%), iso-geranial (0.1 to 2.2%), alpha-terpineol (0.1 to 0.3%), nerol (0.1 to 1.2%), **neral (25 to 34%),** piperitenone (trace amount to 0.02%), **geranial (35 to 41%),** beta-caryophyllene (0.1 to 1%), geraniol (trace amount to 1.6%)

Subtle Connections

Colors: Yellow (*opposite: violet*), orange (*opposite: blue*), red (*opposite: green*)

Chakras: Solar plexus, sacral, base

Gemstones: Citrine (*opposite: amethyst*), carnelian (*opposite: lapis lazuli/ aquamarine*), jasper (*opposite: aventurine*)

Energy: Yang

Element: Fire

Actions and Uses

General actions: Antiseptic, deodorant, disinfectant, environmental disinfectant, insecticidal, stimulant

Skin: Acne, dermatitis, excessive perspiration, greasy skin, spots; insect repellent

Potential psycho-emotional and spiritual support: Eases feelings of anxiety, depression and low mood, fatigue and lethargy; helps with insomnia, memory loss; stimulant; uplifting

MELISSA / LEMON BALM
(Melissa officinalis)

Geographical location: This herb is native to south and central Europe, the Mediterranean region, central and western Asia, Iran, northern Africa, and North America and is cultivated in Hungary, Egypt, and Italy as an herb and in Northern Ireland for its essential oil. The main essential oil–producing countries are Bulgaria, Italy, the United Kingdom, and the United States.

Plant description: A sweet, lemon-scented herb related to mint, lemon balm grows in clumps 24 to 59 inches (60 to 150 centimeters) high, with square stems, aerial branches, bright green, serrated, ovate or heart-shaped leaves arranged oppositely on the stem, and spikes of tiny white, yellow, or pink flowers. The aerial parts of the plant are picked from early summer onward. The optimum time for harvest is just before the flowers open, when the concentration of volatile oil is at its highest. The plant is propagated from seed or cuttings in the spring. The nectar-rich flowers attract bees (the name *melissa* is Greek for "honeybee").

Botanical family: Lamiaceae (Labiatae)

Extraction method: Steam distillation of the leaves and flowering tops. The essential oil is often codistilled with lemon, citronella, may chang, or other lemon-scented oils. Melissa-like essential oils are more commonly sold sometimes as imitations of genuine melissa; however, genuine melissa oil is very expensive and not always available. Purchase from a reputable supplier.

Appearance of essential oil: Clear to pale yellow mobile liquid

Odor of essential oil: Type: citrus; strength: medium; characteristics: sweet, citrus, citronella, herby, grassy, with fresh, lemony notes and weak, citrusy dry-out notes

Compatible essential oils for blending: Chamomile, geranium, lavender, neroli, peppermint, floral and citrus oils

Safety data: Nontoxic; degrades rapidly once oxidized, which increases the propensity for irritation and sensitization. Melissa is often distilled or mixed with other essential oils (see above) and various other isolates and synthetics; for example, synthetic citral and citronellal may be used as adulterants. Apply topically in moderation, use with caution, and do not use on sensitive skin (Tisserand and Young 2014, 350).

Perfume note: Top to middle

Principal chemical constituents: CAS No: 8014-71-9

beta-myrcene (0.01 to 0.3%), cis-beta-ocimene (0.01 to 0.2%), trans-beta-ocimene (0.1 to 2%), 3-octanone (trace amount to 0.3%), 6-methyl-5-hepten-2-one (1 to 4%), cis-, trans-rose oxide (trace amount to 0.1%), nonanal (trace amount to 0.15%), 1-octen-3-ol (trace amount to 0.5%), citronellal (0.1 to 2%), beta-caryophyllene (0.3 to 20%), **neral (9 to 27%),** germacrene D (0.5 to 1.50%), **geranial (10 to 40%),** geranyl acetate (0.5 to 4%), geraniol (0.5 to 2%)

Subtle Connections

Colors: Yellow (*opposite: violet*), orange (*opposite: blue*)

Chakras: Solar plexus, sacral

Gemstones: Citrine (*opposite: amethyst*), carnelian (*opposite: lapis lazuli/ aquamarine*)

Energy: Yang

Elements: Wood (air), fire

Actions and Uses

General actions: Antidepressant, antifungal, anti-infectious, anti-inflammatory, antispasmodic, antiviral (herpes), bactericidal, calming, emmenagoge, expectorant, febrifuge, hypertensive, insect repellent, nervine, sedative, sudorific (causes sweating), tonic, vulnerary (wound healing)

Skin: Athlete's foot, cold sores, insect bites; insect repellent

Respiratory system: Asthma, bronchitis, chronic coughs, colds; calms rapid breathing

Muscles and joints: Muscle fatigue, muscle spasm

Fungal infections: Athlete's foot, candida

Potential psycho-emotional and spiritual support: Calming; eases feelings of anxiety, depression and low mood, fear and shock, grief and bereavement, nervousness and hypertension; relieves insomnia; quells anger, panic attacks; raises the spirit; strengthens memory; tonic, uplifting

MYRRH
(Commiphora myrrha, C. erythraea)

Geographical location: Myrrh is a gum resin extracted from the tree species of the genus *Commiphora,* native to northeast Africa, Yemen, Somalia, Eritrea, and eastern Ethiopia. It is also found in trees in Saudi Arabia, Kenya, India, Iran, and Thailand. The main essential oil–producing countries are France (from imported exudes), Ethiopia, Kenya, and Somalia.

Plant description: Myrrh is extracted from small, thorny, deciduous shrubs or small trees that grow up to 15 to 33 feet (5 to 10 meters) high, with knotted branches and trifoliate, scant, small, unequal, aromatic leaves and white flowers, often found growing on parched, rocky hills, and preferring well-drained soil and sunny positions. The tree's bark produces a thick, aromatic, pale yellow, granular liquid resin that flows from wounds or incisions made in the bark; the resin hardens and darkens into a reddish-brown mass. *C. myrrha* produces herabol myrrh resin, while the Arabian species, *C. erythraea,* produces bisabol myrrh resin.

Botanical family: Burseraceae

Extraction method: Steam distillation from the crude tree resin. An absolute is obtained by solvent extraction.

Appearance of essential oil: Pale yellow to reddish-brown, thick, viscous, oily liquid. The absolute presents as a dark reddish-brown, viscous mass.

Odor of essential oil: Type: balsamic; strength: medium; characteristics: balsamic, dry, amber, toffee, metallic, slightly medicated, resinous, mushroomy, with warm-spicy body tones and nondescript dry-out notes. The absolute has warm, rich, spicy, balsamic tones, with lingering warm, spicy, balsamic dry-out notes.

Compatible essential oils for blending: Benzoin, bergamot, cypress, frankincense, geranium, German chamomile, juniper, lavender, mandarin, mints, patchouli, petitgrain, pine, sandalwood, spice oils, thyme

Safety data: Nonirritant, nonsensitizing, though potentially toxic in high concentration due to its beta-elemene and furanodiene content.

Crude resin extracts have been found to cause adverse dermal reactions and some contact sensitivity. Avoid during pregnancy. Avoid on sensitive or damaged skin. The Somalian species, *Commiphora myrrha,* has antioxidant qualities (Tisserand and Young 2014, 357).

Perfume note: Base

Principal chemical constituents: CAS No: 8016-37-3

Somalian myrrh: alpha-pinene (trace amount to 0.2%), delta-elemene (trace amount to 0.9%), beta-bourbonene (trace amount to 0.3%), beta-elemene (2 to 6%), beta-caryophyllnene (0.1 to 0.4%), germacrene A (0.1 to 2%), germacrene D (0.1 to 2%), selinene (0.1 to 2%), germacrene B (1 to 4%), **curzerene (20 to 42%), furanoeudesma-1,3-diene (20 to 25%),** lindestrene (1 to 5%), sesquiterpenone (0.1 to 0.3%), acetyl-8,12-epoxygermacra-1,4-7-11-tetraene (0.5 to 3%), ester curzerenique (0.1 to 3%)

Subtle Connections

Colors: Yellow (*opposite: violet*), orange (*opposite: blue*), red (*opposite: green*)

Chakras: Solar plexus, sacral, base

Gemstones: Citrine (*opposite: amethyst*), carnelian (*opposite: lapis lazuli/ aquamarine*), jasper (*opposite: aventurine*)

Energy: Yang, yin

Elements: Earth, metal (ether)

Actions and Uses

General actions: Anticatarrhal, antifungal, anti-inflammatory, antimicrobial, antiphlogistic (relating to inflammation and fevers), antiseptic, astringent, balsamic (soothing base balm), cicatrizant, emmenagogue, expectorant, stimulant (digestive, pulmonary)

Skin: Athlete's foot, chapped and cracked skin, eczema, mature skin, ringworm, wounds, wrinkles

Muscles and joints: Arthritis

Respiratory system: Asthma, bronchitis, catarrh, coughs, gum infections, gingivitis, mouth ulcers, sore throat

Antifungal: Athlete's foot, candida, oral thrush, ringworm

Potential psycho-emotional and spiritual support: Eases apathy and warms emotional coldness; brings deep emotions to the surface; calming, revitalizing; regulates and calms breathing; sedative; stimulant

MYRTLE
(Myrtus communis)

Geographical location: The aromatic common myrtle is native to North Africa (Morocco, Sahara mountains, Algeria, Israel) and grows throughout the world—in the Mediterranean region, western Asia, and India, as well as being cultivated as a garden shrub in Europe (including southern England) and in the warm regions of North America. A species also grows in South America, Australia, and New Zealand. The essential oil is produced mainly in Corsica, Spain, Tunisia, Morocco, Italy, the former Yugoslavia (now Bosnia, Serbia, Croatia, Montenegro, Macedonia), and France. *Myrtus communis* grows in southern Europe and Mediterranean regions, while *Myrtus nivellei* grows in North Africa and the Sahara mountains.

Plant description: A bushy, medium-sized evergreen shrub or small tree, myrtle grows up to 16.5 feet (5 meters) high, with many tough but slender branches, brownish-red bark, and small, sharply pointed, ovate, dark green aromatic leaves with profuse solitary white fragrant flowers less than an inch (2 centimeters) in width, borne on short stalks that produce purplish-black berries. Myrtle belongs to a large aromatic family that includes eucalyptus and tea tree, as well as bayberry or wax myrtle (*Myrica cerifera*) and Dutch myrtle or English bog myrtle (*Myrica gale*), which are used in herbal medicine (although the essential oil from these species is said to be poisonous). *Myrtus communis* is not to be confused with iris, sometimes called myrtle flower or calamus, myrtle grass, or sweet myrtle.

Botanical family: Myrtaceae

Extraction method: Steam distillation of the leaves and twigs and sometimes the flowers. There are three types of essential oils produced: regular pinene or cineole myrtle; red cineole myrtle, which is mostly grown in North African regions such as Morocco;

and green linalool myrtle, which is mostly grown in Mediterranean regions, especially Corsica.

Appearance of essential oil: Clear to pale yellow or amber liquid

Odor of essential oil: Type: herbal; strength: medium; characteristics: fresh-camphoraceous, fruity, spicy, sweet, herbaceous; similar to eucalyptus, with warm, camphoraceous body tones and faint, herbaceous, nondescript dry-out notes

Compatible essential oils for blending: Bay leaf, bergamot, clary sage, clove and other spices, ginger, hyssop, laurel, lavender, lime, rosemary

Safety data: Nontoxic, nonsensitizing, nonirritant in low dose; may irritate mucous membranes or skin in high dose or with prolonged use. There is potential for drug interaction (particularly with antidiabetic medication), and it is also potentially carcinogenic—do not take orally (Tisserand and Young 2014, 358).

Perfume note: Middle to top

Principal chemical constituents: CAS No: 8008-46-6

alpha-pinene (18 to 57%), limonene (5 to 13%), **1,8-cineole (18 to 38%),** gamma-terpinene (trace amount to 1%), terpinolene (trace amount to 1.5%), linalool (1 to 10%), linalyl acetate (trace amount to 0.2%), beta-caryophyllene (trace amount to 1%), alpha-humulene (trace amount to 1%), estragole (0 to 1.5%), terpinyl acetate (trace amount to 1%), alpha-terpineol (0.1 to 3.5%), geranyl acetate (0.5 to 3%), germacrene B (0.1 to 0.3%), geraniol (0.1 to 0.4%), caryophyllene oxide (0.1 to 0.5%)

Subtle Connections

Colors: Yellow (*opposite: violet*), orange (*opposite: blue*)

Chakras: Solar plexus, sacral

Gemstones: Citrine (*opposite: amethyst*), carnelian (*opposite: lapis lazuli/ aquamarine*)

Energy: Yin, yang

Elements: Water, earth

Actions and Uses

General actions: Analgesic, anticatarrhal, antifungal, anti-infectious, antiseptic (pulmonary), antiviral, astringent, bactericidal, decongestant, expectorant, insecticidal, slightly sedative

Skin: Acne, inflamed skin, oily skin, skin infections

Joints and muscles: Arthritis

Respiratory system: Asthma, bronchitis, catarrhal conditions, chronic cough, sinusitis, sore throat

Immune stimulant: Especially in cases of lung infections and colds

Potential psycho-emotional and spiritual support: Eases distraction, insomnia; sedative; soothes anger, despair, fear, grief; neuro-balancing

NEROLI / ORANGE BLOSSOM
(*Citrus* x *aurantium* var. *amara*)

Geographical location: Neroli essential oil is made from the blossoms of the bitter orange tree, which is native to tropical Asia and is now grown throughout the tropics, subtropics, and the Mediterranean, especially the southern coasts of France and Spain and regions with similar climates, such as North Africa (Morocco, Tunisia, Egypt), as well as in the United States (Florida, California, Arizona, Alabama). The main essential oil–producing countries are Italy, Morocco, and Tunisia.

Plant description: An evergreen tree growing up to 33 feet (10 meters) high, bitter orange has leathery, dark green, glossy leaves and light, sweet-floral citrusy fragranced white flowers. The blossoms are gathered by hand in late April to early May, and again in October during mild seasons.

Botanical family: Rutaceae

Extraction method: Steam distillation of freshly picked blossoms. It takes 1,000 pounds (454 kilograms) of blossoms to extract 1 pound (0.453 kilogram) of essential oil, making distilled neroli very expensive to produce. Solvent extraction yields a concrete, from which an absolute is produced. Both the concrete and absolute contain residues of the solvent and chemical wash-out materials used. This method produces a less expensive product, which is mainly used as a perfume ingredient. The blossoms of sweet orange (*Citrus aurantium* var. *dulcis*) are also used to make an absolute and essential oil called neroli Portugal (or neroli petalae); however, it is less fragrant and considered of inferior quality.

Appearance of essential oil: Pale yellow to amber mobile liquid that darkens with age

Appearance of absolute: Amber to dark brown viscous liquid

Odor of essential oil: Type: floral; strength: medium; *characteristics, distilled:* sweet, characteristically reminiscent of orange flowers, citrusy, mandarin-like, petitgain, herbal, with light, floral, herbaceous, slightly citrusy middle tones and faint, nondescript dry-out notes; *characteristics, absolute:* fresh, delicate but rich, warm, floral fragrance, closer to nature in character than the distilled oil, with lingering, warm, floral-citrus dry-out notes

Compatible essential oils for blending: *Distilled:* benzoin, bergamot, chamomile, clary sage, coriander, geranium, jasmine, lavender, lemon, lime, orange, rose, sandalwood, ylang-ylang; *absolute:* benzoin, jasmine, myrrh, all citrus oils

Safety data: Nontoxic, nonirritant, nonsensitizing, nonphototoxic; rare reports of dermatitis and photosensitivity; frequently adulterated due to its expense (Burfield 2003). Reconstituted oils may be added to the mixture; also large qualities of leaf and twig material may be distilled with the blossoms (Tisserand and Young 2014, 363). Purchase from reputable suppliers who will vouch for the oil's purity and authenticity.

Perfume note: Base to middle. The absolute is classified as a base note due to its tenacious scent depth.

Principal chemical constituents (essential oil): CAS No: 8016-38-4 alpha-pinene (0.1 to 1.5%), sabinine (0.5 to 3%), beta-pinene (5 to 13%), beta-myrcene (1 to 3.5%), **limonene (10 to 18%),** beta-ocimene (Z) (0.1 to 1.5%), beta-ocimene (E) (1 to 7%), **linalool (30 to 48%),** alpha-terpineol (1 to 5%), nerol (0.1 to 1.5%), linalyl acetate (1 to 11%), geraniol (0.1 to 3%), neryl acetate (0.1 to 1%), geranyl acetate (0.1 to 2%), alpha-humulene (trace amount to 1%), nerolidol (E) (0.1 to 3%), farnesol (E) (0.1 to 1%)

Subtle Connections

Colors: Yellow (*opposite: violet*), orange (*opposite: blue*), red (*opposite: green*)

Chakras: Solar plexus, sacral, base

Gemstones: Citrine (*opposite: amethyst*), carnelian (*opposite: lapis lazuli/ aquamarine*), jasper (*opposite: aventurine*)

Energy: Yang, yin
Elements: Fire, wood (air), earth

Actions and Uses

General actions: Antidepressant, antiseptic, antispasmodic, aphrodisiac, bactericidal, cicatrizant, deodorant, fungicidal

Skin: Dry skin, mature skin, scars, sensitive skin, stretch marks, thread veins; improves tone and elasticity

Joints and muscles: Aids muscle tone

Respiratory: Bronchitis

Antifungal: Mild

Potential psycho-emotional and spiritual support: Eases anxiety, depression, and agitation; eases sadness and disappointment, emotional shock and upset; encourages feelings of self-confidence; relieves fatigue, insomnia; instills a sense of peace; calms nervous tension, premenstrual tension; relaxing, tranquilizing (in low dose), stimulating (nerves; in high dose)

NIAOULI
(Melaleuca quinquenervia)

Geographical location: This tree is native to New Caledonia, Papua New Guinea, the French Pacific Islands, and coastal eastern Australia, including Queensland and the Northern Territory. It also grows in Madagascar and was naturalized in the early 1900s in the United States (in Florida, where the climate is similar to that of Australia, but where it is now considered invasive). Niaouli grows in lowland areas, swamps and marshlands, and flood plains and near rivers and estuaries; it can take over marshland and create swamps that pose a threat to native ecosystems if its spread is not curtailed. The main essential oil producing–countries are Australia, Madagascar, and Tasmania.

Plant description: Niaouli is a medium-size evergreen tree with a flexible trunk covered with thick, whitish-beige, papery bark, which lends it its common names: broad-leaved paperbark, paper bark tree, and punk tree. It grows to a height of 26 to 66 feet (8 to 20 meters), with a spread of alternately arranged branches and leathery, dull, grayish-green, wide, ovate, pointed, linear leaves 2 to 4 inches (5 to 10 centimeters) long and 1/4 to 1 inch (0.5 to 2.5 centimeters) wide. Its white or cream sessile (stalkless) flowers are arranged in cylindrical brushes about 2 to 3 inches (4 to 8 centimeters) long and are borne at or near the end of branchlets. The flowers bloom from September to March (spring in Australia) and are a rich source of nectar for fruit bats, insects, and bird species. The leaves have a strong aromatic scent when they are crushed.

Botanical family: Myrtaceae (and it is in the same genus as tea tree)

Extraction method: Steam distillation of leaves and young twigs. There are three types of essential oil produced: cineole, linalool, and nerolidol. The oil is usually redistilled (rectified) to remove irritant aldehydes.

Appearance of essential oil: Clear to lemon yellow with greenish tints

Odor of essential oil: Type: herbal; strength: medium; characteristics: sweet, camphoraceous, eucalyptus, minty, woody, resinous

Compatible essential oils for blending: Cedarwood, eucalyptus, lavender, lemon, marjoram, myrtle, peppermint, pine, rosemary, thyme

Safety data: Nontoxic, nonsensitizing, nonirritant

Perfume note: Top to middle

Principal chemical constituents: CAS No: 8014-68-4

alpha-pinene (7 to 12%), beta-pinene (1 to 5%), beta-myrcene (trace amount to 2%), limonene (5 to 12%), **1,8-cineole (45 to 65%),** gamma-terpinene (trace amount to 1.5%), para-cymene (0.05 to 4%), benzaldehyde (0.05 to 5%), alpha-teripineol (3 to 10%), ledene (trace amount to 1.5%), alpha-, beta-selinene (trace amount to 1.5%), nerolidol (0.05 to 1.5%), viridifloral (2 to 9%)

Subtle Connections

Colors: Yellow (*opposite: violet*), green (*opposite: red*), pink (*opposite: pale aqua-green*)

Chakras: Solar plexus, heart

Gemstones: Citrine (*opposite: amethyst*), aventurine (*opposite: jasper*), rose quartz (*opposite: aquamarine*)

Energy: Yin

Element: Metal (ether)

Actions and Uses

General actions: Analgesic, anticatarrhal, antirheumatic, antiseptic, antispasmodic, bactericidal, cicatrizant, expectorant, stimulant

Skin: Acne, boils, burns, insect bites, skin infections

Joints and muscles: Aching muscles, arthritis

Respiratory system: Asthma, bronchitis, catarrh, coughs, colds, flu, respiratory infections, sinusitis, sore throat

Antifungal: Athlete's foot, candida

Immune system: Flu, herpes, shingles; immune stimulant

Potential psycho-emotional and spiritual support: Aids concentration, clears head; eases depression (caused by illness/infection); reviving

NUTMEG
(Myristica fragrans)

Geographical location: Native to the tropical region of Maluku (the Spice Islands), of eastern Indonesia, this tree is also cultivated in Sri Lanka, the West Indies (especially Grenada), Guatemala, Kerala in southern India, and Brazil. East India, Sri Lanka, and Grenada are the main essential oil–producing countries.

Plant description: A tropical evergreen dioecious (male and female flowers occuring on separate plants) tree that grows up to 65 feet (20 meters) high, nutmeg has a grayish-brown, smooth bark and dense foliage consisting of leathery, slightly aromatic leaves. The small, unscented, dull yellow flowers resemble those of lily of the valley and produce drupes of tough, yellowish, one-seeded peach-shaped fruits when the tree is eight years old. Once mature, the tree produces fruit all year round for up to eighty to a hundred years. The fruits are harvested two or three times a year. When ripe, the fleshy outer covering of the fruit splits open, revealing its oval seed—the nutmeg. The seed is covered in a bright red, lacy aril—mace—which is removed and flattened into strips and dried, ready to be ground or distilled for its essential oil. The nutmeg seeds are air-dried for several weeks; during this period, worms eat the starch and fat content in the nutlike seeds, giving the dried nutmeg its lacerated appearance.

Botanical family: Myristicaceae

Extraction method: Steam distillation of the dried nutmeg seeds. An essential oil is also extracted from the dried aril, or mace.

Appearance of essential oil: Colorless to pale yellow or watery white

Odor of essential oil: Type: spicy; strength: medium; characteristics: sweet warm, spicy, woody, characteristically nutmeg, powdery, pine, old wood, resinous, with terpenic top notes and warm, spicy-woody dry-out notes

Compatible essential oils for blending: Clary sage, coriander, geranium, ginger, lime, mandarin, may chang, orange, petitgrain, rosemary

Safety data: Nontoxic, nonirritant, nonsensitizing—however, use in moderation and in low dose. Avoid during pregnancy.

Perfume note: Top to middle

Principal chemical constituents: CAS No: 8008-45-5

alpha-pinene (11 to 25%), alpha-thujene (trace amount to 1%), camphene (trace amount to 0.5%), **beta-pinene (12 to 18%), sabinene (14 to 45%),** delta-3 carene (0.5 to 2%), beta-myrcene (1 to 4%), alpha-phellandrene (trace amount to 1%), alpha-terpinene (trace amount to 3%), limonene (2 to 7%), beta-phellandrene (trace amount to 3%), gamma-terpinene (2 to 8%), para-cymene (trace amount to 2%), terpinolene (trace amount to 2%), trans-thujanol (trace amount to 0.5%), alpha-copaene (trace amount to 0.5%), **terpinene-4-ol (2 to 11%),** terpenyl acetate (trace amount to 0.5%), safrole (1 to 4%), methyl eugenol (1 to 3%), elemicine (trace amount to 1%), **myristicin (1 to 14%)**

Subtle Connections

Colors: Orange (*opposite: blue*), yellow (*opposite: violet*)

Chakras: Sacral, solar plexus

Gemstones: Carnelian (*opposite: lapis lazuli/aquamarine*), citrine (*opposite: amethyst*)

Energy: Yang

Elements: Fire, earth

Action and Uses

General actions: Analgesic, antiarthritic, antimicrobial, antioxidant, antiseptic, antispasmodic, aphrodisiac, carminative, digestive, emmenagogue, stimulant, tonic

Endocrine system: Estrogen-like

Joints and muscles: Arthritis; stiff, aching, painful muscles; improves circulation and eases pain

Digestive system: Flatulence, indigestion, irritable bowel syndrome, nausea; stimulates digestion (topical application)

Immune system: Bacterial infections

Nervous system: Nervous fatigue, neuralgia

Potential psycho-emotional and spiritual support: Antidepressant; eases feelings of emotional coldness; warming, euphoric, and hallucinogenic in large dose; intensifies dreams; a mental stimulant

ORANGE, BITTER
(Citrus aurantium var. amara)

Geographical location: Bitter orange is native to tropical Southeast Asia and eastern Africa and is now grown throughout the tropics and subtropics, as well as along the Mediterranean coast, especially in Spain; it also grows abundantly in the United States (California), Israel, South America, and Australia. The main essential oil–producing countries are Australia, Brazil, the Dominican Republic, Guinea, the West Indies, Israel, Italy, Spain, and the United States.

Plant description: This evergreen tree grows from 10 to 33 feet (3 to 10 meters) high. The leaves are leathery and aromatic, with a glossy, dark, evergreen surface, paler underneath, dotted with tiny oil glands and long but not very sharp spines. It produces very fragrant white flowers with yellow stamens, borne singularly or in small clusters on the leaf axils. The fruits, which are smaller and darker than sweet oranges, are round, oblate, or oblong-oval, with a thick, bitter-tasting aromatic peel embedded with minute sunken oil glands (the oil is 90% limonene, flavonoids, coumarins, triterpenes, carotene, and pectin). The composition of the volatile oils in the leaves, flowers, and peel varies significantly, producing three different essential oils (petitgrain, neroli or orange blossom, and bitter orange). The tree is well-known for its resistance to disease and is often used as root stock for other citrus trees, including sweet orange. Also known as Seville orange, sour orange, bigarade orange, and marmalade orange, it is a hybrid between *Citrus maxima* (pomelo) and *Citrus reticulata* (mandarin), with many subsequent varieties. *Citrus x aurantium* var. *amara* is cultivated for its essential oils: the blossoms of this species produces neroli and orange floral water and is applied to flavor teas (Earl Grey, for example).

Botanical family: Rutaceae

Extraction method: Cold expression of the outer part of the almost ripe fruit peel

Appearance of essential oil: Clear to pale orange or dark yellow to brownish liquid. Distilled orange is mostly clear.

Odor of essential oil: Type: citrus; strength: medium; characteristics: fresh, orange-like, dry, woody, leafy, with slightly floral undertones and warm, nondescript dry-out notes

Compatible essential oils for blending: Black pepper, cinnamon, clary sage, clove, coriander, frankincense, geranium, grapefruit, jasmine, juniper, lavender, marjoram (sweet), myrrh, neroli, nutmeg, patchouli, petitgrain, rose, sandalwood, vetivert, ylang-ylang

Safety data: Nontoxic, nonsensitizing, nonirritant; low risk of phototoxicity if used in moderation. Older oxidized oils or those with a high dextro-limonene content have an increased potential for sensitization; also, prolonged use in high dose may irritate sensitive skin.

Perfume note: Top

Principal chemical constituents: CAS No: 68916-04-1
alpha-pinene (trace amount to 0.05%), beta-pinene (trace amount to 0.05%), beta-myrcene (1 to 3%), **dextro-limonene (85 to 95%),** ocimene (trace amount to 0.05%), cyclopropane,1,2-dibutyl (trace amount to 0.01%), cis-linalool oxide (trace amount to 0.05%), myrcenol (trace amount to 0.05%), linalool (0.1 to 2%), linalyl butyrate (trace amount to 0.02%), alpha-terpineol (trace amount to 0.02%), 3-carne (trace amount to 0.02%), bergapten (trace amount to 0.08%), nerol (trace amount to 0.02%)

Subtle Connections

Colors: Yellow (*opposite: violet*), orange (*opposite: blue*), red (*opposite: green*)

Chakras: Solar plexus, sacral, base

Gemstones: Citrine (*opposite: amethyst*), carnelian (*opposite: lapis lazuli/ aquamarine*), jasper (*opposite: aventurine*)

Energy: Yang, yin

Elements: Fire, earth, wood (air)

Actions and Uses

General actions: Antifungal, anti-infectious, anti-inflammatory, anti-microbial, antiseptic, antiviral, astringent, bactericidal, decongestant, expectorant, sedative

Skin: Acne; dry skin; dull, congested, oily complexion; supports skin regeneration

Joints and muscles: Sore muscles, water retention

Respiratory system: Bronchitis

Immune system: Immune stimulant

Potential psycho-emotional and spiritual support: Aids mental clarity and concentration; eases agitation, anxiety, mild depression, insomnia, stress-related tension; energizes; stimulant; supports enthusiasm; supports sympathetic nervous system

PALMAROSA
(Cymbopogon martinii)

Geographical location: Palmarosa, also known as Indian geranium, Turkish geranium, motia, and rosha grass, shares similarities with gingergrass, lemongrass, and citronella. It is a wild grass native to the forests and wetlands of Southeast Asia and also India, Pakistan, and Turkey, and it is now grown in Africa, Madagascar, Indonesia, Brazil, and the Comoros Islands. The main essential oil–producing countries are India, Madagascar, and Nepal.

Plant description: A tall, herbaceous, fragrant (it smells sweet and roselike, hence its common name palma*rosa*) tropical grass growing 4 to 10 feet (1.3 to 3 meters) high, palmarosa has a strong, slender, pale green shoot or stem and a flowering top that produces bluish-white panicles that turn red as they mature. It takes three months for this grass to grow and flower. The grass cannot be harvested until the flowers have matured sufficiently; as the flowers become darker and redden, the essential oil is released from the plant's cells. The essential oil extracted from *Cymbopogon martinii* contains a large quantity of geraniol (60 to 85%); geraniol gives palmarosa its distinctive floral, roselike scent. Palmarosa essential oil is sometimes used to "bulk out" (adulterate) rose essential oil, especially Turkish rose.

Gingergrass (*Cymbopogon martinii* var. *sofia*), also known as russa grass, is very closely related to palmarosa, and consequently their names are sometimes used synonymously. However, gingergrass essential oil contains large quanities of limonene and various types of menthadienols, giving it a spice-like scent. In spite of these differences, there is sometimes confusion about which species is being referred to because their names are so similar. To differentiate and resolve confusion, the main chemical constituents of palmarosa and gingergrass are listed below for comparison.

Botanical family: Poaceae (Gramineae)

Extraction method: Steam distillation from the dried grass stems and leaves

Appearance of essential oil: Clear to yellow or amber to pale olive liquid

Odor of essential oil: Type: floral; strength: medium; characteristics: sweet, floral, rosy, citrus, grassy, citronella, tomato, leafy, herbaceous, with rose/geranium-like undertones and faded, citrusy, nondescript dry-out notes

Compatible essential oils for blending: Bergamot, cedarwood, citronella, geranium, petitgrain, rose and other floral oils, rosewood, sandalwood

Safety data: Nontoxic, nonirritant, nonsensitizing. Use in moderation.

Perfume note: Top to middle

Principal chemical constituents: Palmarosa CAS No: 8014-19-5; gingergrass CAS No: 8023-92-5

Palmarosa (*Cymbopogon martinii*): beta-myrcene (0.05 to 3%), limonene (0.01 to 0.15%), cis-beta-ocimene (trace amount to 0.4%), trans-beta-ocimene (trace amount to 1.5%), linalool (trace amount to 2%), beta-caryophyllene (0.5 to 3%), neral (trace amount to 0.5%), geranial (trace amount to 1%), geranyl acetate (8 to 11%), nerol (trace amount to 1%), **geraniol (75 to 85%),**

geranyl caproate (trace amount to 1%), farnesol (trace amount to 1%)
Gingergrass (*Cymbopogon martinii* var. *sofia*): **dextro-limonene (25 to 35%), trans-rho-mentha-1(7),8-dien-2-ol (10 to 15%), cis-rho-mentha-1(7),8-dien-2-ol (10 to 15%), trans-rho-mentha-2,8-dien-1-ol (10 to 15%),** cis-rho-mentha-2,8-dien-1-ol (5 to 8%), rho-menthadienol (3 to 6%), carvone (2 to 5%), cis-carveol (2 to 5%), rho-menthadienol (1 to 4%), rho-menthatrienol (0.5 to 3%), rho-mentha-1(7),2,8-triene (0.5 to 3%)

Subtle Connections
Colors: Orange (*opposite: blue*), yellow (*opposite: violet*), green (*opposite: red*), pink (opposite: *pale aqua-green*)
Chakras: Sacral, solar plexus, heart
Gemstones: Citrine (*opposite: amethyst*), carnelian (*opposite: lapis lazuli/aquamarine*), aventurine (*opposite: jasper*), rose quartz (*opposite: aquamarine*)
Energy: Yang, yin
Elements: Fire, earth

Actions and Uses
General actions: Analgesic, antifungal, anti-infectious, anti-inflammatory, antimicrobial, antiseptic, antiviral, bactericidal, cicatrizant, circulatory stimulant, decongestant, expectorant, febrifuge, hydrating, vulnerary (wound healing)
Skin: Acne, dermatitis, dry skin, eczema, psoriasis, scars; regulates sebum, stimulates cellular/skin regeneration
Muscles and joints: Arthritis
Antifungal: All candida species
Potential psycho-emotional and spiritual support: Eases mild depression and anxiety, stress and agitation; relieves fatigue, headache, and migraine; grounding and uplifting

PATCHOULI
(Pogostemon cablin)

Geographical location: A flowering plant in the mint family, patchouli is native to tropical regions of Asia, where it is also widely cultivated, especially in China, Indonesia, India, Malaysia, Mauritius, the Taiwan Region, the Philippines, Thailand, and Vietnam, as well as in western Africa and South America. The essential oil is distilled in Europe and the United States from imported dried leaves. Other essential oil–producing countries include Brazil, China, India, Indonesia, Malaysia, and Sri Lanka.

Plant description: This perennial, fragrant, shrubby herb grows up to over 3 feet (1 meter) in height, with sturdy, erect, hairy, square stems and large, furry, oval, fragrant leaves and spikes bearing small white or pale pink to light purple flowers. The shoots and leaves are picked two or three times a year; the leaves are usually partially fermented before distillation.

Botanical family: Lamiaceae (Labiatae)

Extraction method: Steam distillation of the young, fresh, dried and partially fermented leaves.

Patchouli is sometimes adulterated with gurjun balsam (*Dipterocarpus* spp.) oil, copaiba balsam oil, cedarwood oil, or the distillate residue from patchouli, vetivert, camphor, and vegetable oils, among others. The better-quality patchouli oil (Indonesian) is sometimes bulked out with cheaper Chinese oil (Tisserand and Young 2014, 382).

Appearance of essential oil: Dark brownish-orange or yellowish-amber viscous liquid

Odor of essential oil: Type: woody; strength: medium; characteristics: rich, sweet, herbaceous, mossy-woody, earthy, weedy, balsamic, spicy, minty to slightly camphoraceous-spicy, dry-woody, tenacious, with lingering dry-out notes

Compatible essential oils for blending: Bergamot, cedarwood, clary sage, clove, geranium, lavender, mandarin, myrrh, neroli, rose, spikenard, vetivert

Safety data: Nontoxic, nonirritant, nonsensitizing. Assure authenticity and purity with your essential oil supplier.

Perfume note: Base to middle

Principal chemical constituents: CAS No: 8014-09-3

beta-pinene (trace amount to 0.2%), delta-elemene (trace amount to 0.2%), beta-patchoulene (1.5 to 3.5%), alpha-copaene (trace amount to

1%), **alpha-guaiene (11 to 16%)**, beta-caryophyllene (2 to 5%), **alpha-patchoulene (6 to 11%)**, seychellene (2.5 to 5%), gamma-patchoulene (trace amount to 1%), alpha-humulene (trace amount to 0.7%), aciphyllene (guai-4,11-diene) (1 to 3%), **alpha-bulnesene (13 to 21%)**, caryophyllene oxide (trace amount to 0.02%), norpatchoulenol (0.3 to 1%), **patchoulol (27 to 35%)**, pogostol (1 to 2.5%)

Subtle Connections

Colors: Orange (*opposite: blue*), violet (*opposite: yellow*)
Chakras: Sacral, third eye
Gemstones: Carnelian (*opposite: lapis lazuli/aquamarine*), amethyst (*opposite: citrine*)
Energy: Yin, yang
Element: Earth

Actions and Uses

General actions: Antiallergic, antidepressant, anti-infectious, anti-inflammatory, antimicrobial, antiseptic, antitoxic, antiviral, astringent, bactericidal, deodorant, fungicidal, skin healing
Skin: Abscesses, chapped and cracked skin, dermatitis, eczema, hair (dandruff), impetigo, insect bites, oily hair (scalp) and skin, scars, sores, wounds, wrinkles (mature skin); insect repellent
Respiratory system: Calms and regulates flow of breathing
Fungal infections: Candida species (nails), ringworm (fungal nail infection, athlete's foot), *Epidermophyton floccosum* infections (groin, feet)
Immune system: Immune support
Other: PMS, menopause; endocrine stimulant
Potential psycho-emotional and spiritual support: Eases confusion and indecision, anxiety, depression, low mood, agitation, apathy, nervous exhaustion, nervous tension, panic attacks, premenstrual tension; regulates and calms breathing; sedative at low dose, stimulant at high dose; relieves stress and stress-related conditions; supports meditation and a sense of spirituality

PEPPER, BLACK
(Piper nigrum)

Geographical location of growth: *Piper nigrum* is native to southwest India and is cultivated extensively in eastern India, Sri Lanka, and other tropical countries. Vietnam is the largest producer, providing a third of the world's black pepper crop; other major producers are India, Indonesia, Malaysia, China, and Madagascar. The dried pepper fruits, or peppercorns, are imported and distilled in Europe and the United States.

Plant description: A perennial woody climber or flowering vine, black pepper can grow up to 33 feet (10 meters) high by means of its aerial roots. It is cultivated for its fruit. The vine has heart-shaped or oval, alternately arranged leaves that are dark green on the upper side and whitish green on the underside, and flower spikes that grow from the stem and produce small white flowers and drupes of small, round fruits or berries, which turn from green to yellowish red as they mature. The fruit is harvested from plants that are at least three years old. Black peppercorns are picked just before they are ripe; the fruit drupes are boiled to cleanse them, then laid out in the sun to dry or dried by machine (some producers separate the fruit berries from their stalks and dry them in the sun). Essential oils are found in the leaves and fruits. An essential oil is produced from both black and green pepper fruits from the same species.

Botanical family: Piperaceae

Extraction method: Steam distillation of the dried, crushed peppercorns

Appearance of essential oil: Colorless to pale yellow with bluish tints

Odor of essential oil: Type: spicy; strength: medium; characteristics: fresh, warm, spicy, terpenic, peppery, woody, with herbaceous undertones and mellow-peppery dry-out notes

Compatible essential oils for blending: Basil, bergamot, cypress, frankincense, grapefruit, lavender, lemon, marjoram, may chang, orange, rose, rosemary, sandalwood; blends well with florals, fruits, and spices

Safety data: Nontoxic, nonsensitizing, nonirritant; has a propensity for oxidation, which can render the oil sensitizing. Store in a cool, dark place and ensure the lid is tightly secured.

Perfume note: Middle

Principal chemical constituents: CAS No: 8006-82-4

alpha-pinene (1 to 16%), beta-pinene (4 to 12%), sabinene (1 to 13%), delta-3-carene (trace amount to 15%), beta-myrcene (trace amount to 3%), alpha-terpinene (trace amount to 0.5%), **limonene (14 to 25%),** beta-phellandrene (trace amount to 2%), alpha-cubebene (trace amount to 2%), delta-elemene (trace amount to 2%), alpha-copeane (trace amount to 3%), **beta-caryophyllene (9 to 30%),** alpha-humulene (0 to 1%), germacrene D (trace amount to 0.3%), beta-selinene (trace amount to 0.1%), alpha-selinene (trace amount to 1%), beta-bisabolene (trace amount to 5%), caryophyllene oxide (trace amount to 1%)

Subtle Connections

Colors: Yellow (*opposite: violet*), green (*opposite: red*), pink (*opposite: pale aqua-green*), blue (*opposite: orange*)

Chakras: Solar plexus, heart, throat

Gemstones: Citrine (*opposite: amethyst*), aventurine (*opposite: jasper*), rose quartz (*opposite: aquamarine*), lapis lazuli/aquamarine (*opposite: carnelian*)

Energy: Yang

Element: Fire

Actions and Uses

General actions: Analgesic, antimicrobial, antiseptic, antispasmodic, bactericidal, circulatory stimulant, febrifuge

Skin: Bruises, chilblains

Joints and muscles: Arthritis, muscle aches and pains, muscle tone, sprains

Respiratory system: Bronchitis, catarrh, sinusitis, tonsillitis

Immune system: Antiviral

Potential psycho-emotional and spiritual support: Aids alertness; eases transitions and life changes; relieves cold feelings, adds warmth to indifference; mental stimulant

PEPPERMINT
(Mentha x piperita)

Geographical location: Indigenous to Europe and the Middle East, peppermint is a cultivated hybrid plant created from a cross between *Mentha spicata* (spearmint) and *Mentha aquatica* (water mint). Grown commercially and in gardens throughout Europe, Asia, and North America, this plant is now found in habitats worldwide, especially alongside water (streams and ditches). The main essential oil–producing countries are Australia, China, India, Italy, Japan, and the United States.

Plant description: Peppermint is a seedless, or sterile, herbaceous hybrid plant propagated via its roots or rhizome spread. It grows from 12 to 35 inches (30 to 90 centimeters) tall. Its stem is smooth and square-shaped in cross-section and produces broad, dark green leaves with reddish veins and coarsely toothed edges; both stem and leaves are covered with a soft, fine hair. Whorls of small white or purple flowers are borne on spikes that grow from the stem during mid- to late summer.

Botanical family: Lamiaceae (Labiatae)

Extraction method: Steam distillation of the fresh leaves and flowers. Plants distilled in June contain more menthol; those distilled closer to flowering, in September, contain more menthone; the flowers are rich in menthone and menthofurane.

Appearance of essential oil: Colorless to pale green or pale yellow

Odor of essential oil: Type: minty; strength: medium; characteristics: cool, penetrating, pungent, pepperminty, grassy-minty, with a creamy-minty-balsamic undertone and dry-herbaceous dry-out notes

Compatible essential oils for blending: Benzoin, eucalyptus, geranium, lavender, lemon, marjoram, rosemary, and other mints

Safety data: Nontoxic, nonsensitizing (but potentially neurotoxic and sensitizing if applied in high dose). Menthol, a constituent of peppermint, is a dermal irritant that can influence (increase/decrease) dermal permeability of other chemicals. Avoid on sensitive or damaged skin. Use in moderation as a precaution, as peppermint essential oil constituents can vary tremendously depending on species and conditions of growth, length of distillation time, and so on. Peppermint essential oil is often adulterated with corn mint (*Mentha arvensis*) oil. Tisserand and Young (2014, 387) warn that peppermint oil should be avoided altogether in cases of cardiac fibrillation and in people with a glucose-6-phosphate dehydrogenase (G6PD) deficiency, a metabolic condition.

Perfume note: Middle to top

Principal chemical constituents: CAS No: 8006-90-4

alpha-pinene (trace amount to 1%), sabinene (trace amount to 0.3%), beta-pinene (trace amount to 0.7%), myrcene (trace amount to 0.3%), para-cymene (trace amount to 0.1%), limonene (1 to 2.5%), eucalyptol (1 to 5%), **menthone (15 to 32%),** menthofuran (trace amount to 9%), iso-menthone (0.1 to 8.5%), neo-menthone (0.1 to 10%), **menthol (25 to 45%),** pulegone (trace amount to 5%), carvone (trace amount to 0.4%), piperitone (trace amount to 2%), methyl acetate (1 to 10%), beta-bourbonene (trace amount to 3%), beta-elemene (trace amount to 0.2%), beta-caryophyllene (0.1 to 4%), germacrene D (0.1 to 4.5%)

Subtle Connections

Colors: Yellow (*opposite: violet*), green (*opposite: red*), pink (*opposite: pale aqua-green*)

Chakras: Solar plexus, heart

Gemstones: Citrine (*opposite: amethyst*), aventurine (*opposite: jasper*), rose quartz (*opposite: aquamarine*)

Energy: Yang, yin

Elements: Wood (air), earth

Actions and Uses

General actions: Analgesic, antifungal, anti-infectious, anti-inflammatory, antimicrobial, antiparastic, antiseptic, antispasmodic, antiviral, astringent, bactericidal, cephalic, expectorant, febrifuge, nervine, vasoconstrictive

Skin: Acne, dermatitis, inflammation, itchy skin, psoriasis, ringworm, sunburn, toothache

Respiratory system: Asthma, bronchitis, coughs, sinusitis; clears nasal passages and stimulates breathing

Joints and muscles: Joint and muscle pain

Digestive system: Irritable bowel syndrome (topical compress)

Potential psycho-emotional and spiritual support: Eases breathing, panic attacks, mild depression, racing thoughts and mental chatter, tension headache; improves concentration; eases mental fatigue and exhaustion, memory loss, migraine, nervous stress, vertigo; refreshing and invigorating; sedative and calming in low dose

PETITGRAIN / ORANGE LEAF
(Citrus aurantium var. amara)

Geographical location: Petitgrain is native to southern China and northeast India and cultivated in Paraguay, France, North Africa, and Haiti. France produces the best-quality petitgrain essential oil (used mainly as a perfume ingredient), although Paraguay also produces an intensely perfumed essential oil. Petitgrain is also known as orange leaf oil and mandarin leaf oil.

Plant description: An evergreen, aromatic tree growing up to 33 feet (10 meters) high—but only 19 feet (6 meters) when growing wild—petitgrain has a smooth brown trunk, stout branches, and leathery, dark green leaves, with fragrant blossoms and small, bitter orange fruits. An essential oil is extracted from both the blossoms (neroli) and the fruits (bitter orange). Petitgrain essential oil is extracted from the leaves and twigs. A type of petitgrain is also produced from lemon, sweet orange, mandarin, and bergamot trees.

Botanical family: Rutaceae

Extraction method: Steam distillation of the leaves and twigs

Appearance of essential oil: Clear to pale yellow or yellow to amber liquid

Odor of essential oil: Type: floral; strength: medium; characteristics: floral, sage, neroli, citrus, sweet, fresh, floral, woody-orange, green-mossy, with dry-herbaceous dry-out notes

Compatible essential oils for blending: Clove, benzoin, bergamot, bitter orange, geranium, grapefruit, jasmine, lavender, mandarin, neroli, palmarosa, rosemary, sandalwood, spikenard

Safety data: Nonirritant, nontoxic, nonsensitizing, nonphototoxic. Petitrain bigarade may be adulterated with cheaper Paraguayan oil (Tisserand and Young 2014, 375). Petitgrain oils (*Citrus* spp.) may also be adulterated with the addition of other citrus leaf oils and fractions, fatty aldehydes, linalyl acetate, and orange terpenes. Paraguayan oil is often adulterated with the synthetically derived chemicals linalool, linalyl acetate, alpha-terpineol, geranyl and neryl acetates, and trace amounts of pyrazines (Burfield 2003). Assure authenticity and purity with your essential oil supplier.

Perfume note: Top to middle

Principal chemical constituents: CAS No: 8014-17-3

alpha-pinene (trace amount to 0.3%), beta-pinene (trace amount to 2%), sabinene (trace amount to 0.3%), delta-3-carene (0.1 to 0.6%), myrcene (0 to 3%), limonene (0 to 2%), cis-beta-ocimene (0 to 1%), trans-beta-ocimene (0.1 to 3%), neral (trace amount to 1%), terpinolene (0 to 1%), **linalool (20 to 30%), linalyl acetate (36 to 57%),** beta-caryophyllene (0 to 1%), alpha-terpineol (3 to 8%), neryl acetate (0.1 to 3%), geranial (0.1 to 0.1%), geranyl acetate (2 to 6%), nerol (trace amount to 2%), geraniol (0.01 to 5%)

Subtle Connections

Color: Yellow (*opposite: violet*)
Chakra: Solar plexus
Gemstone: Citrine (*opposite: amethyst*)
Energy: Yin, yang
Elements: Earth, wood (air)

Actions and Uses

General actions: Antiarthritic, anti-infectious, anti-inflammatory, antiseptic, antispasmodic, deodorant, toner
Skin: Acne, chapped and cracked skin, dry skin, excessive perspiration, greasy hair and skin, dry/oily scalp, scars
Respiratory system: Asthma, colds, flu, hay fever, respiratory infections, stress-related shallow breathing; eases breathing
Joints and muscles: Arthritis, joint inflammation
Fungal infections: Candida and *Microsporum* species (ringworm and

other fungal infections of the skin, hair, scalp, and body, e.g., athlete's foot)

Immune system: Chronic fatigue syndrome, myalgic encephalomyelitis; immune stimulant

Other: PMS, menopause

Potential psycho-emotional and spiritual support: Eases anger, agitation, anxiety, apathy, nervous tension, depression and low mood, sense of hopelessness; relieves hyperactivity, insomnia, mental and nervous exhaustion; restores mental clarity; nervous system sedative; relieves premenstrual tension, stress and stress-related conditions

PINE NEEDLE, SCOTCH
(Pinus sylvestris)

Geographical location: Scotch pine is native to the United Kingdom (thriving in heathlands and planted in Scotland for its timber) and the mountainous regions of Europe, western Asia (from the Arctic Circle in Scandinavia to the Anatolia region that embraces Turkey); it is cultivated in New Zealand, the eastern United States, Canada, Russia, the Baltic states, Scandinavia, and Europe and is now found throughout the northern hemisphere. It is mainly cultivated for its wood (and also for the Christmas tree trade). The main essential oil–producing countries are Canada, France, and the United States.

Plant description: A tall, evergreen, coniferous tree growing from 100 to 147 feet (35 to 45 meters) high, Scotch pine can live up to seven hundred years. The bark is scaly red, orange, and brown. Bluish-green (becoming dark green to yellowish-green in the winter), needlelike, slightly twisted leaves grow in pairs on short side shoots stemming from twigs and branches. Both the male and female trees' flowers grow on the same tree (i.e., they are monoecious) and are pollinated by the wind. The male flowers are comprised of a cluster of yellow anthers at the base of the shoots. Small, reddish-purple, globular female flowers grow at the tips of new shoots. When fertilized, these flowers turn green and develop into pointed-oval to conical cones (i.e., the fruits) that mature the following year, when they turning grayish brown, with a raised, circular bump at the center of each scale. The needles are gathered in the summer. The stems are usually harvested when the tree is felled. The needles on young trees grow longer than those on old trees.

There are numerous species of pine that yield an essential oil from their heartwood, twigs, and needles and also produce turpentine. The essential oil from Scotch pine is one of the most therapeutically safe and useful. Other species that produce pine oil from needles and terminal branches include black pine (*Pinus nigra*), sea or ocean pine (*Pinus palustris*), ponderosa pine (*Pinus ponderosa*), dwarf or mountain pine (*Pinus mugo*), gray pine (*Pinus divarticata*), red or Norway pine (*Pinus resinosa*), and white pine (*Pinus strobus*). Huon pine (*Dacrydium franklinii*) is not used in aromatherapy.

Botanical family: Pinaceae

Extraction method: Steam distillation of the dried needles

Appearance of essential oil: Colorless to pale yellow or straw yellow

Odor of essential oil: Type: earthy; strength: medium; characteristics: earthy, dry, weedy, pine-like, woody, resinous, with turpentine-like tones

Compatible essential oils for blending: Cedarwood, eucalyptus, lavender, lemon, marjoram, may chang, niaouli, peppermint, rosemary, sage

Safety data: Nontoxic, nonsensitizing, nonirritant when stored correctly; it oxidizes very quickly and so must be kept in cool, dark place (preferably the fridge) with the lid tightly secured and used within twelve months. Add antioxidant ingredients to blends, especially those prepared for long-term use. Discard small amounts of oil remaining in the bottle. Scotch pine needle essential oil is often adulterated with turpentine oil and mixtures of terpenes (Tisserand and Young 2014, 398).

Perfume note: Middle

Principal chemical constituents: CAS No: 8023-99-2

alpha-pinene (25 to 55%), camphene (0.1 to 3%), beta-pinene (10 to 35%), delta-3-carene (0.1 to 32%), beta-myrcene (0.1 to 4%), limonene (0.1 to 4%), beta-pinocamphone (trace amount to 1%), bornyl acetate (trace amount to 0.2%), trans-beta-ocimene (0 to 1%), beta-caryophyllene (0.1 to 4%), terpinene-4-ol (trace amount to 0.2%), alpha-terpineol (trace amount to 1%), delta-cadinene (trace amount to 0.5%)

Subtle Connections

Color: Yellow (*opposite: violet*)
Chakra: Solar plexus
Gemstone: Citrine (*opposite: amethyst*)
Energy: Yin, yang
Elements: Metal (ether), earth

Actions and Uses

General actions: Analgesic, antimicrobial, antineuralgic, antiseptic (especially pulmonary), antiviral, bactericidal, decongestant, deodorant, expectorant, hypertensive, insecticidal, restorative, stimulant (adrenals, circulatory and nervous systems)

Skin: Cuts, eczema, excessive perspiration, lice, psoriasis, ringworm, skin congestion, sores

Joints and muscles: Arthritis, gout, joint and muscular aches and pains, sciatica, stiffness, water retention

Respiratory system: Asthma, bronchitis, catarrh, sinusitis, sore throat; cleanses respiratory tract, increases mucus secretion and expulsion

Immune system: Immune stimulant

Potential psycho-emotional and spiritual support: Bracing; clears head; eases debility, sense of hopelessness, fatigue, nervous exhaustion; refreshes and stimulates a tired mind; relieves stress-related conditions

ROSEMARY
(Rosmarinus officinalis)

Geographical location: Native to the Mediterranean and Caucasus (the area situated between eastern Europe and Asia), rosemary is also cultivated in China, Morocco, Tunisia, the Middle East, Russia, France, Spain, Portugal, Bosnia, Serbia, Croatia, Montenegro, Macedonia, and the United States. The essential oil is produced worldwide.

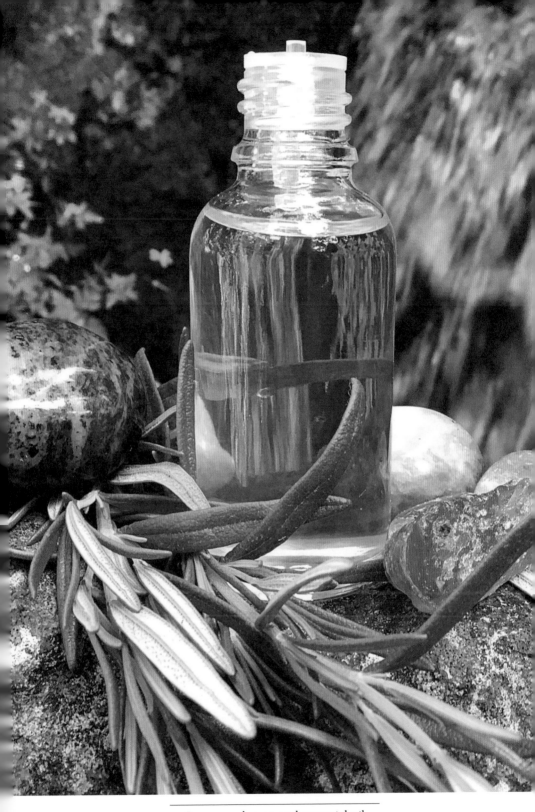

Rosemary leaves and essential oil

Plant description: An evergreen bushy perennial herb or shrub, rosemary can grow up to 6 feet (2 meters) high and 6 feet (2 meters) wide, with strongly aromatic green and silverish-green, needlelike leaves and purplish-white, purple, pink, or blue two-lipped flowers with protruding stamens. It is propagated from seeds or cuttings in the spring and prefers warm, modestly sheltered locations. The branches are gathered and dried during the summer after flowering. The whole plant is strongly aromatic. The name *rosemary* is derived from the Latin *ros,* "dew," and *marinus,* "sea," hence "dew of the sea." *R. officinalis* is the type used for essential oil production, and there are many cultivars and chemotypes (for example, the camphor, cineole, verbenone, and beta-myrcene chemotypes).

Botanical family: Lamiaceae (Labiatae)

Extraction method: Steam distillation of the fresh flowering tops or the whole plant (which produces a poorer quality)

Appearance of essential oil: Colorless or pale yellow

Odor of essential oil: Type: herbal; strength: medium; characteristics: strong, fresh, herbal, camphoraceous, woody, minty, balsamic, medicinal, phenolic, with woody-balsamic undertones and dry-herbaceous dry-out notes. Oxidized or poor-quality essential oils have a strong camphoraceous scent.

Compatible essential oils for blending: Basil, cedarwood, cinnamon and other spice oils, citronella, frankincense, grapefruit, lavender, peppermint, petitgrain, pine, thyme

Safety data: Nontoxic, nonirritant, nonsensitizing. Use in moderation, especially the camphor-type rosemary. Do not use on babies or infants; 1,8-cineole is reported to cause serious poisoning in children when accidently ingested (Tisserand and Young 2014, 409). Avoid using on sensitive, damaged, or traumatized skin.

Perfume note: Middle

Principal chemical constituents: CAS No: 8000-25-7

alpha-pinene (9 to 14%), camphene (2.5 to 10%), beta-pinene (4 to 9%), beta-myrcene (1 to 2%), limonene (1 to 4%), **1,8-cineole (38 to 55%),** gamma-terpinene (trace amount to 2%), para-cymene (0.5 to 2.5%), camphor (5 to 15%), linalool (0.3 to 2%), bornyl acetate (0.1 to 2%), beta-caryophyllene (0.1 to 4%), terpinene-4-ol (trace

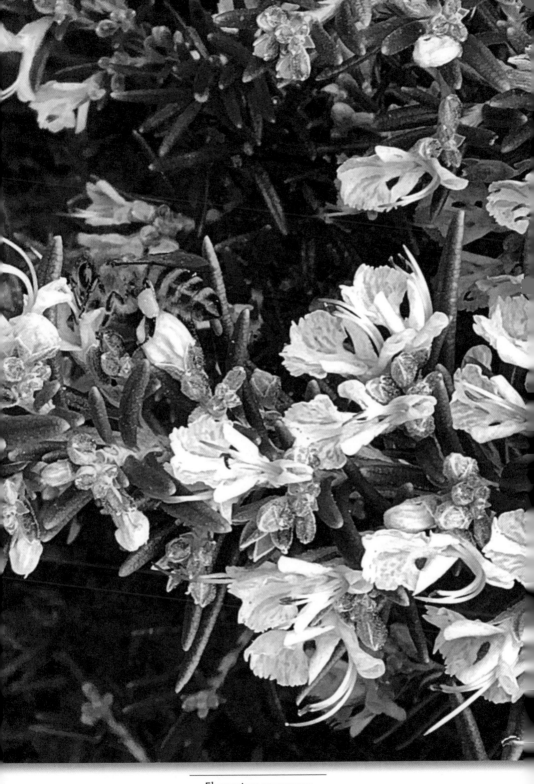

Flowering rosemary

amount to 1%), alpha-terpineol (1 to 2.5%), borneol (1 to 9%), methyl eugenol (trace amount to 0.5%)

Subtle Connections

Colors: Yellow (*opposite: violet*), blue (*opposite: orange*)
Chakras: Solar plexus, throat
Gemstones: Citrine (*opposite: amethyst*), carnelian (*opposite: lapis lazuli/ aquamarine*)
Energy: Yang
Element: Fire

Actions and Uses

General actions: Analgesic, antibacterial, antifungal, anti-infectious, anti-inflammatory, antimicrobial, antiparasitic, antiseptic, antispasmodic, antiviral, astringent, cephalic, cicatrizant, circulatory stimulant, decongestant, diuretic, emmenagogue, expectorant, nervine, vulnerary (wound healing)

Skin: Acne, congested and puffy skin, dandruff, dermatitis, edema, greasy hair, lice; promotes hair growth, repels insects

Joints and muscles: Arthritis, muscle pains and cramp, myalgia, sprains; supports connective tissue regeneration

Respiratory: Asthma, bronchitis, colds, coughs, infections, sinusitis, tonsillitis

Potential psycho-emotional and spiritual support: Enlivens the brain and clears the head; aids in opening the throat chakra, finding your voice; aids memory; aphrodisiac; eases debility, mild depression, headache, lethargy, mental fatigue, migraine, nervous exhaustion; restorative, stimulating; tonic

ROSE OTTO
(Rosa x damascena, R. centifolia)

Geographical location: Originally native to the Asia and the Middle East, rose otto has a long historical association dating back thousands of years in Japan, Morocco, Tunisia, and Iran. The name *rose otto* is derived from "attar of roses" (*attar* means "fragrance") and dates back to the seventeenth century. The largest producers of rose otto today are Afghanistan, Bulgaria, and Turkey, then France and India and, to a lesser degree, the Middle East. India specializes in producing rose otto absolutes and concretes. *Rosa* x *damascena* is strictly a cultivated species. The main essential oil–producing countries are Afghanistan, Bulgaria, China, France, India, Russia, and Turkey.

Plant description: *Rosa* x *damascena* (commonly known as damask rose and rose of Castile) is a hybrid derived from *Rosa gallica* (French rose) and *Rosa moschata* (musk rose) and was originally cultivated hundreds of years ago. It is a deciduous, informally shaped shrub growing up to 7 feet (2.2 meters) high, with curved prickles and stiff bristles protruding from its stem, pinnate leaves, and relatively small pink to light red, highly fragrant, numerously petaled flowers that grow in clusters. *Rosa centifolia* (also known as Provence rose or cabbage rose), a derivative of *Rosa* x *damascena,* was originally cultivated in Holland between the seventeenth and nineteenth centuries. It is similar in stature to damask rose, although slightly shorter, growing up to 6 feet (2 meters), with long, drooping, cane-like stems, greenish-gray pinate leaves, and multipetaled, highly fragrant, globular, pink or sometimes white to dark reddish-purple flowers. Both cultivars sport numerous hybrids.

Botanical family: Rosaceae

Extraction method: Water or steam distillation of the fresh petals; labor-intensive to produce (flowers must be hand-picked), with a relatively low yield of essential oil per volume of plant material, rendering the oil very expensive. For example, 250 pounds (113 kilograms) of petals produce just one ounce of rose otto essential oil.

Appearance of essential oil: Pale yellow or olive yellow, depending on the color of the petals. The oil crystallizes/solidifies at low temperatures.

Appearance of absolute: Deep orangish-red or reddish-brown to olive-green viscous liquid

Odor of essential oil: Type: floral; strength: medium; characteristics: complex; rich, intense, sweet, powerful, beeswax-like, highly floral; rosy, with waxy, floral, spicy, green, metallic body notes, then tenacious, warm, floral, spicy dry-out notes

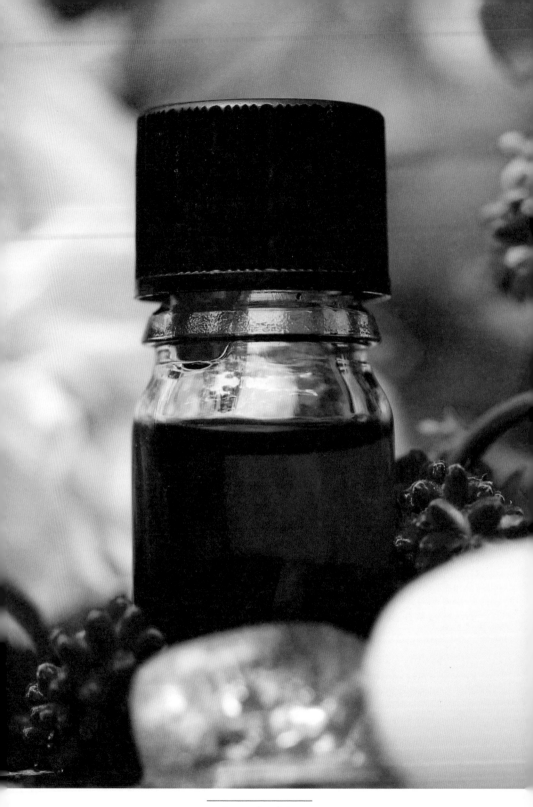

Rose absolute

Odor of absolute: Intense, sweet, floral, rose, waxy, honey, spicy, green, cortex, geranium, metallic, with rich, spicy, sweet, floral body notes and warm, floral, honey-like dry-out notes; used extensively in perfumery

Compatible essential oils for blending: Benzoin, bergamot, chamomile, clary sage, clove, frankincense, geranium, jasmine, lavender, neroli, palmarosa, patchouli, sandalwood (and most other essential oils)

Safety data: The essential oil is nonirritant, nontoxic, nonsensitizing (highly perfumed, though; use in reduced dose). Although it contains methyleugenol, which is considered potentially carcinogenic, evidence suggests that the presence of geraniol apparently counteracts the effect of this compound. Cheaper, nature-identical synthetic reconstructions are created using damascones, beta-ionone plus (–)-citronellol, and other rose alcohols, plus rose steroptenes; also, occasionally the oil is adulterated with beta-phenylethyl alcohol, rhodinol fractions, and cheaper rose oils (Morocco, Crimea) (Burfield 2003), as well as ethanol, 2-phenylethanol, and fractions of geranium oil (Tisserand and Young 2014, 405–06). Absolutes should be regarded as perfume, having irritant and sensitizing potential. Assure authenticity and purity with your essential oil supplier.

Perfume note: Base (very tenacious) to middle (with intense but fleeting top notes)—a complex scent

Principal chemical constituents (essential oil): CAS No: 8007-01-0 alpha-pinene (trace amount to 0.4%), cis-rose oxide (trace amount to 0.3%), trans-rose oxide (trace amount to 0.2%), pentadecane (trace amount to 0.3%), linalool (0.1 to 3.5%), beta-elemene (trace amount to 0.1%), alpha-pinene (trace amount to 0.4%), alpha-guaiene (trace amount to 0.4%), beta-caryophyllene (trace amount to 1%), terpinene-4-ol (trace amount to 0.4%), citronellyl acetate (trace amount to 2%), neral (trace amount to 2%), alpha-terpineol (trace amount to 0.3%), germacrene D (trace amount to 2%), heptadecane (trace amount to 1%), alpha-bulnesene (trace amount to 0.4%), neryl acetate (trace amount to 0.3%), geranial (0.1 to 3%), geranyl acetate (0.1 to 3%), **citronellol (15 to 36%), nerol (3 to 12%), geraniol (15 to 30%),** nonadecane C19 (1 to 8%), methyleugenol (0.1 to 4%), alpha-pinene (trace amount to 0.4%), heneicosane (trace amount to 3%), eugenol (trace amount to 2%), farnesol (trace amount to 2%)

Subtle Connections: Essential Oil

Colors: Yellow (*opposite: violet*), green (*opposite: red*), pink (*opposite: pale aqua-green*)

Chakras: Solar plexus, heart

Gemstones: Citrine (*opposite: amethyst*), aventurine (*opposite: jasper*), rose quartz (*opposite: aquamarine*)

Energy: Yin

Elements: Metal (ether), water

Subtle Connections: Absolute

Colors: Red (*opposite: green*), orange (*opposite: blue*)

Chakras: Base, sacral, heart

Gemstones: Jasper (*opposite: aventurine*), carnelian (*opposite: lapis lazuli/aquamarine*)

Energy: Yin, yang

Elements: Earth, wood (air), fire

Actions and Uses

General actions: Analgesic, anti-infectious, anti-inflammatory, antimicrobial, antioxidant, antiseptic, antispasmodic, antiviral, aphrodisiac, astringent, bactericidal, hydrating, skin-healing, tonic

Skin: Abscesses, acne, dermatitis, dry scalp, dry skin, eczema, herpes simplex, mature skin, oily skin (balancing), shingles

Respiratory system: Chronic asthma, coughs, hay fever, mouth ulcers, sore throat

Joints and muscles: Tonic to smooth muscle tissue

Immune system: Chronic fatigue syndrome, myalgic encephalomyelitis; immune stimulant

Circulatory system: Regulates blood pressure

Other: Endocrine stimulant (hormone-like); headaches, migraine, painful periods, PMS, menopause

Potential psycho-emotional and spiritual support: Aphrodisiac; eases depression (especially postnatal) and low mood, agitation, anger, anxiety, fear, paranoia, grief, bereavement and sense of loss, headache (tension and hormonal), migraine, hypersensitivity; hypnotic; relieves insomnia (in low dose), jealousy, mood swings (especially hormonal), nervous tension, panic attacks, premenstrual tension and menopausal symptoms, resentment and disappointment, sadness and despair; sedative at low dose, stimulant at high dose; eases shock, stress, and stress-related tension and conditions

SAGE, CLARY
(Salvia sclarea)

Geographical location: Clary sage is native to southern Europe, especially the northern Mediterranean basin, and some areas in northern Africa and central Asia. It is cultivated worldwide, especially in northern and central Europe, Morocco, Russia, the United Kingdom, and the United States. English, French, and Moroccan oils are regarded as being the best quality for perfumery. The main essential oil–producing countries are Bulgaria, France, Italy, Morocco, Russia, Spain, and the United Kingdom.

Plant description: Sage is a biennial or short-lived perennial herb, shrub, or subshrub that grows up to 3.3 feet (1 meter) and produces strongly scented, wrinkled, green with a hint of purple, hairy leaves oppositely arranged along square stems, with long racemes of tubular, two-lipped, pink-flecked white blossoms or pale pink flowers with pinkish-mauve bracts that open in late spring and summer. The plants are harvested after the first fifteen months of growth, then two to three times a year. Clary sage is closely related to garden sage (*Salvia officinalis*) and Spanish sage (*Salvia lavandulaefolia*), which are both used to produce an essential oil. Other types of sage include meadow clary (*Salvia pratensis*) and wild clary sage (*Salvia verbenaca*).

Botanical family: Lamiaceae (Labiatae)

Extraction method: Steam distillation of the flowering tops and leaves

Appearance of essential oil: Colorless to pale yellow or yellowish green to brownish yellow

Odor of essential oil: Type: herbal; strength: medium; characteristics: fresh, herbal, tea, green, woody, weedy, dry, spicy, sage, powdery, with resinous-balsamic, herbaceous-woody body notes and dry-herbaceous dry-out notes

Compatible essential oils for blending: Bergamot, cardamom, cedarwood, coriander, frankincense, geranium, grapefruit, jasmine, juniper, lavender, lemon, lime, mandarin, orange, pine, rose, sandalwood

Safety data: Nontoxic, nonsensitizing, nonirritant; euphoric. Do not use clary sage while drinking alcohol; it can induce a narcotic effect and exaggerate drunkenness. Avoid during pregnancy.

Perfume note: Middle to top

Principal chemical constituents: CAS No: 8016-63-5

alpha-pinene (trace amount to 0.5%), beta-pinene (trace amount to 0.5%), beta-myrcene (trace amount to 1%), cis-beta-ocimene (trace amount to 0.3%), trans-beta-ocimene (trace amount to 0.4%), alpha-copaene (trace amount to 1%), **linalool (6 to 16%), linalyl acetate (62 to 78%),** beta-caryophyllene (trace amount to 2%), alpha-terpineol (trace amount to 1.5%), germacrene D (1.5 to 12%), neryl acetate (trace amount to 0.4%), geranyl acetate (trace amount to 1%), geraniol (trace amount to 0.4%), sclareol oxide (0.4 to 3%)

Subtle Connections

Colors: Yellow (*opposite: violet*), green (*opposite: red*), pink (*opposite: pale aqua-green*)

Chakras: Solar plexus, heart

Gemstones: Citrine (*opposite: amethyst*), aventurine (*opposite: jasper*), rose quartz (*opposite: aquamarine*)

Energy: Yin

Elements: Earth, metal (ether)

Actions and Uses

General actions: Anticonvulsive, antiseptic, antispasmodic, astringent, bactericidal, cicatrizant, deodorant, emmenogogue, hypertensive, nervine

Skin: Acne, boils, dandruff, hair loss, inflammation, oily skin; supports cell regeneration

Joints and muscles: Aching, painful muscles, spasms, and cramps

Respiratory system: Asthma, colds, throat infections

Potential psycho-emotional and spiritual support: Aids creativity and dreams; aphrodisiac; euphoric; bracing during difficult times; eases depression, anxiety, fatigue, migraine; mildly intoxicating; relieves nervous tension; sedative

SANDALWOOD
(Santalum album, S. spicatum)

Geographical location: Sandalwood is native to and cultivated in tropical Asia, especially India, Bangladesh, Pakistan, Nepal, Sri Lanka, Malaysia, Indonesia, Vietnam, and the Taiwan Region; it is also found in Hawaii, New Guinea, and Australia. India is the main essential-oil producer of *Santalum album* (white sandalwood); the region of Mysore exports the highest-quality oil, and some oil is distilled in Europe and the United States from imported wood. Unfortunately, Indian *Santalum album* has been overharvested and is now classified as an endangered species. *Santalum spicatum* is cultivated in Australia and provides an alternative, although this species is also reaching a critical point due to its popularity and the demand for the oil, as well as a consequence of drought and climate change in the region. Cultivated plantation-grown and managed sandalwood trees are preferable to wild-growing trees and produce ecologically viable and sustainable essential oils. *Eucaria spicata* is currently a viable alternative to *S. spicatum*. The main essential oil–producing countries are Australia, India, and Vietnam.

Plant description: Sandalwood is a semiparasitic (it obtains some nutrients from the roots of other neighboring trees and is part of the same botanical family as mistletoe), slow-growing tree with heavy, yellow, fine-grained, very fragrant wood that retains its scent for decades. It grows up to 30 feet (10 meters) high and has a brownish-gray trunk and many smooth, slender branches with lanced-shaped, leathery leaves and clusters of small, pale yellow to pinkish-purple flowers that produce small, almost black fruits. The Indian species must mature for thirty years before being harvested for its essential oil and wood; Australian sandalwood, which is obtained from cultivated and managed sources, must mature for fifteen years before harvest. Australian sandalwood (*S. spicatum* as well as *Eucaria spicata*) produces a very similar oil to *S. album,* but with a dry, bitter top note. Balsam torchwood (also known as West Indian sandalwood or West Indian rosewood) and amyris (*Amyris balsamifera*) are poor substitutes and bear no botanical relation to Indian sandalwood.

Botanical family: Santalaceae

Extraction method: Steam (or hydro) distillation of the pulverized heartwood or milled sawdust. The wood (or sawdust) is soaked for forty-eight hours, then slow-distilled over two to three days, then redistilled and rectified to remove undesirable compounds such as N-fufuryl pyrrol (Burfield 2003).

Appearance of essential oil: Pale yellow to dark golden or greenish to mild brown, clear, viscous liquid.

Odor of essential oil: Type: woody; strength: medium; characteristics: dry, woody, balsamic, sweet, myrrh, creamy, with nondescript top notes and soft, sweet, woody, balsamic, fatty-floral, very tenacious middle notes and faint dry-out notes

Compatible essential oils for blending: Bergamot, black pepper, clove, jasmine, lavender, mandarin, myrrh, orange, patchouli, rose, vetivert, ylang-ylang

Safety data: Nontoxic, nonsensitizing, nonirritant. Australian sandalwood holds some risk of interaction with certain drugs metabolized by CYP2D6 enzymes (i.e., liver enzymes). Commercial sandalwood is extracted using hydrodistillation and solvents, so traces of solvent remain in the oil and may cause sensitization or irritation (Tisserand and Young 2014, 420).

Perfume note: Base to middle

Principal chemical constituents: *Santalum album:* CAS No: 8006-87-9 / *Santalum spicatum:* CAS No: 8024-35-9

Santalum spicatum: alpha-sedrene (trace amount to 0.1%), alpha-santalene (trace amount to 0.5%), alpha-tans-bergamotene (trace amount to 1%), epi-beta-santalene (trace amount to 0.5%), beta-santolene (trace amount to 1%), gamma-curcumene (trace amount to 0.3%), beta-bisabolene (trace amount to 0.2%), beta-curcumene (trace amount to 0.5%), alpha-curcumene (trace amount to 0.3%), cendrolasine (trace amount to 1.5%), nerolidol (0.01 to 3%), guaiol (trace amount to 0.3%), epi-beta-bisabolol (trace amount to 1%), alpha-santalal (trace amount to 1%), **epi-alpha-bisabolol (2 to 13%), Z-alpha-santalol (15 to 25%), Z-alpha-trans-bisabolol (2 to 10%), farnesol (2 to 15%),** epi-beta-santalol (0.5 to 4%), **Z-beta-santalol (5 to 20%),** Z-gamma-curcumene-12-ol (0.5 to 6%), Z-alpha-curcumene-12-ol (0.5 to 8%), Z-lanceol (1 to 10%), nuciferol (0.5 to 7%)

Subtle Connections

Colors: Orange (*opposite: blue*), yellow (*opposite: violet*), green (*opposite: red*), pink (*opposite: pale aqua-green*)

Chakras: Sacral, solar plexus, heart

Gemstones: Carnelian (*opposite: lapis lazuli/aquamarine*), citrine (*opposite: amethyst*), aventurine (*opposite: jasper*), rose quartz (*opposite: aquamarine*)

Energy: Yin

Elements: Water, earth, metal (ether)

Actions and Uses

General actions: Anti-inflammatory, anti-infectious, antimicrobial, antiseptic (especially for the urinary and pulmonary systems), antispasmodic, astringent, bactericidal, cicatrizant, diuretic, expectorant, insecticidal

Skin: Acne, mature skin; dry, cracked, and chapped skin; greasy skin; infected wounds; aids moisturization; stimulant (circulatory); soothes inflammation and infection of the mouth and genital/urinary orifices (in a mouthwash or douche)

Joints and muscles: Cramps and muscle spasms; improves circulation

Respiratory system: Bronchitis, catarrh, dry cough, laryngitis, sore throat

Immune system: Immune stimulant

Potential psycho-emotional and spiritual support: Aids meditation, calms and harmonizes the mind (racing thoughts and mental clutter); aphrodisiac; sedative; eases mild depression, nervous tension, and end-of-life agitation; relieves insomnia, stress-related conditions; tonic

SPIKENARD
(Nardostachys jatamansii, N. grandiflora)

Geographical location: *Nardostachys jatamansii* and *N. grandiflora* are native to the mountains of India and now grow in the high-altitude regions of Nepal and China. Biblical and ayurvedic scriptures and other historical texts testify to the growth, production, and use of spikenard in the Middle East, Europe, and India. The essential oil is distilled and produced mainly in the United States, Nepal, and India, with some production in Europe. It is also known as nard, nardin, and muskroot and is traditionally used as a perfume, incense, and herbal sedative. Overexploitation of wild spikenard in Nepal means that managed cultivation of the plant is encouraged in this region in preference to wild-harvesting. *Aralia racemosa* is a native herb that grows in North America and is known as American spikenard (also small spikenard, Indian root, spiceberry) and belongs to the ginseng or Araliaceae botanical family. Its roots, which are edible, are used as a medicine to alleviate colds, coughs, asthma, and arthritis and are applied as an herb but not as an essential oil.

Plant description: A tender, flowering herb or plant growing up to a little over 3 feet (1 meter) in height, spikenard has pink, bell-shaped flowers clustered in umbels on top of a long green stem, with dark to light green elongated or oval-shaped leaves and underground rhizome roots. It is related to valerian, with similar, although less pungent, odorous and sedating qualities. The roots are often traded as valerian. Ensure that your supplier obtains the oil from a sustainable source.

Botanical family: Valerianaceae

Extraction method: Steam distillation of the dried, crushed rhizomes and roots

Appearance of essential oil: Pale orange-yellow-green to reddish-orange viscous liquid

Odor of essential oil: Type: woody; strength: medium; characteristics: very sweet, intense, woody, spicy, animal, valerian root, ginger, cardamom, with tones of fresh-cut grass; becomes less intense and delicately woody, with undertones of spice, fresh pea, and hay, with sweet and tenaciously lingering dry-out notes of fresh pea and hay

Compatible essential oils for blending: Black pepper, cypress, frankincense, geranium, lavender, orange, patchouli, petitgrain, pine, rose, turmeric, vetivert

Safety data: Nontoxic, nonirritant, nonsensitizing

Perfume note: Base

Principal chemical constituents: Major constituents between species vary considerably from region to region (Satyal et al. 2016).

Nardostachys grandiflora CAS No: 8022-22-8

Nepalese: alpha-pinene (trace amount to 0.3%), beta-pinene (trace amount to 0.7%), 1,8-cineole (trace amount to 0.1%), methyl myrtenate (trace amount to 0.3%), cis-myrtenyl acetate (trace amount to 0.4%), beta-patchoulene (0.1 to 3%), beta-elemene (trace amount to 0.6%), alpha-gurjunene (0.1 to 3%), aristolene (trace amount to 2%), nardoguanidiene C (trace amount to 2%), calarene (0.5 to 10%), beta-vatirenene (0.1 to 5%), 6,9-guanidiene (0.5 to 2.5%), valerena-4,7(11)-diene (1 to 8%), gamma-gurjunene (trace amount to 0,4%), laurene (0.1 to 3%), valencene (trace amount to 2%), nardol A (1 to 10%), **1(10)-aristolen-9-beta-ol (0.5 to 12%), valeranone jatamansone (0.3 to 8%), valerenal (0.3 to 6%), cis-valerinic acid (0.3 to 6%)**

Indian: **alpha-selinene (5 to 10%),** selinene isomer (0.5 to 4%), alpha-caryophyllene (0.1 to 3%), beta-caryophyllene (0.1 to 4%), alpha-gurjunene (0.1 to 3%), cubebol (0.1 to 3.5%), **nardol (6 to 11%),** gamma-gurjunene (0.1 to 3%), calamenene (0.1 to 1.5%), **dihydro-B-ionene (4 to 8%),** nardol isomer (1 to 5%), 7-hexadecene (0.1 to 2%), (E)-nerolidol, dextro-ledene epoxy (trace amount to 1.5%), propionic acid (0.5 to 4%), **formic acid (5 to 10%)**

Subtle Connections

Colors: Orange (*opposite: blue*), yellow (*opposite: violet*), green (*opposite: red*), pink (*opposite: pale aqua-green*)

Chakras: Sacral, heart, throat

Gemstones: Carnelian (*opposite: lapis lazuli/aquamarine*), citrine (*opposite: amethyst*), aventurine (*opposite: jasper*), rose quartz (*opposite: aquamarine*)

Energy: Yang, yin

Elements: Fire, wood (air), earth

Actions and Uses

General actions: Anti-infectious, anti-inflammatory, bactericidal, deodorant, fungicidal, rejuvenating, tonic

Skin: Inflammation, mature skin, rashes (skin conditions caused by nervousness)

Respiratory system: Panic attacks; calms the flow of breathing

Circulatory system: Improves circulation

Potential psycho-emotional and spiritual support: Balances sympathetic nervous system with parasympathetic nervous system (tonic to the sympathetic nervous system, regulates the parasympathetic nervous system); calms restlessness; eases anxiety, grief, bereavement; grounds feelings of hatred; relieves heartache, headache, migraine, hyperactivity, hysteria, impatience, insomnia; inspires a sense of peace and spirituality; eases intolerance, irritability, nervous tension, panic attacks, premenstrual tension and menopausal symptoms, stress and stress-related conditions; sedative

TEA TREE
(Melaleuca alternifolia)

Geographical location: Also known as paperback tree, tea tree is native to Australia, flourishing in moist, low-lying, swampy areas found in the subtropical coastal regions around northeastern New South Wales and southern Queensland. It also grows in China, South Africa, Zimbabwe, and Kenya. Although other *Melaleuca* species have been cultivated elsewhere, *M. alternifolia* does not naturally occur and is not produced outside Australia. There are six identified chemotypes of *M. alternifolia,* including a terpinen-4-ol chemotype, a terpinolene chemotype, and four 1,8-cineole chemotypes. Each type produces an essential oil with distinct chemical compositions, but no obvious difference has been observed to date in the bioactive capability between these. Terpinen-4-ol has antimicrobial and anti-inflammatory properties; 1,8-cineole is an irritant (and this component is deliberately reduced in some commercial tea tree essential oils). Tea tree is usually grown from seed on commercial plantations and harvested for distillation after one to three years of intense growth. Australia is the main essential oil–

producing country (accounting for 80 percent of global distribution). China is the next-highest producer of tea tree oil, although this is mostly for the country's internal market. South Africa, Zimbabwe, and Kenya also produce tea tree essential oil. The commercial demand for tea tree oil has grown exponentially over the last decade.

Plant description: Tea tree is a shrub or small tree growing from 6.6 to 23 feet (2 to 7 meters) tall, with green to dark green ovate or lanceolate, cypressy, needlelike leaves. The bark is often flaky. It produces white to yellow or greenish to pink and red, many-spiked sessile flowers comprised of small petals on long and tightly bundled central stamens, which mature to produce woody, cup-shaped seed capsules or fruits.

Botanical family: Myrtaceae

Extraction method: Steam distillation of the leaves and terminal twigs and branches

Appearance of essential oil: Clear to pale yellow or yellowish-green liquid

Odor of essential oil: Type: spicy; strength: medium; characteristics: fresh, strong, citrusy, spicy, nutmeg-like, piney, camphoraceous, slightly metallic (yet with hints of sweetness), with warm, camphoraceous, medicinal body tones and dry-out notes of weak or little character. The oil is prone to alter during storage, with para-cymene levels increasing and alpha- and gamma-terpinene levels declining (Carson et al. 2006).

Compatible essential oils for blending: Cinnamon, clary sage, clove, eucalyptus, geranium, grapefruit, lavender, lemon, mandarin, marjoram, nutmeg, pine, rosemary

Safety data: Nontoxic, nonirritant; possible sensitization in some people

Perfume note: Top to middle

Principal chemical constituents: CAS No: 68647-73-4

alpha-pinene (1 to 3%), sabinene (0.05 to 0.3%), beta-myrcene (trace amount to 1.5%), alpha-terpinene (5 to 13%), limonene (0.5 to 4%), 1,8-cineole (1 to 15%), **gamma-terpinene (10 to 22%),** para-cymene (0.1 to 5%), terpinolene (1 to 5%), alpha-gurjunene (trace amount to 0.5%), **terpinen-4-ol (30 to 48%),** aromadendrene (trace amount to 5%), alpha-terpineol (1 to 5%), ledene (trace amount to 0.6%), delta-cadinene (trace amount to 0.7%), globulol (trace amount to 3%), viridifloral (trace amount to 2%)

Subtle Connections

Colors: Yellow (*opposite: violet*), green (*opposite: red*), pink (*opposite: pale aqua-green*)

Chakras: Solar plexus, heart

Gemstones: Citrine (*opposite: amethyst*), aventurine (*opposite: jasper*), rose quartz (*opposite: aquamarine*)

Energy: Yin predominantly, yang

Elements: Metal (ether) predominantly, fire

Actions and Uses

General actions: Analgesic, antifungal, anti-infectious, anti-inflammatory, antimicrobial, antiseptic, antiviral, bactericidal, decongestant, expectorant, immune-boosting, insecticide, skin-healing

Skin: Abscesses, acne, athlete's foot, burns, herpes simplex, insect bites, oily skin, pimples, ringworm, shingles (with added geranium); cleansing

Respiratory system: Asthma, bronchitis, catarrh, colds, coughs, ear-nose-throat infections, gum disease, hay fever, mycosis, sinusitis, sore throat, tonsillitis, upper respiratory-tract infections

Antifungal: *Candida* spp., *Epidermophyton* spp., *Malassezia* spp., *Microsporum* spp., *Trichophyton* spp. (ringworm, athlete's foot, candida)

Antimicrobial: Alters permeability of invasive microbial cells, penetrating, disrupting, and destroying cell (Carson et al. 2006).

Immune system: Chronic fatigue syndrome, myalgia encephalomyelitis; immune stimulant

Potential psycho-emotional and spiritual support: Aids concentration, clears and stimulates the mind; eases apathy, nervous exhaustion, shock; revitalizing, stimulating

THYME
(Thymus vulgaris, T. zygis)

Geographical location: Thyme is native to southern Europe and Asia. Originally cultivated from wild thyme (*T. serpyllum*), it is now found throughout the world, including Israel, Algeria, Morocco, Tunisia, the United States, and South Africa. The main essential oil–producing countries are Algeria, Bulgaria, France, Germany, Greece, Israel, Morocco, Portugal, Spain, and the United States.

Plant description: A perennial, low-growing, woody-based or stemmed evergreen subshrub, common or garden thyme grows from 6 to 12 inches (15 to 30 centimeters) high and up to 16 inches (40 centimeters) wide, with many branches and small, oppositely arranged, highly aromatic grayish-green linear to ovate leaves and terminal clusters or whorls of purple, pink, or white two-lipped tubular (bee-loving) flowers that bloom in late spring to early summer. Cultivated thyme is propagated by root division or from seed and grows best in light, chalky soil. The aerial parts of the plant are harvested in the summer. It is gathered in the wild in Spain; however, many species of thyme grown in this region are overharvested and consequently endangered (Burfield 2003).

Botanical family: Lamiaceae (Labiatae)

There are many subspecies or chemotypes of thyme with various chemical structures. The main essential oil–producing species and chemotypes are *T. vulgaris* (thymol, terpinen-4-ol, geraniol), *T. zygis* and *T. serphyllum* (carvacrol, thymol, linalool, linalyl acetate), and *T. satureioides* (thymol, corneol, gamma-terpineol, and alpha-terpineol).

Extraction method: Steam distillation of the fresh or partially dried leaves and flowering tops. Red thyme oil is the first, crude distillate (the red color is caused by traces of metals, mainly iron, reacting with thymol during distillation in metal containers). White thyme oil is produced by subsequent redistillation or rectification. Thyme essential oil is sometimes adulterated with thymol, para-cymene, and other essential oils, or with synthetic thymol; red thyme is often entirely synthetic (Tisserand and Young 2014; Burfield 2003).

Appearance of essential oil (red thyme): Red to reddish-brown or orange liquid

Appearance of essential oil (white thyme): Clear to pale yellow or straw-colored liquid

Odor of essential oil: Type: herbal; strength: high; characteristics, *red thyme:* pungent, phenolic, camphoraceous, medicinal, with warm, resinous, green-herbaceous, spicy-wood body notes and herbaceous-spicy to mild dry-out notes; *white thyme:* fresh, powerful, thyme-like, herbaceous, camphoraceous, medicinal, phenolic, terpenic, fruity, spicy, with herbaceous-spicy middle notes and mild dry-out notes

Compatible essential oils for blending: Bergamot, cardamom, cinnamon, grapefruit, lavender, lemon, marjoram, melissa, nutmeg, orange, pine, rosemary

Safety data: Nonsensitizing and nontoxic; use in moderation; may cause skin irritation in high dose (especially red thyme); may inhibit blood clotting. Ensure authenticity and genuineness of essential oil. Apply topically in 1% dilution (1 drop of essential oil in 5 ml base medium).

Perfume note: Top to middle

Principal chemical constituents: CAS No: 8007-46-3

Thymus zygis ct. linalool: alpha-pinene (1 to 5%), alpha-thujene (0.05 to 0.2%), camphene (0.05 to 2%), sabinene (0.05 to 2%), **beta-myrcene (5 to 10%), alpha-terpinene (2 to 9%),** limonene (2 to 4%), gamma-terpinene (0.5 to 5%), para-cymene (0.5 to 2%), alpha-terpinolene (0.01 to 1%), trans-sabinene hydrate (5 to 10%), **linalool (30 to 50%), terpinene-4-ol (5 to 15%),** alpha-terpineol (0.1 to 2%), borneol (0.5 to 3%), germacrene D (trace amount to 1%)

Thymus zygis ct. thymol (red): alpha-pinene (0.5 to 3%), alpha-thujene (0.05 to 2%), camphene (0.1 to 1%), beta-pinene (0.1 to 0.3%), beta-myrcene (1 to 3%), alpha-terpinene (0.5 to 3%), limonene (0.1 to 0.5%), **gamma-termpinene (4 to 11%), para-cymene (14 to 28%),** trans-thujanol (0 to 0.5%), linalool (3 to 7%), beta-caryophyllene (0.5 to 2%), **thymol (37 to 55%), carvacrol (0.5 to 6%)**

Subtle Connections

Colors: *Thymus zygis* ct. linalool—orange (*opposite: blue*), yellow (*opposite: violet*), pale aqua-green (*opposite: pink*); *Thymus zygis* ct. thymol (red thyme)—red (*opposite: green*)

Chakras: Sacral, solar plexus, base

Gemstones: Carnelian (*opposite: lapis lazuli/aquamarine*), citrine (*opposite: amethyst*), aquamarine (*opposite: rose quartz*), jasper (*opposite: aventurine*)

Energy: Yin, yang

Elements: Water, earth

Actions and Uses

General actions: Antifungal, anti-inflammatory, antimicrobial, antioxidant, antiseptic, antispasmodic, antitussive, antitoxic, bactericidal, balsamic (soothing base balm), calming, cicatrizant, circulatory stimulant, decongestant, diuretic, emmenagogue, immune-boosting, nervine

Skin: Abscesses, acne, bruises, cuts, dermatitis, eczema, insect bites, lice, gum infections, oily skin; apply in very diluted solution

Joints and muscles: Arthritis; cellulitis; edema; gout; muscular aches, pains, and sprains; poor circulation

Respiratory system: Asthma, bronchitis, colds, coughs, sinusitis, sore throat, tonsillitis

Immune system: Infectious diseases, thymus and immune stimulant

Potential psycho-emotional and spiritual support: Aids concentration and memory, aphrodisiac, calming, eases mild depression and lifts low mood, aids in letting go of anger and frustration, encourages release of mental blocks, eases headache, strengthens and supports higher heart/throat chakra, relieves insomnia, strengthening to the nervous system, eases stress and stress-related conditions, tonic, uplifting

TURMERIC
(Curcuma longa)

Geographical location: Tumeric is native to India and is now cultivated throughout subtropical regions of the world, including

China, Indonesia, Jamaica, Haiti, Guatemala, and Hawaii. The roots are imported to Europe and the United States for distillation.

Plant description: A perennial herbaceous, flowering plant that grows to a bit over 3 feet (1 meter) in height, turmeric bears long, simple leaves with long leaf stems that emerge from branching rhizomes that are buried just beneath the soil. Small yellowish-orange flowers are borne in the axils of waxy bracts. The thick, aromatic rhizomes are between 1 and 3 inches (2.5 and 7.5 centimeters) long and are a deep orange inside, becoming brown and scaly as they age. The roots are boiled, cleaned, and then sun-dried for five to seven days. Turmeric is very similar to ginger—they are in the same family—but less irritant.

Botanical family: Zingiberaceae

Extraction method: Steam distillation of chopped rhizomes

Appearance of essential oil: Orangish yellow

Odor of essential oil: Type: spicy; strength: medium; characteristics: fresh, spicy, spicy-woody, sweet, orange, ginger, rooty, with lingering sweet-earthy, softly spicy body and dry-out notes

Compatible essential oils for blending: Cardamom, cinnamon, clary sage, ginger, grapefruit, rose, ylang-ylang

Safety data: Nontoxic, nonsensitizing, nonirritant; may become slightly irritant with age

Perfume note: Base to middle

Principal chemical constituents: CAS No: 8024-37-1

alpha-oinene (trace amount to 0.3%), delta-3-carene (trace amount to 2%), myrcene (trace amount to 0.3%), alpha-phellandrene (0.5 to 13%), alpha-terpinene (trace amount to 0.2%), limonene (trace amount to 0.5%), beta-phellandrene (trace amount to 0.2%), 1,8-cineole (trace amount to 7%), gamma-terpinene (trace amount to 5%), para-cymene (trace amount to 2%), terpinolene (trace amount to 0.4%), beta-caryophyllene (trace amount to 2%), trans-beta-farnesene (trace amount to 1%), alpha-humulene (trace amount to 1%), alpha-zingiberene (3 to 17%), beta-bisabolene (1 to 2.5%), beta-sesquiphellandrene (1 to 10%), **alpha-turmerone (15 to 40%), beta-turmerone (10 to 20%), ar-turmerone (10 to 20%),** trans-alpha-atlantone (trace amount to 2%)

Subtle Connections

Colors: Orange (*opposite: blue*), yellow (*opposite: violet*)

Chakras: Sacral, solar plexus

Gemstones: Carnelian (*opposite: lapis lazuli/aquamarine*), citrine (*opposite: amethyst*)

Energy: Yang

Elements: Fire, earth

Actions and Uses

General actions: Analgesic, antiarthritic, anti-inflammatory, antioxidant, bactericidal, stimulant

Joints and muscles: Arthritis, muscular aches and pains

Potential psycho-emotional and spiritual support: Antianxiety; eases debility, nervous exhaustion; grounding yet stimulating; warming, comforting, and gently brightening mood, emotions, and spirit; gently dispels feelings of stagnation

VALERIAN
(Valeriana officinalis, V. jatamansi)

Geographical location: This perennial flowering plant is native to Europe and northern Asia, naturalized in North America, and cultivated in Belgium, China, France, Hungary, the Netherlands, Russia, the United Kingdom, Bosnia, Serbia, Croatia, Montenegro, and Macedonia. The main essential oil–producing countries are Nepal and China.

Plant description: An upright herbaceous plant, valerian grows up to 5 feet (1.5 meters) high and has a hollow stem; scented, pinnate, dark leaves; and rounded clusters of pink or purplish-white or white-scented flowers that bloom in the summer. The roots are highly aromatic, grayish in color, short, and thick, and they protrude above ground. The flowers and roots are used in perfumery and in the production of essential oils. There are many species growing throughout the world, each with a slightly different chemical and odor profile. Valerian is in the same botanical family as spikenard.

Botanical family: Valerianaceae

Extraction method: Steam distillation of the rhizomes. The chemical composition of the essential oil varies considerably according to the geographical location of growth (for example, Indian valerian, Japanese valerian, European valerian) and also factors such as cultivar, time of harvest, and the age of the plant. European valerian comprises fifty-two-plus identified chemical constituents, many of which are present in minute quantity, whereas Indian valerian comprises eighteen-plus constituents, which are present in higher quantities.

Appearance of essential oil: Olive-green to brown viscous liquid

Odor of essential oil: Type: herbal; strength: medium; characteristics: pungent, fresh, green top notes that quickly give way to warm, woody, balsamic, rooty, animal, musky notes, with tenacious base notes sometimes likened to peas or smelly socks (the later transcended by its therapeutic value)

Compatible essential oils for blending: Cedarwood, chamomile, grapefruit, lavender, mandarin, orange, patchouli, petitgrain, pine, rosemary

Safety data: Nontoxic, nonirritant, nonsensitizing

Perfume note: Base

Principal chemical constituents: CAS No: 8008-80-6

Nepalese valerian (*Valeriana officinalis*): methyl isovalerate (1 to 6%), alpha-pinene (trace amount to 1%), limonene (trace amount to 0.5%), 1,8-cineole (trace amount to 0.05%), furfural (0.1 to 3%), beta-patchoulene (0.1 to 0.5%), linalool (trace amount to 0.1%), calarene (1 to 5%), seychelene (0.1 to 2%), **isovaleric acid (40 to 52%),** alpha-bulnesene (1 to 3%), 3-methylvaleric acid (1 to 10%), maaliol (1 to 6%)

Indian valerian (*Valeriana jatamansi*): alpha-pinene (0.1 to 2%), beta-pinene (0.1 to 4%), camphene (0.1 to 3%), alpha-muurolene (0.1 to 2.5%), alpha-patchoulene (1 to 5%), 8-acetoxy-patchouli alcohol (1 to 5%), beta-caryophyllene (0.1 to 2%), **patchouli alcohol (30 to 45%),** viridifloral (1 to 6%), delta-guaiene (1 to 11%), alpha-guaiene (1 to 5%), seychellene (1 to 9%), valericene (trace amount to 2%), gamma-patchouline (trace amount to 2%), bornyl acetate (trace amount to 2%), methyl carvacrol (0.1 to 3%), methyl thymol (0.1 to 2%), kessane (0 to 2%)

Subtle Connections

Colors: Red (*opposite: green*), orange (*opposite: blue*), green (*opposite: red*), pink (*opposite: pale aqua-green*)

Chakras: Base, sacral, heart

Gemstones: Jasper (*opposite: aventurine*), carnelian (*opposite: lapis lazuli/aquamarine*), aventurine (*opposite: jasper*), rose quartz (*opposite: aquamarine*)

Energy: Yin, yang

Elements: Earth, wood (air)

Actions and Uses

General actions: Antispasmodic, bactericidal, hypotensive, sedative, tranquilizer

Joints and muscles: Muscle spasms

Potential psycho-emotional and spiritual support: Eases feelings of anxiety and tension; hypnotic; relieves insomnia, nervousness, restlessness, stress-related conditions; tranquilizing

VETIVERT
(Vetiveria zizanioides)

Geographical location: This perennial grass is native to India and widely cultivated throughout tropical regions of the world, including Haiti, Réunion, and Java. Indonesia, China, Haiti, and Java are the major producers of the essential oil, most of which, due to its remarkable fixative properties, is prepared for the perfume industry (vetivert apparently features as an ingredient in 90 percent of all Western perfumes). Réunion produces a high-quality Bourbon vetivert. Other essential oil–producing countries include Brazil, Mexico, El Salvador, and Madagascar.

Plant description: Vetivert has tall stems and long, thin, rigid leaves growing in clumps (or bunches) up to 5 feet (1.5 meters) high and bearing brownish-purple flowers. The dense network of slender, hairy roots extends anywhere from 6.6 to 13 feet (2 to 4 meters) deep, providing good anchorage, while also aiding in the plant's drought resistance. The grass and roots are harvested after developing for twelve to eighteen months. Valerian is grown to protect soil from erosion, to provide animal feed, and for its essential oil, used in perfumery and for aesthetic and medicinal applications.

Botanical family: Poaceae (Gramineae)

Extraction method: Steam distillation of the roots and rootlets, which are washed, dried, and chopped. The chemical composition of the extracted essential oil is highly complex and cannot be reproduced synthetically.

Appearance of essential oil: Yellowish-brown to deep brownish-red viscous liquid

Odor of essential oil: Type: woody; strength: medium; characteristics: sweet, earthy, woody top notes, with rich, complex, burnt, smoky, woody, rooty, balsamic, amber body notes that have hints of grapefruit and tenacious woody and earthy dry-out notes. The scent is said to improve with aging.

Compatible essential oils for blending: Clary sage, frankincense, grapefruit, jasmine, lavender, lemongrass, mandarin, orange, patchouli, rose, sandalwood, spikenard, ylang-ylang

Safety data: Nontoxic and nonirritant. Generally nonsensitizing, though there are rare reports of sensitization in hypersensitive persons.

Perfume note: Base

Principal chemical constituents: CAS No: 8016-96-4

ylangene (trace amount to 0.2%), alpha-funebrene (trace amount to 0.2%), beta-elemene (trace amount to 0.1%), beta-cedrene (trace amount to 0.1%), 6,9-guaiadiene (trace amount to 0.2%), preziza-7-ene (trace amount to 0.5%), gurjunene isomer (trace amount to 0.1%), khusimene (trace amount to 0.1%), alpha-humulene (trace amount to 0.05%), gamma-muurolene (0.1 to 2%), calarene (trace amount to 0.6%), copacamphene (trace amount 0.6%), sativene (trace amount to 0.5%), cadinene isomer (trace amount to 2%), valencene isomer (trace amount to 2%), alpha-vetispirene (trace amount to 2%), delta-cadinene (trace amount to 0.5%), cadina-1,4-diene (trace amount to 0.3%), eudesmatriene isomer (trace amount to 0.3%), beta-vetispirene (trace amount to 0.3%), dehydro-aromadendrene (trace amount to 0.2%), cyperene isomer (trace amount to 0.5%), beta-vetivene (0.5 to 3%), alpha-calacorene (trace amount to 0.3%), khusimone (trace amount to 0.5%), cadinatriene isomer (trace amount 0.5%), eudesmol isomer (0.1 to 2%), levojunenol (0.1 to 2%), elemol (trace amount to 0.7%), 10,epi-gamma-eudesmol (trace amount to 0.5%), alpha-muuralol (0.1 to 2.5%), valerianol (0.1 to 2%), alpha-eudesmol (trace amount to 0.5%), beta-eudesmol (trace amount to 0.5%), beta-bisabolol isomer (trace amount to 2%), bicyclovetivenol (trace amount to 2%), zizanol (trace amount to 2%), **vetivenol (trace amount to 1.5%), vetiselinenol (1 to 4%), beta-vetivone (2 to 4%), khusimol (9 to 15%), alpha-vetivone (2 to 4%), isovalencenol (10 to 16%),** Z-gamma-curcumene-12-OL (trace amount to 2%), khusenic acid (trace amount to 1%)

Subtle Connections
Colors: Red (*opposite: green*), orange (*opposite: blue*)
Chakras: Base, sacral
Gemstones: Jasper (*opposite: aventurine*), carnelian (*opposite: lapis lazuli/aquamarine*)
Energy: Yin
Elements: Earth, water

Actions and Uses
General actions: Antiarthritic, antifungal, anti-inflammatory, antimicrobial, antiparasitic, antiseptic, antispasmodic, antiviral, bactericidal, calming, expectorant, nervous-system sedative, tonic
Skin: Acne, dry or oily skin, inflammation, mature skin; stimulates circulation
Respiratory system: Due to calming effect on nervous system, calms and regulates the flow of breathing
Joints and muscles: Aching and painful muscles, arthritis, sprains, strains
Antifungal: *Trycophyton* species (ringworm, athlete's foot, etc.)
Immune system: Chronic fatigue syndrome, myalgic encephalomyelitis; immune stimulant
Other: PMS, menopause
Potential psycho-emotional and spiritual support: Reduces symptoms of withdrawal when coming off pharmaceutical drugs (especially tranquilizers); eases anxiety, confusion, indecision, debility, depression

and low mood, hyperactivity, hypersensitivity, impatience, insomnia, intolerance, irritability, mental exhaustion, nervous tension, panic attacks, premenstrual tension, stress and stress-related conditions; encourages feelings of tranquility; sedative to the nervous system; grounding

YARROW
(Achillea millefolium)

Geographical location: This upright perennial herb is native to the temperate regions of North America, Asia, and Europe and is cultivated in New Zealand and Australia. It now grows wild in most temperate regions throughout the world and can be found in meadows and along borders such as roads. The main essential oil–producing countries are Africa, France, Germany, Hungary, Bosnia, Serbia, Croatia, Montenegro, Macedonia, the United Kingdom, and the United States.

Plant description: Yarrow produces a simple single stem or several stems that grow to over 3 feet (about 1 meter) in height, which are supported by a rhizomatous root spread. Its finely dissected, almost feathery or lacy leaves are evenly distributed along the stem. Disk or ray, ovate to round, white or pinkish-white flowers appear as a dense, flat-topped cluster. This plant spreads via its roots. The flowering aerial parts are picked in summer. Yarrow is an ancient herbal plant used traditionally to heal wounds and stem bleeding. It belongs to the same botanical family as chamomile.

Botanical family: Asteraceae (Compositae)

Extraction method: Distillation of the dried herb

Appearance of essential oil: Bluish to dark olive-green liquid

Odor of essential oil: Type: herbal; strength: high; characteristics: fresh, green, sweet (almost sickly), intense, medicinal, phenolic, and fruity, with herbaceous, slightly camphoraceous body notes and warm, hay-like, tobacco-like dry-out notes; very similar to German chamomile

Compatible essential oils for blending: Bergamot, cedarwood, eucalyptus, grapefruit, juniper, peppermint, pine, Roman chamomile, rosemary, valerian, vetivert

Safety data: Nonsensitizing, nonirritant when applied in moderation. Chamuzulene inhibits the activity of the enzymes CYP1AZ, CYP2D6, and CYP3A4, which means there may be interaction between yarrow essential oil and drugs metabolized by these enzymes (Tisserand and Young 2014, 476).

Perfume note: Middle

Principal chemical constituents: CAS No: 977000-16-6 (herb leaves); CAS No: 8022-07-9 (herb flowers)

Bulgarian *Achillea millefolium:* santoline triene (trace amount to 0.2%), alpha-thujene (trace amount to 0.3%), alpha-pinene (1 to 3%), camphene (trace amount to 0.3%), **beta-pinene (10 to 15%), sabinene (10 to 15%),** beta-myrcene (trace amount to 0.8%), alpha-terpinene (trace amount to 1.5%), limonene (trace amount to 0.6%), beta-phellandrene (trace amount to 0.2%), 1,8-cineole (1 to 3%), cymene (trace amount to 1%), terpinolene (trace amount to 8%), **artemisia ketone (1 to 4%),** camphor (trace amount to 0.7%), 1-terpinol-4-ol (1 to 2.5%), bornyl acetate (trace amount to 2%), **beta-caryophyllene (5 to 12%),** alpha-humulene (trace amount to 3%), alpha-caryophyllene (trace amount to 2%), **germacrene D (15 to 24%),** caryophyllene oxide (0.5 to 2%), **chamazulene (5 to 10%)**

Subtle Connections

Colors: Green (*opposite: red*), pink (*opposite: pale aqua-green*), blue (*opposite: orange*)

Chakras: Heart, throat

Gemstones: Aventurine (*opposite: jasper*), lapis lazuli/aquamarine (*opposite: carnelian*), rose quartz (*opposite: aquamarine*)

Energy: Yin

Elements: Water, metal (ether)

Actions and Uses

General actions: Anti-inflammatory, antiseptic, antispasmodic, astringent, cicatrizant, expectorant, hypotensive

Skin: Acne, burns, eczema, inflammation, itchy rashes, scar tissue (use in moderation); stems bleeding

Joints and muscles: Arthritis, neuralgia, pain

Respiratory: Infections, sinus congestion

Potential psycho-emotional and spiritual support: Relieves insomnia, stress and stress-related conditions, tension; supports intuition; uplifts spirit and mood

YLANG-YLANG
(Cananga odorata)

Geographical location: *Cananga odorata* is native to the Philippines, Malaysia, Indonesia, and other areas of tropical Asia; it is also grown in Madagascar, Melanesia, Micronesia, Polynesia, and the island nation of Comoros. The main essential oil–producing countries are Madagascar and Comoros.

Plant description: This tall, slim, tropical, evergreen, smooth-barked tree or woody climber grows to a height of 80 feet (25 meters) and has alternate, smooth, glossy, wavy-edged, oval, pointed leaves 5 to 8 inches (13 to 20 centimeters) long. The tree produces drooping, long-stalked flowers all year round, which have six narrow, yellow to greenish-yellow or sometimes (but rarely) pink or mauve petals that yield a highly fragrant essential oil, and dark green, oval fruits that ripen to black. Originally the wild flowers had no fragrance and were thus likely to have been composed of different chemical constituents. However, selection and cloning produced the scent we know today. *Ylang-ylang* means "flower of flowers." It is in the same botanical family as cananga (*Cananga odorata* f. *macrophylla*), though cananga is less floral, with greener notes.

Botanical family: Annonaceae

Extraction method: Steam distillation of the freshly picked flowers. The first distillate (about 40%) is called ylang-ylang extra and is considered to be the superior grade; subsequent distillation produces oils respectively graded 1, 2, and 3. Ylang-ylang "complete" is another classified version and comprises the whole or unfractionated oil, but it is often created by blending ylang-ylang 1 and 2 together. An absolute and a concrete are produced by solvent extraction and are preferred in perfumery for their long-lasting floral, balsamic effects.

Appearance of essential oil: Clear to pale yellow oily liquid

Odor of essential oil: Type: floral; strength: medium; characteristics: strong, sweet, heavy, floral, jasmine, lily, spicy, and medicated notes, with floral, fruity-spicy middle tones, then sweet, balsamic, floral, medicated dry-out notes

Compatible essential oils for blending: Bergamot, bitter orange, black pepper, cedarwood, clary sage, frankincense, galbanum, grapefruit, jasmine, lavender, lemon, lime, mandarin, rose, sandalwood, vetivert; blends well with most woods, florals, and fruits; forms a tenacious base note in perfume blends

Safety data: Nontoxic, nonirritant, nonsensitive. Use in moderation. Avoid use on hypersensitive, diseased, or damaged skin.

Perfume note: Base to middle

Principal chemical constituents: CAS No: 8006-81-3

Madagascar extra *Cananga odorata*: alpha-pinene (trace amount to 0.3%), beta-myrcene (trace amount to 0.2%), 1,8-cineole (trace amount to 1%), prenyl acetate (0.5 to 2.5%), 3-hexen-1-ol acetate (trace amount to 0.2%), **methyl-para-cresol (7 to 16%)**, alpha-copaene (trace amount to 0.3%), **linalool (15 to 24%)**, beta-elemene (trace amount to 0.2%), **beta-caryophyllene (2 to 9%), methyl benzoate (4 to 9%)**, estragole (trace amount to 0.4%), alpha-humulene (trace amount to 2%), **germacrene D (5 to 20%), benzyl acetate (5 to 14%)**, alpha-muurolene (trace amount to 0.3%), geranial (trace amount to 0.1%), E,E-alpha-farnesene (1 to 5%), **geranyl acetate (7 to 14%)**, geraniol (1 to 3%), prenyl benzoate (trace amount to 0.5%), cinnamyl acetate (0.5 to 3%), alpha-muurol (trace amount to 0.3%), farnesyl acetate (0.5 to 3%), farnesol (0.5 to 3%), benzyl benzoate (3 to 8%), benzyl silacylate (1 to 4%)

Subtle Connections

Colors: Orange (*opposite: blue*), yellow (*opposite: violet*)

Chakras: Sacral, solar plexus

Gemstones: Carnelian (*opposite: lapis lazuli/aquamarine*), citrine (*opposite: amethyst*)

Energy: Yin, yang

Elements: Earth, wood (air)

Actions and Uses

General actions: Antidepressant, anti-infectious, antiseptic, circulatory stimulant, hypotensive, nervine; regulates and balances sebum

Skin: Acne; dry, oily, and combination skin; insect bites

Respiratory system: Hyperventilation

Potential psycho-emotional and spiritual support: Aphrodisiac; euphoric; tonic; eases mild depression, nervous tension, fear and feelings of panic, shock; calms anger and rage; relieves insomnia, stress, and stress-related conditions; relaxes the central nervous system

Glossary

alkaloids: Any of numerous nitrogen-containing organic compounds with toxic or medicinal properties that occur naturally in certain plants; examples include caffeine and nicotine

biosynthesis: The manufacture by living organisms of complex organic compounds such as proteins, fats, etc., from simpler molecules

bitters: A specific group of herbs that can affect physiological reactions in the body, working as astringents, tonics, relaxers, stomachics, and internal cleansers; especially used to improve digestion and soothe inflammation. Herbs in this category include angelica, chamomile, dandelion, goldenseal, horehound, milk thistle, rue, and yarrow. Bitters have a sharp taste (like that of quinine or hops). Liquids prepared from bitter herbs or roots are used to aid digestion or stimulate appetite or to flavor drinks.

carbohydrate: Any of a group of organic compounds that consist of carbon, hydrogen, and oxygen. They are present in the cells of all living organisms and are formed in plants during photosynthesis.

carcinogen: Any substance or agent capable of causing cancer in a living tissue that is exposed to it, e.g., ionizing radiation, many chemical compounds, and some viruses

CAS number: Abbreviation for Chemical Abstracts Service. The abbreviation CAS, or CAS RNs, appears with unique numerical identifiers, or codes, that are assigned to every chemical described in scientific literature, including elements, isotopes, organic and inorganic compounds, ions, organometallics, metals, or materials of "unknown, variable composition, or biological origin." The system was created by the American

Chemical Society (ACS). The numbers in this system of identification have no bearing on the chemicals identified other than simply for the purpose of listing and cataloging. All essential oils are denoted by a unique CAS catalog identification number.

cellulose: A complex carbohydrate that is the main constituent of plant cell walls and is used in the manufacture of paper, rope, textiles (e.g., cotton and linen) and plastics (e.g., cellophane)

chloroplasts: Any of many specialized membrane-bound structures containing the green pigment chlorophyll, found in the cytoplasm of photosynthetic cells of all green plants

chromoplasts: Organelles responsible for pigment synthesis and storage in specific photosynthetic eukaryotes, giving plants their distinctive colors; found in fruits, flowers, and roots and in stressed and aging leaves

cicatrizant: An agent that promotes healing by formation of scar tissue

ciliate: Any of numerous microscopic, single-celled organisms that typically possess cilia and are found free-living in all kinds of aquatic and terrestrial habitats and as parasites

cotyledon: In flowering plants, one of the leaves produced by the embryo, providing the initial food source for the plant

cuticle: The waxy, waterproof, protective layer that covers all the parts of a plant exposed to the air except for the stomata; the protective layer of horny, noncellular material that covers the epidermis of many invertebrates and forms the exoskeletons of arthropods

cytoplasm: The part of a living cell, excluding the nucleus, that is enclosed by the cell membrane and contains a range of organelles

dicotyledon (dicot): Any member of the angiosperms, or flowering plants, that has a pair of leaves or cotyledons in the embryo of the seed

distillate: A concentrated extract, the product of distilling

diuretic: A drug or other substance that increases the volume of urine produced and excreted.

drupe: A fleshy fruit containing one or more seeds that are surrounded by an inner protective layer, e.g., plum, cherry, peach, holly

emmenagogue: A substance that induces or assists menstruation

enzyme: A substance produced by a living organism that acts as a catalyst to bring about a specific biochemical reaction such as fermentation of sugar in fruit or cereals; also called ethyl alcohol

epidermis: The outermost layer of a plant or animal that serves to protect the underlying tissues from infection, injury, and water loss

epithelium: The cell tissue that covers the outer surface of the body and closed cavities within it

ester: An organic chemical compound formed by the reaction of an alcohol with an organic acid, with the loss of a water molecule

ethers: Any of a group of organic chemical compounds formed by the dehydration of alcohols that are volatile and highly flammable and contain two hydrocarbon groups linked by an oxygen atom

expectorant: Causing the coughing up of phlegm

exude: To release or give out (an odor or substance); to ooze out slowly; the substance expressed

flavonoid: Any of a group of organic compounds, including numerous water-soluble plant pigments, that are responsible for most of the red, pink, and purple colors found in higher plants. Flavonoid groups include flavonols, flavones, flavanones, isoflavones, catechins, anthocyanidins, and chalcones.

furanocoumarins/furocoumarins: Oxygen-containing cyclic structures associated with phototoxicity upon exposure to ultraviolet light

genus (pl. *genera*): In taxonomy, any of the groups into which a family is divided and that in turn is subdivided into one or more species; a class divided into several subordinate classes

glucoside: Any of various derivatives of glucose in which the first hydroxyl group is replaced by another group, and which yields glucose when treated with enzymes or acids

glycosides: Any of a class of compounds with two hydroxyl groups on adjacent carbon atoms, and so intermediate between *glyc*erine and alcoh*ol*

gums: Any of various substances found in certain plants, especially trees, that produce a sticky solution or gel when added to water; used in confectionery, gummed envelopes, etc.

hemicellulose: A type of polysaccharide found in plant cell walls that is broken down more easily than cellulose; the main component of cell walls

hydrocarbon: A compound whose molecules are made up of only atoms of hydrogen and carbon

hydrolate: A term that describes the condensed steam used to infuse water with the essence of beneficial plants; also referred to as *aromatic water* and *hydrosol* (although not strictly correct)

hydrophilic: Referring to a substance that absorbs, attracts, or has an affinity for water

hydrosol: A colloidal suspension in water achieved by steeping material in water to absorb or soak out hydrophilic and volatile chemicals (with the original material removed or strained), leaving a colliodal mixture, emulsion, or suspension

isodiametric: Having equal diameters

ketones: Any of a class of organic compounds characterized by a carbonyl group attached to two carbon atoms; present in essential oils and often considered very powerful and potentially toxic (e.g., thujone)

lactones: Organic compounds characterized by the presence in their molecules of an ester functional group as part of a ring system in their chemical structure

lacuna: In botany, any air space in the center of a plant stem or root; an intracellular space; a cavity; a depression in a pitted surface

leucoplast: A starch-forming body in protoplasm; a colorless plastid in the cells of roots, storage organs, and underground stems, serving as a point around which starch forms

lignin: The complex polymer that cements together the fibers within the cell walls of plants, making them woody and rigid

lumen (pl. *lumina*): The space or cavity enclosed by the walls of a vessel or tubular organ, e.g., within a blood vessel or intestine or the space within a cell wall

metabolic: Relating to an organism's metabolism; exhibiting metamorphosis

metabolism: The sum of all the chemical reactions that occur within the cells of a living organism, including both anabolism and catabolism of complex organic compounds

metabolite: A molecule that participates in the biochemical reactions that take place in the cells of living organisms

mitochondria: Specialized oval structures consisting of a central matrix surrounded by two membranes, found in the cytoplasm of eukaryotic cells; more prevalent in the cells of muscle tissue

molecule: The smallest particle of an element or compound that can exist independently and participate in a reaction, consisting of two or more atoms bonded together

monocotyledon: A flowering plant with an embryo that bears a single seed leaf, or cotyledon

monoterpene: A terpene of the molecular formula $C_{10}H_{16}$ (comprising two isoprene units)

mucolytic: Dissolving or breaking down mucus

oleoresin: Oily resin obtained from the sap of various plants and trees, especially conifers, often aromatic and usually in the form of a brittle, translucent, solid, or viscous liquid

organelle: In the cell of a living organism, any of various different types of membrane-bound structures, each of which has a specialized function, e.g., mitochondria, ribosomes, and chloroplasts

ovule: In flowering plants, characteristic of spermatophytes, the structure that develops into a seed after fertilization

oxidation: A chemical reaction in which oxygen combines with an element or compound or in which hydrogen is removed from a compound; the loss of one or more electrons by an atom, ion, or molecule, causing a chemical change in a substance

oxide: Any compound of oxygen and another element, often formed by burning that element or one of its compounds in oxygen or air—e.g., 1,8-cineole, the most commonly occurring oxide found in essential oils

parenchyma: A tissue composed of thin-walled, relatively unspecialized cells that serves mainly as a packing tissue

perisperm: Nutritive tissue in a seed derived from the nucleus

phenols: Aromatic compounds with one or more hydroxyl groups directly attached to the benzene nucleus

phloem: The plant tissue that is responsible for the transport of sugars and other nutrients from the leaves to all other parts of the plant

photosynthesis: The process whereby green plants manufacture carbohydrates from carbon dioxide and water, using the light energy from the sun trapped by the pigment chlorophyll, in specialized structures known as chloroplasts. Oxygen is a by-product of photosynthesis.

phytoplankton: That part of plankton—the minute plant or animal life found in a body of water—that is composed of microscopic plants

plasma: A gas that has been heated to a very high temperature so that most of its atoms or molecules are broken down into free electrons and positive ions

plastid: Any of various highly specialized, membrane-bound structures found within the cytoplasm of plant cells, e.g. chloroplasts

polymer: A very large molecule consisting of a long chain of monomers linked end-to-end to form a series of repeating units

respiration: A metabolic process in plants and animals whereby compounds are broken down to release energy, incorporated into ATP, commonly (but not exclusively) requiring oxygen, and with carbon dioxide as an end product

rhizome: A thick, horizontal, underground stem that produces roots and leafy shoots

saponin: A glucoside extracted from plants, e.g., soapwort, which gives a soapy lather

sesquiterpene: A terpene with the molecular formula $C_{15}H_{24}$ (three isoprene units)

sessile: A flower or leaf that is attached directly to the base of a plant, not raised up on a stalk

sperm: In botany, denoting a seed

starch: A carbohydrate that occurs in all green plants that serves as an energy store, usually in the form of small, white granules in seeds, tubers, etc.

steroids: Any of a large group of fat-soluble organic compounds such as sterols, some sex hormones, bile acids, etc., that have a complex molecular structure (seventeen carbon atoms arranged in four rings) and that are important both physiologically and pharmacologically

stoma (pl. *stomata*): One of many tiny pores found on the stems and leaves of vascular plants, each of which has two guard cells for the control and regulation of its functions, and which are the sites where water loss from the plant and gaseous exchange between plant tissue and the atmosphere takes place

suspension: A liquid or gas that contains small, insoluble solid particles that are more or less evenly dispersed throughout it

taxonomy: The theory and techniques of describing, naming, and classifying living and extinct organisms on the basis of the similarity of their anatomical and morphological features and structures

terpene: Any of three classes of unsaturated hydrocarbons based on the isoprene (formula C_5H_8) unit that are present in plant resins and also form the main constituents of essential oils such as rose and jasmine

tonic: A medicine that increases strength, energy, and the general well-being of the body; anything that is refreshing or invigorating

trichome: Any outgrowth, such as a prickle, hair, or scale, from the epidermis of a plant

trimerous: Having three parts or being in a group of three

tuber: A swollen, rounded, underground stem or rhizome such as a potato, where food is stored, allowing the plant to survive from one growing season to the next, which may also have buds or "eyes" on the surface, which can develop into new plants

vascular: Relating to the blood vessels of animals or the sap-conducting tissues (xylem and phloem) of plants

volatile: Changing quickly from a solid or liquid into a vapor

vulnerary: Used in the healing or treating of wounds

xylem: The woody tissue that transports water and mineral nutrients from the roots to all other parts of a plant and also provides structural support

Bibliography

Acimovic, Milica G., Snezana D. Pavlovic, Anna O. Varga, Vladimir M. Filipovic, Mirjana T. Cvetkovic, Jovana M. Stankovic, Ivana S. Cabarkapa. 2017. "Chemical Composition and Antibacterial Activity of *Angelica archangelica* Root Essential Oil." *Natural Product Communications* 12, no. 2: 205–6.

Agency for Toxic Substances and Disease Registry (ATSDR). 2011. "Benzene FAQ." Department of Health and Human Services. www.atsdr.cdc.gov.

Ahmad, S. H., A. A. Malek, H. C. Gan, T. L. Abdullah, A. A. Rahman. 1998. "The Effect of Harvest Time on the Quantity and Chemical Composition of Jasmine (*Jasminum multiflorum* L.) Essential Oil." *International Society for Horticultural Science* 454: 355–64.

Ahmed, Salman, Haroon Khan, Michael Aschner, Hamed Mirzae, Ezra K. Akkol, Raffael Capasso. 2020. "Anticancer Potential of Furanocoumarins: Mechanistic and Therapeutic Aspects." *International Journal of Molecular Science* 21, no. 16: 5622.

Bag, Anwesa, and Rabi R. Chattopadhyay. 2015. "Evaluation of Synergistic Antibacterial and Antioxidant Efficacy of Essential Oils of Spices and Herbs in Combination." *PLoS ONE* 10, no. 7: e0131321.

Bassolé, Imael Henri N., Aline Lamien-Meda, Bale Bayala, Souleymane Tirogo, Chlodwig Franz, Johannes Novak, Roger C. Nebié, Mamoudo H. Dicko. 2010. "Composition and Antimicrobial Activities of *Lippia multiflora* Moldenke, *Mentha piperita* L., and *Ocimum basilicum* L. Essential Oils and Their Major Monoterpene Alcohols Alone and in Combination." *Molecules* 15, no. 11: 7825–39.

Battaglia, Salvatore. 2003. *The Complete Guide to Aromatherapy* (2nd ed.). Brisbane, Australia: International Centre of Holistic Aromatherapy.

Becker, Shannon. 2018. "Essential Oils to Prevent the Spread of Flu." Tisserand Institute. https://tisserandinstitute.org.

Bensouila, Janetta, and Philippa Buck. 2006. *Aromadermatology: Aromatherapy in the Treatment and Care of Common Skin Conditions*. Oxon, UK: Radcliffe Publishing.

Benveniste, Jacques. 1988. "Doctor Jacques Benveniste Replies." *Nature* 344, no. 291.

Bousbia, N., Abert M. Vian, B. Y. Meklatic, F. Chemata. 2010. "Microwave Hydrodiffusion and Gravity (MHG): A Solvent-Free Extraction of Essential Oils." *Journal of Chromotography A*. 1190, no. 1–2: 14–17.

Bowles, E. Joy. 2002. *The Basic Chemistry of Aromatherapeutic Essential Oils*. Self-published.

Brady, Nyle C., and Ray R. Weil. 2016. *Elements of the Nature and Properties of Soils* (15th ed.). London: Pearson.

Burfield, Tony. 2003 (October 11). "The Adulteration of Essential Oils—and the Consequences to Aromatherapy and Natural Perfumery Practice." Presented to the International Federation of Aromatherapists Annual AGM, London.

Bush, Dr. Zach. 2020 (May 26). "Humanity, Consciousness, and Covid 19." Interview with Josh Trent, the Wellness Force. YouTube.

———. 2020 (June 16). "Embracing the Connection between Agriculture and Health, with Zach Bush." *Regenerative Agriculture Podcast*.

———. 2021 (May 7). "GMOs: Engineering the Nature out of Humanity." Webinar replay with Dr. Zach Bush. YouTube.

Caddy, Rosemary. 2005. *Aromatherapy: Essential Oils in Colour*. Rochester, Kent, UK: Amberwood Publishing Limited.

Carson, C. F., K. A. Hammer, T. V. Riley. 2006. "*Melaleuca alternifolia* (Tea Tree) Oil: A Review of Antimicrobial and Other Medicinal Properties." *Clinical Microbiology Reviews* 19, no. 1: 5–62.

Catty, Suzanne. 2001. *Hydrosols: The Next Aromatherapy*. Rochester, Vt.: Healing Arts Press.

Chevallier, Andrew. 2001. *Encyclopedia of Medicinal Plants*. London: Dorling Kindersley.

Chouhan, Sonam, Kanika Sharma, Sanjay Guleria. 2017. "Antimicrobial Activity of Some Essential Oils—Present Status and Future Perspectives." *Medicines* (Basel) 4, no. 3: 58.

Clarke, Sue. 2002. *Essential Oil Chemistry for Safe Aromatherapy*. London: Churchill Livingstone.

Cseke, Leland J., Peter B. Kaufman, Ara Kirakosyan. 2007. "The Biology of Essential Oils in the Pollination of Flowers." *Natural Product Communications* 2, no 12: 1317–36.

Cushnie, Tim T. P., and Andrew J. Lamb. 2005. "Antimicrobial Activity of Flavonoids." *International Journal of Antimicrobial Agents* 26, no. 5: 343–56.

———. 2011. "Recent Advances in Understanding the Antibacterial Properties of Flavonoids." *International Journal of Antimicrobial Agents* 38, no. 2: 99–107.

Damian, Peter, and Kate Damian. 1995. *Aromatherapy, Scent and Psyche: Using Essential Oils for Physical and Emotional Well-Being.* Rochester, Vt.: Healing Arts Press.

Da Silva, Joyce Kelly R., Pablo Luis B. Figueiredo, Kendall G. Byler, William N. Setzer. 2020. "Essential Oils as Antiviral Agents, Potential of Essential Oils to Treat SARS-CoV-2 Infection: An In-Silico Investigation." *International Journal of Molecular Science* 21, no. 10: 3426.

Del Giudice, Luigi, Domenica R. Massardo, Paolo Pontieri, Cinzia M. Bertea, Domenico Mombello, Elisabetta Carat, Salvatore M. Tredici, et al. 2008. "The Microbial Community of Vetiver Root and Its Involvement into Essential Oil Biogenesis." *Environmental Microbiology* 10, no. 10: 2824–41.

Doyle, James A. 2006. "Seed Ferns and the Origin of Angiosperms." *Journal of the Torrey Botanical Society* 133, no. 1: 169–209.

Farmer's Footprint. 2021. "Regeneration: The Beginning." Farmer's Footprint website, https://farmersfootprint.us/watch/.

Francis, George W., and Yen Thuy Hoang Bui. 2015. "Changes in Composition of Aromatherapeutic *Citrus* Oils during Evaporation." *Journal of Evidenced-Based Alternative and Complementary Medicine* 2015, no. 421695.

Friedman, Mendal. 2006. "Overview of Antibacterial, Antitoxin, Antiviral, and Antifungal Activities of Tea Flavonoids and Teas." *Molecular Nutrition and Food Research* 51, no. 1: 116–34.

García-García, Rebecca, Aurelio López-Malo, Enrique Palou. 2011. "Bactericidal Action of Binary and Ternary Mixtures of Carvacrol, Thymol, and Eugenol against *Listeria innocua.*" *Journal of Food Science* 76, no. 2: M95–M100.

Gattefossé, Rene-Maurice. 1937, 1995. *Gattefosse's Aromatherapy.* Walden, UK: C. W. Daniel Company Ltd.

Gerber, Richard. 2001. *Vibrational Medicine: The Handbook of Subtle Energy Therapies.* Rochester, Vt.: Bear and Co.

Gienger, Michael. 2004. *Crystal Power, Crystal Healing: The Complete Handbook.* London: Cassell Illustrated.

Giles, Martin, Jian Zhao, Min An, Samson Agboola. 2010. "Chemical Composition and Antimicrobial Properties of Essential Oils of Three

Australian *Eucalyptus* Species." *Journal of Food Chemistry* 119, no. 2: 731–37.

Gimble, Theo. 1994. *Healing with Colour and Light.* London: Gia Books.

———. 2005. *Healing Energies of Colour.* London: Gia Books.

Godfrey, Heather Dawn. 2018. *Essential Oils for Mindfulness and Meditation.* Rochester, Vt.: Healing Arts Press.

———. 2019. *Essential Oils for the Whole Body: The Dynamics of Topical Application.* Rochester, Vt.: Healing Arts Press.

Gomes, Marcelo P., Elise Smedbol, Annie Chalifour, Louise Henault-Ethier, Michel Lebrecque, Laurent Lapage, Marc Lucotte, Philippe Juneau. 2014. "Alteration of Plant Physiology by Glyphosate and Its By-product Aminomethylphosphonic Acid: An Overview." *Journal of Experimental Botany* 65, no. 17: 4691–703.

Good Scents Company Information System. www.thegoodscentscompany.com.

Grieve, Maude. 1931. *A Modern Herbal,* vol. II. New York: Dover.

Griffin, Robert D. 1981. *The Biology Coloring Book.* New York: Harper Perennial.

Harris, Rhiannon. 2002. "Synergism in the Essential Oil World." *International Journal of Aromatherapy* 12, no. 4: 179–86.

Hendawy, Saber Fayez, Mohamed Salah Hussein, Heba M. Amer, Ahmed E. El-Gohary, Wagdi Saber Soliman. 2017. "Effect of Soil Type on Growth, Productivity, and Essential Oil Constituents of Rosemary, *Rosmarinus officinalis.*" *Asian Journal of Agriculture and Biology* 5, no. 4: 303–11.

Hossain, Farah, Peter Follett, Khang Dang Vu, Medhi Harich, Stephane Salmieri, Monique Lacroix. 2016. "Evidence for Synergistic Activity of Plant-Derived Essential Oils against Fungal Pathogens of Food." *Food Microbiology* 53 (Pt B): 24–30.

Jeliazkov, Valtcho D., Santosh Shiwakoti, Ekaterina A. Jeliazkova, Tess Astatkie. 2016 (Aug. 25). "Chemical Profile and Bioactivity of Essential Oil Fractions as a Function of Distillation Time." *Medicinal and Aromatic Crops, Phytochemistry, and Utilization* (ACS Symposium Series, vol. 1218).

Kapit, Wynn, and Lawrence M. Elson. 1993. *The Anatomy Coloring Book* (2nd ed.). New York: HarperCollins.

Keener, Amanda. 2019. "Exosomes Make Their Debut in Plant Research." *The Scientist.* Available online.

Kerr, John. 2002. "The Use of Essential Oils in Healing Wounds." *International Journal of Aromatherapy* 12, no. 4: 202–6.

Krumbec, Erika. 2014 (September 8). "When to NOT Use Essential Oils (Essential Oils Can Cause Seizures in Kids)." Naturopathicpediatrics.com.

Kusmirek, Jan. 2002. *Liquid Sunshine: Vegetable Oils for Aromatherapy.* Glastonbury, UK: Floramicus.

Langeveld, Wendy T., Edwin J. A. Veldhuizen, Sara A. Burt. 2013. "Synergy between Essential Oil Components and Antibiotics: A Review." *Critical Reviews in Microbiology* 40, no. 1: 76–94.

Lawless, Julia. 1995. *The Illustrated Encyclopedia of Essential Oils: The Complete Guide to the Use of Oils in Aromatherapy and Herbalism.* London: Element.

LeFevre, Amnesty, Samuel D. Schillcutt, Samir K. Saha, A. S. M. Nawshad Uddin Ahmed, Mak-Azad Chowdhury, Paul A. Law, et al. 2010. "Cost-Effectiveness of Skin Barrier-Enhancing Emollients among Preterm Infants in Bangladesh." *Bulletin of the World Health Organization* 88, no. 2: 104–12.

Leliaert, Frederik, David R. Smith, Herve Moreau, Matthew D. Herron, Heroen Verbruggen, Charles F. Delwiche, Oliver De Clerck. 2012. "Phylogeny and Molecular Evolution of the Green Algae." *Critical Reviews in Plant Sciences* 31, no. 1: 1–46.

Luqman, Suaib, Gauraav R. Dwivedi, Mahendra P. Darokar, A. Kalra, Suman P. S. Khanuja. 2008. "Antimicrobial Activity of *Eucalyptus citriodora* Essential Oil." *International Journal of Essential Oil Therapeutics* 2: 69–75.

Market Analysis Report. 2020 (May). "Essential Oils Market Size, Share and Trends Analysis Report by Application (Food and Beverages, Spa and Relaxation), by Product (Orange, Peppermint), by Sales Channel, and Segment Forecasts—2020 to 2027." Grand View Research (website).

Maury, Marguerite. 1989. First published in 1961. *Marguerite Maury's Guide to Aromatherapy: The Secrets of Life and Youth: A Modern Alchemy.* London: C. W. Daniel Co. Ltd.

Moyjay, Gabriel. 2000. *Aromatherapy for Healing the Spirit: A Guide for Restoring Emotional and Mental Balance through Essential Oils.* Rochester, Vt.: Inner Traditions.

Nazzaro, Filomena, Florinda Fratiani, Laura de Martino, Raffaele Coppola, Vincenzo de Feo. 2013. "Effect of Essential Oils on Pathogenic Bacteria." *Pharmaceuticals* (Basel) 6, no. 12: 1451–74.

NHR Organic Oils. Chemical analysis. Available online, www.nhrorganicoils .com.

Nunez, L., and M. D. Aquino. 2012. "Microbicide Activity of Clove Essential Oil (*Eugenia caryphylleta*)." *Brazilian Journal of Microbiology* 43, no. 4: 1255–60.

Onawunmi, G. O., W. A. Yisak, E. O. Ogunlana. 1984. "Antibacterial Constituents in the Essential Oil of *Cymbopogon citratus* (DC) Stapf." *Journal of Ethnopharmacology* 12, no. 3: 279–86.

Perini, J. F., W. P. Silvestre, F. Agostini, D. Toss, G. F. Pauletti. 2017. "Fractioning of Orange (*Citrus sinensis* L.) Essential Oil Using Vacuum Fractional Distillation." *Separation Science and Technology* 52, no. 8: 1397–403.

Peterfalvi, Agnus, Eva Miko, Tama Nagy, Barbara Reger, Diana Simon, Attila Miseta, Boldizsar Czeh, Laszio Szereday. 2019. "Much More Than a Pleasant Scent: A Review on Essential Oils Supporting the Immune System." *Molecules* 24, no. 24: 4530.

Pollack, Gerald. 2016. "Water, Cells and Life: The Fourth Phase of Water." TEDx Talks (Nov 21, 2016). Available on YouTube.

Price, Len, and Shirley Price. 2004. *Understanding Hydrolates: The Specific Hydrosols for Aromatherapy—a Guide for Health Professionals*. London: Churchill Livingstone.

Rohloff, Jens, Stiener Dragland, Ruth Mordal, Iversen Tor-Henning. 2005. "Effect of Harvest Time and Drying Method on Biomass Production, Essential Oil Yield, and Quality of Peppermint (*Menth* x *piperita* L.)." *Journal of Agriculture Food Chemistry* 53, no. 10: 4143–48.

Rohwer, Forrest, David Prangishvili, Debbie Lindell. 2009. "Roles of Viruses in the Environment." *Society for Applied Microbiology* 11, no. 11: 2771–74.

Satyal, Prabodh, Brittany L. Murray, Robert L. McFeeters, William N. Setzer. 2016. "Essential Oil Characterization of *Thymus vulgaris* from Various Geographical Locations." *Foods* 5, no. 4: 70.

Satyal, Prabodh, and William N. Setzer. 2020. "Chemical Compositions of Commercial Essential Oils from *Coriandrum sativum* Fruits and Aerial Parts." *Natural Product Communications* 15, no. 7.

Scala, Alessandra, Silke Allmann, Rosanna Mirabella, Michele A. Haring, Robert C. Shuurink. 2013. "Green Leaf Volatiles: A Plant's Multifunctional Weapon against Herbivores and Pathogens." *International Journal of Molecular Science* 14, no. 9: 17781–811.

Schnaubelt, Kurt. 1995. *Advanced Aromatherapy: The Science of Essential Oil Therapy*. Rochester, Vt.: Healing Arts Press.

Senatore, Felice. 1996. "Influence of Harvesting Time on Yield and Composition of the Essential Oil of a Thyme (*Thymus pulegioides* L.) Growing Wild in Campania (Southern Italy)." *Journal of Agriculture and Food Chemistry* 44, no. 5: 1327–32.

Sharma, Saurabh, and Rakesh Kumar. 2018. "Influence of Harvesting Stage and Distillation Time of Damask Rose (*Rosa damascena* Mill.) Flowers on Essential Oil Content and Composition in the Western Himalayas." *Journal of Essential Oil Bearing Plants* 21, no. 1: 92–102.

Sheng-Ji, Pei. 2001. "Ethnobotanical Approaches of Traditional Medicine Studies: Some Experiences from Asia." *Pharmaceutical Biology* 39, suppl. 1: 74–79.

Sheppard-Hanger, Sylla. 1995. *The Aromatherapy Practitioner Reference Manual.* Tampa, Fla.: Atlantic Institute of Aromatherapy.

Silvestre, Wendal P., Femanda R Medeiros, Fabiana Agostini, Daniel Toss, Gabrielle F. Pauletti. 2019. "Fractionation of Rosemary (*Rosmarinus officinalis* L.) Essential Oil Using Vacuum Fractional Distillation." *Journal of Feed Science and Technology* 56: 5422–34.

Smith, Lewis. 2007. "Fossil from a Forest That Gave Earth Its Breath of Fresh Air." *Times* (London). Available online at www.thetimes.co.uk.

Soil Association. Undated. "Seven Ways to Save Our Soils." Available online at www.soilassociation.org.

Soil Health Institute. 2020. *Living Soil* film. Available at Livingsoilfilm.com.

Sumorek-Wiadro, Joanna, Adrian Zajac, Aleksandra Maciejczyk, Joanna Jakubowicz-Gil. 2020. "Furanocoumarins in Anticancer Therapy—For and Against." *Fitoterapia* 142: 104492.

Svoboda, Katrina R., and Thomas G. Svoboda. 2000. *Secretory Structures of Aromatic and Medicinal Plants.* Powys, UK: Microscopix Publications.

Tisserand, Robert, and Tony Balacs. 1995. *Essential Oil Safety: A Guide for Health Professionals.* London: Churchill Livingstone.

Tisserand, Robert, Marco Valussi, Andrea Cont, Joy Bowles. 2021. "Debunking Functional Group Theory: Not Supported by Current Evidence and Not a Useful Educational Tool." Tisserand Institute. Available at the Tisserand Institute website.

Tisserand, Robert, and Rodney Young. 2014. *Essential Oil Safety: A Guide for Health Care Professionals* (2nd ed.). London: Churchill Livingstone.

Tölke, Elizabeth D., Julien B Bachelier, Elimar A. de Lima, Marcelo Jose P Ferreira, Diego Demarco, Sandra M. Carmello-Guerreiro. 2018. "Osmophores and Floral Fragrance in *Anacardium humile* and *Mangifera indica* (Anacardiaceae): An Overlooked Secretory Structure in Sapindales." *AoB PLANTS* 10, no. 6: ply062.

Valnet, Jean. 1990. *The Practice of Aromatherapy.* Rochester, Vt.: Healing Arts Press.

Vasey, Christopher. 2018. *Natural Antibiotics and Antivirals: 18 Infection-Fighting Herbs and Essential Oils.* Rochester, Vt.: Healing Arts Press.

Vasireddy, Lakshmi, Lewis E. H. Bingle, Mark S. Davies. 2018. "Antimicrobial Activity of Essential Oils against Multidrug-Resistant Clinical Isolates of the *Burkholderia cepacia* complex." *PLoS ONE* 13, no. 8: e0201835.

Virgin, Herbert. 2013. "Interactions between the Mammalian Virome, Disease Susceptibility Genes, and the Phenome." NASEM Health and Medicine Division: You Tube Lecture.

Wang, Xin, Yi Shen, Diran Thakur, Jinzhi Han, Jian-Guo Zhang, Fei Hu, Zhoa-Jun Wei. 2020 (25 September). "Antibacterial Activity and Mechanisms of Ginger Essential Oil against *Escherichia Coli* and *Staphylococcus aureus.*" *Molecules* 25, no. 17: 3955.

Watts, Geoff. 2004. "Jacques Benveniste." *British Medical Journal* 329, no. 7477: 1290.

Whitman, William B., David C. Coleman, William J. Wiebe. "Prokaryotes: The Unseen." *Proceedings of the National Academy of Sciences* 95, no. 12: 6578–83.

Williams, David G. 2000. *Lecture Notes on Essential Oils.* London: Eve Taylor.

———. 2006. *The Chemistry of Essential Oils: An Introduction for Aromatherapists, Beauticians, Retailers and Students.* Dorset, England: Micelle Press.

Young, Paul. 1999. *The Botany Coloring Book.* New York: HarperCollins.

Younis, Adna, Atif Riaz, Aslam Khan, Asif Ali Khan. 2009. "Effect of Time of Growing Season and Time of Day for Flower Harvest on Flower Yield and Essential Oil Quality and Quantity of Four *Rosa* Cultivars." *Floriculture and Ornamental Biotechnology* (Global Science Books). Available online at www .globalsciencebooks.info.

Zheljazkov, Valtcho. D., Charles L. Cantrell, Tess Astatkie, Ekaterina Jeliazkova. 2013. "Distillation Time Effect on Lavender Essential Oil Yield and Composition." *Journal Oleo Science* 62, no. 4: 195–99.

Index

about this book, 2–4

absolutes, 28, 90–95, 99, 104

accidental ingestion, 161

acids, 125–26

acid value test, 106

alcohols, 118, 119–20, 129

aldehydes, 120, 130

alkaloids, 13

analytical testing methods, 104–8

   acid value, 106

   Chemical Abstracts Services, 107–8

   gas liquid chromatography, 106–7

   mass spectrometry, 107

   optical rotation, 105–6

   refraction, 105

   specific gravity, 104–5

anatomy of plants, 48–52

   flowers, 51–52

   fruits and seeds, 52

   root system, 48–49

   shoot system, 50

animal cells, 38

anions, 111

Annonaceae family, 53, 69

antimicrobials/antivirals

   room fumigation using, 138

synergistic blends of, 133, 134–36, 137

   whole essential oils as, 136–37

Apiaceae family, 53–54, 68, 70

Aristotle, 39

aromatherapy

   essential oils to avoid in, 29

   use of essential oils in, 71

Art of Aromatherapy, The (Tisserand), 176

Asteraceae family, 54, 68

atoms, 110–11

Ayurveda, 173

bacteria, 41, 136, 147

bark and wood oils, 21–22

basil, 27–28, 183–85

being, state of, 145–46

Benveniste, Jacques, 86

benzoin, 95, 185–87

bergamot, 187–90

Betulaceae family, 54–55, 68

biodiversity

   explanation of, 31–32

   future of, 71–75

bitter orange, 27, 149, 182, 269–71

black pepper, 276–77

blends
    antimicrobial/antiviral, 133,
        134–36, 137
    creating synergy with optimal,
        138–40
    factors in effectiveness of, 139–40
blue color, 168–69
blue green color, 169
botanical families, 53–68
botany, 39
bulbs, 48, 50, 70
Burseraceae family, 55, 68, 69
Bush, Zach, 2, 72, 73

cajeput, 190–92
calendula, 99–100, 152
Caprifoliaceae family, 55–56, 70
caraway, 192–93
carbohydrates, 7–8, 9, 11
carbon dioxide
    absorbed by plants, 8, 9
    extraction of oils using, 95–97
cardamom, 194–95
carrot seed, 196–97
CAS number, 107–8
cations, 111
cedarwood Atlas, 75, 198–200
chakras, 166, 167, 171
chamomile
    German, 96, 183, 200–202
    Roman, 153, 167, 183, 202–5
chaste tree, 205–6
chemotypes, 43
children, 150–57. See also infants
    diffusion of oils for, 154–56

oil safety precautions with, 157
    topical use of oils on, 152–54
Chinese medicine. See traditional
    Chinese medicine (TCM)
chloroplasts, 7
cinnamon leaf/bark, 27, 207–9
Cistaceae family, 56, 70
citronella, 209–11
citrus fruits, 88–89
citrus trees, 26–27
clary sage, 293–95
climate biomes, 32–36
clove bud, 211–13
cold pressing, 89
colors, 166–67, 168–71
compounds, 113
conifers, 44, 45
coriander, 213–15
cultivars, 43
Cupressaceae family, 56, 68
cypress, 149, 167, 178, 179, 215–17

dicots, 45, 47, 49
diffusion of oils, 154–56, 159
Dioscorides, 39
Dipterocarpaceae family, 56–57,
    69
distillation methods, 28, 78–88
    folding process, 85
    fractional distillation, 84
    hydrodiffusion, 81–83
    hydrodistillation, 79–80
    hydrosols and, 85–87
    rectification, 83–84
    steam distillation, 80–81
diterpenes, 115, 117–18

ecological sustainability, 72–74

ecosystems, 31

electrons, 110–11

elements, 110, 112, 172–74

emotional states, 149, 178

enfleurage method, 100–101

English lavender, 241–45

environmental conditions, 23

epidermal cells, 18

essential oils

    antimicrobial/antiviral, 133, 134–37

    avoidance of specific, 29

    botanical families and, 53–68

    children and use of, 150–57

    climate biomes and, 33–36

    constituents of, 114–32

    ethical sourcing of, 74–75

    evaluation of, 102, 103–8

    extraction of, 25–26, 28, 77–101

    fragrance characteristics of, 176–77

    global production of, 71–72

    harvesting plants for, 24

    hormones and, 13

    how they work, 1–2

    immunity and, 146–47

    industrial use of, 71

    measurement of, 163–64

    parts of plants containing, 14, 15–22, 26, 78

    plant anatomy related to, 48–52

    psycho-emotional influence of, 147–50

    quick reference to plants and, 68–70

    role of, within plants, 5, 14–15, 30

    safety considerations for, 157, 158–62

    scent profiles of, 128–32

    storage methods for, 102–3

    subtle dynamics of, 165–79

    synergistic blends of, 133–36, 137, 138–40

    therapeutic use of, 71, 72

Essential Oils for Mindfulness and Meditation (Godfrey), 3, 150n

Essential Oils for the Whole Body (Godfrey), 3, 137n, 150n

esters, 121–22, 131

estragole, 27–28

ethers, 123, 132

ethical sources, 74–75

eucalyptus, 75, 217–19

eugenol, 27

eukaryotes, 37, 40–41

evaluation process, 102, 103–8

    analytical testing and, 104–8

    oil qualities and, 103–4

evening primrose oil, 152

exosomes, 143–44

expression process, 77, 88–89

extraction methods, 28, 77–101

    carbon dioxide extraction, 95–97

    distillation, 78–88

    enfleurage, 100–101

    expression, 77, 88–89

    illustrated overview of, 79

    maceration, 97–100

    oil concentration and, 25–26

    solvent extraction, 90–95

eyes, flushing, 161–62

Fabaceae family, 57, 69, 70

fennel, 219–21

five elements, 172–74

flavonoids, 13, 98

flowers

    essential oils in, 21, 51, 68–70

    parts and functions of, 51–52

folded oils, 85

forma, 43

fractional distillation, 84

fragrance notes, 174–77

frankincense/olibanum, 75, 149, 178, 179, 222–24

fruits

    essential oils in, 21, 52, 69–70

    parts and functions of, 52

fumigation process, 138

fungi, 41, 70

furanocoumarins, 125

furans, 124

galbanum, 75, 224–26

gas liquid chromatography (GLC), 106–7

gemstones, 167–71

genes, 31

Geraniaceae family, 57–58, 70

geranium, 149, 226–28

Gerard, John, 39

German chamomile, 96, 183, 200–202

ginger, 229–30

gingergrass, 272

glandular trichomes, 18

glyphosates, 73, 74

GMOs, 73

Grace, Janey Lee, ix–x

grapefruit, 133, 230–32

grass, essential oils in, 69

green color, 169

Grieve, Maude, 92–93

Hamamelidaceae family, 58, 70

hand sanitizer, 138

health/wellness

    cornerstones of, 141, 144

    essential oils for, 146–50

    hygiene related to, 146

    microbiome support for, 143–45

    state of being and, 145–46

helichrysum/immortelle, 232–34

herbs, 24, 37, 68

heterogeneous mixtures, 114

heteronuclear molecules, 113

hexane, 90, 91

homogeneous mixtures, 114

homonuclear molecules, 113

hormones, 13

hybrids, 43

hydrocarbons, 114, 115

hydrodiffusion, 81–83

hydrodistillation, 79–80

hydrosols, 83, 85–87

hygiene, 146

hyssop, 235–36

immunity, 143–47. *See also* health/wellness

    essential oils and, 146–47

    good hygiene and, 146

    microbiome and, 143–45

    state of being and, 145–46

infants. *See also* children

    essential oils and, 150–51

    massage and skin care for, 151–52

internal ingestion, 158, 161
ions, 111
isoprenes/isoprenoids, 115

jasmine, 237–38
jojoba oil, 152
juniper berry, 238–40

ketones, 120–21, 130

lactones, 125
Lamiaceae family, 58, 68, 70
Lauraceae family, 59, 68, 69
lavender, 42–43, 149, 153–54, 161,
    241–45
leaves, essential oils in, 21
lemon, 154, 245–48
lemon balm/melissa, 256–58
lemongrass, 133, 248–50
lichen, 62, 70
Liliaceae family, 59, 69, 70
limbic system, 148
Linnaeus, Carl, 39

maceration process, 97–100
Malvaceae family, 59–60, 68, 70
mandarin, 149, 154, 250–52
marigold-infused olive oil, 152
marjoram, sweet, 252–55
mass spectrometry (MS), 107
matter, forms of, 109–13
Maury, Marguerite, 2
may chang, 255–56
measuring essential oils, 163–64
melissa/lemon balm, 256–58
metabolism, plant, 12–14, 22

microbiome, 143–45
mixtures, 113–14
Modern Herbal, A (Grieve), 92
molecules, 31, 113
Monimiaceae family, 60, 70
monocots, 45, 46, 49
monoterpenes, 115, 116–17, 128
Myristicaceae family, 60–61, 69
myrrh, 75, 149, 259–61
Myrtaceae family, 61, 69
myrtle, 261–63

neroli, 27, 154–55, 181–82, 263–65
neutrons, 110–11
niaouli, 265–67
nitrogen, 127
nonrenewable energy, 11
nonvascular plants, 44, 45
notes, fragrance, 174–77
nutmeg, 267–69

Oleaceae family, 61–62, 70
olive oil, 152
optical rotation test, 105–6
orange, bitter, 27, 149, 182, 269–71
orange blossom, 86, 263–65
orange color, 170
orange leaf, 280–82
oregano, 253
osmophores, 17
oxidation, 104, 106
oxides, 123–24, 132
oxygen, 7–8, 9, 22, 30

palmarosa, 271–73
Parmeliaceae family, 62, 70

patchouli, 273–75

pepper, black, 276–77

peppermint, 278–80

periodic table, 112

peroxides, 126

petitgrain, 27, 181, 280–82

phenolic ethers, 27–28

phenols, 122–23, 131, 159n

photolysis, 7

photons, 6, 7, 8, 10

photosynthesis, 6–11

   human animal and, 10

   overview of phases in, 8–9

   requirements for, 22

phytohormones, 13

Pinaceae family, 62–63, 69

pine needle, Scotch, 75, 282–84

pink color, 169–70

Piperaceae family, 63, 69

plants

   anatomy of, 48–52

   cells of animals vs., 38

   climate biomes and, 33–36

   ecological sustainability of, 72–74

   environmental conditions and, 23

   essential oil–bearing, 53–68

   evolution of, 36–37

   harvesting for essential oils, 24

   identifying and labeling, 39–43

   metabolic activity in, 12–14, 22

   parts with essential oils, 14, 15–22, 26, 78

   quick reference to essential oils and, 68–70

   requirements for growth of, 22–23

   role of essential oils in, 5, 14–15, 30

sugar types present in, 11

vascular vs. nonvascular, 44–47

Plinus, 39

Poaceae family, 63, 69, 70

pregnant women, 150–51

primary metabolism, 12

prokaryotes, 37, 39, 40–41

protons, 110–11

quarks, 110

rectification, 83–84

red color, 170–71

refraction test, 105

respiration, 8, 9

Roman chamomile, 153, 167, 183, 202–5

room fumigation, 138

roots

   essential oils in, 21, 48, 70

   parts and functions of, 48

   various types of, 49

Rosaceae family, 64, 70

rosemary, 284–88

rose oil, 92, 93–94, 149, 155–56, 178, 179

rose otto, 93, 288–93

rosewater, 86

rosewood, 75

Rutaceae family, 64–65, 69, 70

safety considerations, 158–62

   accidents and reactions, 161–62

   storage and care, 159–60

   use of oils, 158–59, 161

   young children and, 157

safflower oil, 152

sage, clary, 293–95

sandalwood, 75, 295–97

Santalaceae family, 65, 69

saponins, 13

scent detection, 147–49

scent observation, 104

scent profiles, 128–32

Schisandraceae family, 65–66, 69, 70

Scotch pine, 75, 282–84

secondary metabolism, 12

secretory cavities, 17

secretory ducts, 17

secretory structures, 15, 16–17

Secrets of Life and Youth, The (Maury), 2

seeds

  essential oils in, 21, 52, 68–69

  parts and functions of, 52

  vascular plants with, 44–45

sesquiterpenes, 115, 117, 129

shoot system of plants, 50

shrubs, essential oils in, 70

single secretion-containing cells, 16

skin reactions, 162

solar energy, 6–7, 8

solvent extraction, 28, 90–95

Spanish marjoram, 253

spearmint, 156

species, 31

  divisions of plant, 43

  examples of classifying, 42

specific gravity test, 104–5

spices, 68–69

spike lavender, 241–45

spikenard, 75, 178, 179, 298–300

spores, plants with, 44

state of being, 145–46

steam distillation, 28, 80–81

stems, essential oils in, 21

storage methods, 102–3, 159–60

subspecies, 91

subtle dynamics, 165–79

  chakras, 171

  colors, 166–67, 168–71

  five elements, 172–74

  fragrance notes, 174–77

  gemstones, 167–71

  yin and yang, 172, 173, 174

sulfur, 126

sunflower oil, 152

sustainability, 72–75

sweet marjoram, 252–55

synergy, 133–40

  antimicrobial/antiviral blends and, 133, 134–36, 137

  creating optimal blends using, 138–40

  enhancing the potential for achieving, 140

  explanation and examples of, 133–34

taxonomy, 39

tea tree, 161, 300–302

terpenes, 13, 81–82, 113, 115–18

terpenoids, 13, 118–27

Theophrastus, 39

thyme, 303–5

Tiliaceae family, 66, 70

Tisserand, Robert, 91, 176

topical application, 152–54, 158, 159, 161

traditional Chinese medicine (TCM), 165, 166, 172–73, 179
trees
  chaste, 205–6
  citrus, 26–27
  essential oils from, 68–70
  tea, 300–302
  turmeric, 305–7

valerian, 75, 307–9
variety, botanical, 43
vascular plants, 44–47
vegetable oils, 151–52
Verbenaceae family, 66–67, 68
vetivert, 75, 149, 309–12
Violaceae family, 67, 68

violet color, 168
viruses, 143, 146
volatile organic compounds, 12

wellness. *See* health/wellness
wild marjoram, 253
witch hazel, 86, 87
wood and bark oils, 21–22

yarrow, 312–14
yellow color, 170
yin and yang, 172, 173, 174
ylang-ylang, 314–16

Zingiberaceae family, 67, 69, 70
Zygophyllaceae family, 67–68, 69

About the Author

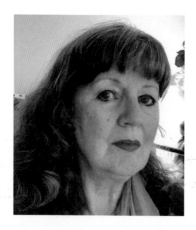

Heather studied at the University of Salford, where she was awarded a joint honors degree in counseling and complementary medicine and master's certificates in integrated mindfulness and supervision of counseling and therapeutic relationships. She also gained a postgraduate teaching certificate from Bolton Institute. She worked at the College of Health and Social Care (now the School of Health and Society) at the University of Salford for a number of years, fulfilling multiple roles. She served as a program lead and lecturer in integrated therapy, complementary therapy, aromatherapy, communication, and professional skills.

Heather has had a number of articles and research papers published in associated professional journals, including the *International Journal of Clinical Aromatherapy* (IJCA). A fellow of the International Federation of Aromatherapists (IFA), she was chair of education in 2013 and supports the IFA's educational program in an advisory capacity. She is also a member of the Federation of Holistic Therapists (FHT). Through her private practice, Heather continues to provide professional training, essential oil therapy treatments, professional supervision for therapists, professional development, and introductory workshops. Visit her website at

www.aromantique.co.uk